MAYO CLINIC ON BETTER HEARING AND BALANCE

Christopher D. Bauch, Ph.D.

Medical Editor

Mayo Clinic
Rochester, Minnesota

Mayo Clinic on Better Hearing and Balance provides reliable information on treating and managing hearing and balance problems. Much of the information comes directly from the experience of ear, nose and throat specialists and audiologists at Mayo Clinic. This book supplements the advice of your physician, whom you should consult for individual medical problems.

This book does not endorse any company or product. MAYO, MAYO CLINIC and the Mayo triple-shield logo are marks of Mayo Foundation for Medical Education and Research.

All rights reserved. No part of this book may be reproduced or used in any form or by any means, electronic or mechanical, including photocopying and recording, or by any information storage and retrieval system, without permission in writing from the publisher, except by a reviewer, who may quote brief passages in review.

For bulk sales to employers, member groups and health-related companies, contact Mayo Clinic Health Solutions, 200 First St. SW, Rochester, MN 55905, or send an email to SpecialSalesMayoBooks@Mayo.edu.

Published by Mayo Clinic

© 2014 Mayo Foundation for Medical Education and Research (MFMER)

Library of Congress Control Number: 2013952776

Second Edition

4 5 6 7 8 9 10

Image credits

CREDIT: © MAYO FOUNDATION FOR MEDICAL EDUCATION AND RESEARCH (MFMER)

NAME: 153917510.JPG/PAGE: 19/CREDIT: © ISTOCK/THINKSTOCK — NAME: 170082501.JPG/PAGE: 26–27/CREDIT: © MONKEY BUSINESS/THINKSTOCK — NAME: 162312389.JPG/PAGE: 28/CREDIT: © ISTOCK/THINKSTOCK — NAME: 97829449.JPG/PAGE: 34–35/CREDIT: © MONKEY BUSINESS/THINKSTOCK — NAME: 78813006.JPG/PAGE: 36/CREDIT: © FUSE/THINKSTOCK — NAME: 156957296.JPG/PAGE: 51/CREDIT: © ISTOCK/THINKSTOCK — NAME: 78752316.JPG/PAGE: 53/CREDIT: © FUSE/THINKSTOCK — NAME: 97892605.JPG/PAGE: 66/CREDIT: © ISTOCK/THINKSTOCK — NAME: 170083394.JPG/PAGE: 69/CREDIT: © MONKEY BUSINESS/THINKSTOCK — NAME: 133298142.JPG/PAGE: 75/CREDIT: © ISTOCK/THINKSTOCK — NAME: 120543972.JPG/PAGE: 84/CREDIT: © ISTOCK/THINKSTOCK — NAME: 145157652.JPG/PAGE: 93/CREDIT: © ISTOCK/THINKSTOCK — NAME: 86487906.JPG/PAGE: 103/CREDIT: © JUPITERIMAGES/CREATAS/THINKSTOCK — NAME: 78807867.JPG/PAGE: 108/CREDIT: © FUSE/THINKSTOCK — NAME: 102915301.JPG/PAGE: 115/CREDIT: © FUSE/THINKSTOCK — NAME: 80471782.JPG/PAGE: 117/CREDIT: © ISTOCK/THINKSTOCK — NAME: 172587282.JPG/PAGE: 121/CREDIT: © WAVEBREAK MEDIA/THINKSTOCK — NAME: 109592686.JPG/PAGE: 125/CREDIT: © HUNSTOCK/THINKSTOCK — NAME: 172588626.JPG/PAGE: 129/CREDIT: © WAVEBREAK MEDIA/THINKSTOCK — NAME: 136610999.JPG/PAGE: 130/CREDIT: © ISTOCK/THINKSTOCK — NAME: 120876634.JPG/PAGE: 135/CREDIT: © ISTOCK/THINKSTOCK — NAME: 90366633.JPG/PAGE: 151/CREDIT: © ISTOCK/THINKSTOCK — NAME: DV1051011.JPG/PAGE: 155/CREDIT: © DIGITAL VISION/THINKSTOCK — NAME: 119743251.JPG/PAGE: 156/CREDIT: © ISTOCK/THINKSTOCK — NAME: 92034793.JPG/PAGE: 185/CREDIT: © ISTOCK/THINKSTOCK

THE IMAGES ON PAGE 127 APPEAR COURTESY OF PAWS WITH A CAUSE.

THE IMAGES ON PAGES 170, 172 AND 181 APPEAR COURTESY OF COCHLEAR AMERICAS.

THE IMAGES ON PAGES 189 AND 193 APPEAR COURTESY OF ULTRATEC.

Editorial staff

Medical Editor
Christopher D. Bauch, Ph.D.

Managing Editor
Jennifer L. Duesterhoeft

Product Manager
Christopher C. Frye

Editorial Director
Paula M. Marlow Limbeck

Art Director
Richard A. Resnick

Editorial Research
Anthony J. Cook
Amanda K. Golden
Deirdre A. Herman
Erika A. Riggin

Proofreading
Miranda M. Attlesey
Donna L. Hanson
Julie M. Maas

Production
Downtown Bookworks Inc., New York
Sara N. DiSalvo, project manager
Laura J. Smyth, designer

Indexing
Steve Rath

Contributing Editors and Reviewers
Ann B. Anderson, Au.D.
David M. Barrs, M.D.
Charles W. Beatty, M.D.
Michael J. Cevette, Ph.D.
Melissa D. DeJong, Au.D.
Colin L.W. Driscoll, M.D.
Millicent S. Garry, Au.D.
David B. Hawkins, Ph.D.
Cynthia A. Hogan, Ph.D.
Kathryn A. Kerst
Larry B. Lundy, M.D.
Brian A. Neff, M.D.
Sarah R. Oakley, Au.D., C.C.C.-A
Janet S. Shelfer, Au.D.
Neil T. Shepard, Ph.D.
Douglas P. Sladen, Ph.D.
Katherine H. Teece, Au.D.
Linsey S. Wagner, Au.D.
David A. Zapala, Ph.D.

Administrative Assistant
Beverly J. Steele

Preface

Hearing loss and dizziness are two of the most common reasons to visit your doctor. Hearing loss may be present at birth (congenital) or hereditary. Dizziness may be a solitary symptom, or it may be the most debilitating of multiple symptoms. Frequently, hearing loss and balance problems are complications of illness or disease, medication, trauma, noise exposure, and the normal process of aging.

This book describes the sensitive structures and exquisite functions of the ear, which is so fundamental to good hearing and balance. Attention is focused on many common ear disorders and the ear-related problems of tinnitus and dizziness. Explanations are provided for diagnostic tests, medical treatment, surgery, habilitation and rehabilitation. This content helps you become a more informed participant in effective prevention and treatment strategies.

When hearing loss cannot be alleviated medically, many devices are available to help you communicate more easily. Hearing aids, cochlear implants and assistive listening devices are discussed in separate chapters. The treatment and management of balance problems are discussed in the final chapter.

Audiologists and ear, nose and throat specialists at Mayo Clinic facilities in Minnesota, Florida and Arizona have reviewed the content of this book for accuracy and completeness. The result is a practical resource to assist you in protecting and preserving your hearing, maintaining your mobility and balance, and minimizing the impact of hearing loss, dizziness and imbalance on your daily life.

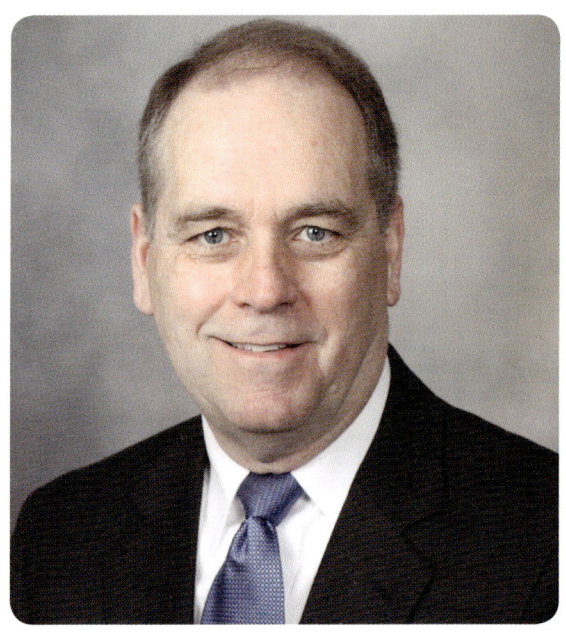

Christopher D. Bauch, Ph.D.
Medical Editor

Table of contents

Part 1 — Understanding common hearing problems 9

Chapter 1 — How you hear 11
Structure of the ear 12
Characteristics of sound 17
Sound pathways 20
Types of hearing loss 23
Compensating for hearing loss 25

Chapter 2 — Getting a hearing exam 29
Who provides ear care? 30
Schedule for hearing exams 32
Typical hearing exam 36
Understanding your audiogram 49
The speech spectrum 53

Chapter 3 — Problems of the outer ear and middle ear ... 55
Outer ear problems 56
Eardrum problems 61
Middle ear problems 64

Chapter 4 — Problems of the inner ear 77
Presbycusis 78
Noise-induced hearing loss 80
Sudden deafness 85
Other causes of hearing loss 86
Research on the horizon 95

Chapter 5	**Tinnitus**	**97**
	Unraveling the mystery	98
	Types	99
	Diagnosis	102
	Management	104

Part 2   **The management of hearing loss 109**

Chapter 6	**Living with hearing impairment**	**111**
	Quality of life	112
	Improving social interaction	119
	Finding support	128
Chapter 7	**Hearing aids**	**133**
	Setting priorities	134
	How hearing aids work	136
	Hearing aid styles	138
	Other selection considerations	145
	Buying a hearing aid	149
	Wearing your hearing aid	154
	Maintenance	161
Chapter 8	**Cochlear implants**	**163**
	Cochlear implants and hearing aids	164
	How cochlear implants work	165
	Implant candidates	167
	Contributing factors	171
	Benefits	172
	The implant procedure	173
	Adjusting to an implant	179
	Stay positive	181

Chapter 9	**Other options to communicate better**	**183**
	Assistive listening devices	184
	Telephone devices	188
	Text messaging	194
	Assistive listening systems	196
	Captioning	201
	Alerting devices	203
	On the horizon	205
	Many options	206
Chapter 10	**Problems with balance**	**207**
	Keeping yourself balanced	208
	Causes of dizziness	212
	Diagnostic tests	213
	Vestibular disorders	220
	Vestibular rehabilitation	231
	Staying active	236
	Additional resources	237
	Index	241

Part 1

Understanding common hearing problems

Chapter 1

How you hear

In 1802 the famed German composer Ludwig van Beethoven wrote a letter to his brothers about his deteriorating hearing: "I am compelled to live as an exile. If I approach near to people, a feeling of hot anxiety comes over me lest my condition should be noticed."[1]

It's striking that such feelings belonged to a composer whose music, more than two centuries later, still brings so much listening enjoyment to people around the world.

But if you're experiencing problems with hearing, you — like Beethoven — may feel uncomfortable when you're in social situations and conversing with others. Not being able to hear clearly can be frustrating, to say the least, as you try to maintain the conversation and go about your day.

Hearing loss can cause social isolation because you may find it easier to withdraw from group activities rather than participate in them. Such behavior might in turn cause people to think of you as timid or disconnected and give up trying to communicate with you.

Then again, if you have hearing loss, you have plenty of company. About 17 percent of Americans — 36 million — have some degree of hearing loss, ranging from mild to profound.

Older adults are most affected, as hearing tends to deteriorate with age. An estimated one-third of Americans ages 65 to 74, and approximately half of those age 75 and older, have a hearing impairment. But hearing loss can occur at any age due to factors such as noise exposure, trauma, genetics and illness.

1 Eaglefield-Hull, A., ed. Beethoven's Letters. New York: Dover Publications; 1972:38.

Worldwide, the number of people with disabling hearing loss is estimated at 360 million — a figure much higher when mild hearing loss is included.

Many people refuse to acknowledge their hearing loss. Estimates are that only about 1 person in 5 who would benefit from a hearing aid actually wears one. Many choose to persevere without any assistance.

According to a study from the National Council on Aging, people with hearing impairment who don't use hearing aids are more likely to feel sad or anxious, be less active socially, and feel greater emotional insecurity than are those with hearing impairment who do use hearing aids. The study also reported that hearing aid users maintained better relationships with their families.

There's even evidence to suggest that, in addition to the emotional and social consequences of hearing loss, some cognitive functions may be affected. Specifically, a recent study reported a relationship between hearing loss and the risk of developing dementia.

Hearing aids have come a long way since the conspicuous ear trumpets of the 18th and 19th centuries. In fact, astounding improvements in hearing technology have been made in the last few decades. More options for treating hearing loss are available. And some of these options are not even noticeable to onlookers. The key is to find a treatment that fits your needs and lifestyle.

In the chapters that follow, you'll find pertinent information about hearing loss — why it occurs, how it's diagnosed, how it can be treated and how you can live with it. You'll also learn about dizziness and problems with balance, conditions that sometimes are associated with hearing difficulties. This knowledge will help you live an active life despite any changes that may occur to your hearing.

Structure of the ear

The ears are pretty amazing acoustic devices, as yet unmatched by human ingenuity or invention. In a person with normal hearing, the ears, in combination with the brain, can almost instantly transform sound waves from the external world into the recognizable voice of a loved one, the call of a songbird or a crack of thunder.

Many factors play into this sensory organ, so let's take a systematic look at the important structures that make up the ear. The flap of cartilage on each side of your head may be the most recognizable structure, but that's only the external part of the ear. The organ that you use for hearing is actually composed of three complex, interconnected sections known as the outer ear, middle ear and inner ear.

Outer ear

The outer ear is the part of the organ you can see sticking out from either side of your head. It's made up of folds of skin and cartilage, called the pinna (auricle), and the ear canal. The cupped shape of the pinna (PIN-uh) gathers sound waves from the environment and directs them toward the ear canal.

The ear canal is an inch-long passageway leading to the eardrum. The skin lining the ear canal contains tiny hairs and glands that produce wax, or cerumen (suh-ROO-mun). The hairs and wax serve as cleaning mechanisms for the ear canal by repelling water, protecting against bacteria and keeping foreign objects such as dirt from slipping through the ear canal and reaching the eardrum.

The eardrum (tympanic membrane) is a thin, taut membrane at the end of the ear canal that separates the outer ear from the middle ear. The arrival of sound waves through the ear canal will cause the eardrum to vibrate.

Middle ear

The middle ear is an air-filled cavity located behind the eardrum. The cavity is lodged in the temporal bone of your skull and houses three tiny bones called ossicles (OS-ih-kuls). The ossicles have scientific names, but each is known by a name that best describes its shape: the hammer (malleus), anvil (incus) and stirrup (stapes). See the illustration on page 14.

Together, the ossicles form a bridge between the eardrum and the membrane-covered entrance to the inner ear (oval window). Sound waves are transmitted through the ossicles. Each bone moves back and forth, much as a small lever, to increase the sound level that reaches the inner ear. A tiny muscle is attached to the hammer on one end of the ossicular bridge, and another tiny muscle to the stirrup at the other end.

A narrow channel called the eustachian (u-STAY-shun) tube connects the middle

Parts of the ear

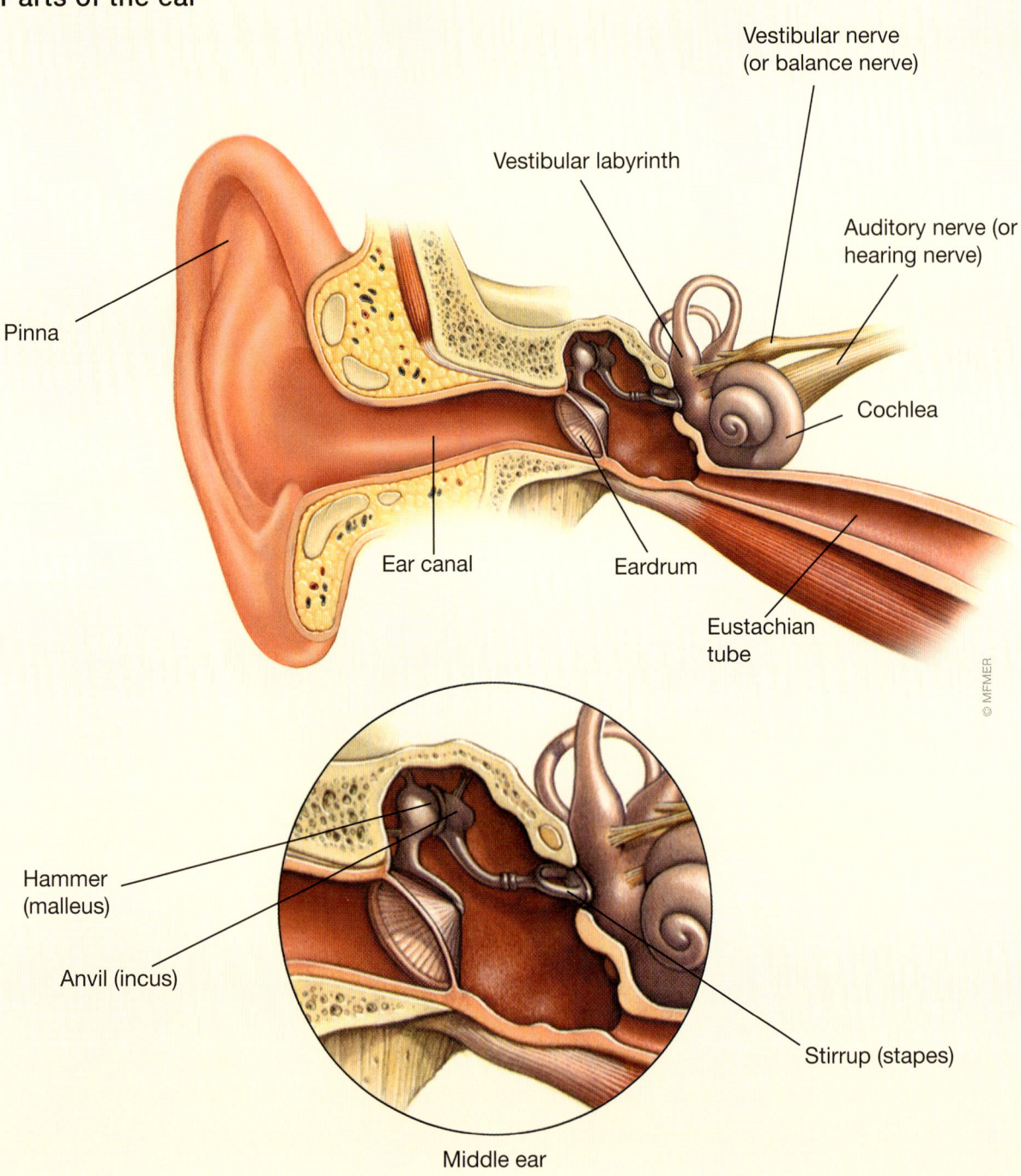

14   Chapter 1: How you hear

ear to the back of the nose and upper part of the throat — an area called the nasopharynx (nay-zoe-FAR-inks).

The eustachian tube normally remains closed until you swallow or yawn. Then it opens briefly to equalize the air pressure within your middle ear to the air pressure that's outside — you may feel and hear a pop when this occurs. Maintaining equal air pressure on both sides of the eardrum allows the membrane to vibrate easily.

In adults, the eustachian tube angles slightly downward to the nasopharynx. In children, because their skulls aren't yet fully developed, the eustachian tube is narrower and more horizontal. This makes it easier for a child's eustachian tube to become blocked and for fluid to build up in the middle ear. Occasionally, this fluid becomes infected, causing pain and inflammation.

Inner ear

The inner ear contains the most sophisticated part of the hearing mechanism: the fluid-filled, snail-shaped cochlea (KOK-lee-uh). The cochlea translates incoming sound waves into signals that can be understood by the brain. See the illustration on page 16.

The spiraling tube of the cochlea would be just over an inch in length if it were stretched out straight, but it naturally curls around almost three times. The whole cochlear structure is no bigger than the size of a pea.

The tube of the cochlea is divided into three chambers that spiral around a bony core. The upper chamber (scala vestibuli) and lower chamber (scala tympani) are filled with a fluid called perilymph. The middle chamber or cochlear duct (scala media) has a different type of fluid called endolymph.

The cochlear duct also contains the organ of Corti, which is vital to the hearing process. Lining the organ of Corti is a strip of tissue called the basilar membrane, on which stand four to five rows of ultrasensitive hair cells topped by tiny tufts of fine hair strands (cilia).

There are two different types of hair cells in the cochlea. Three rows of outer hair cells receive and amplify sound waves from the outer and middle ear. A single row of ultrasensitive inner hair cells receives the amplified sound and then sends the signals to the brain. The longest cilia (found on the outer hair cells) are embedded in an overlying strip of tissue called the tectorial

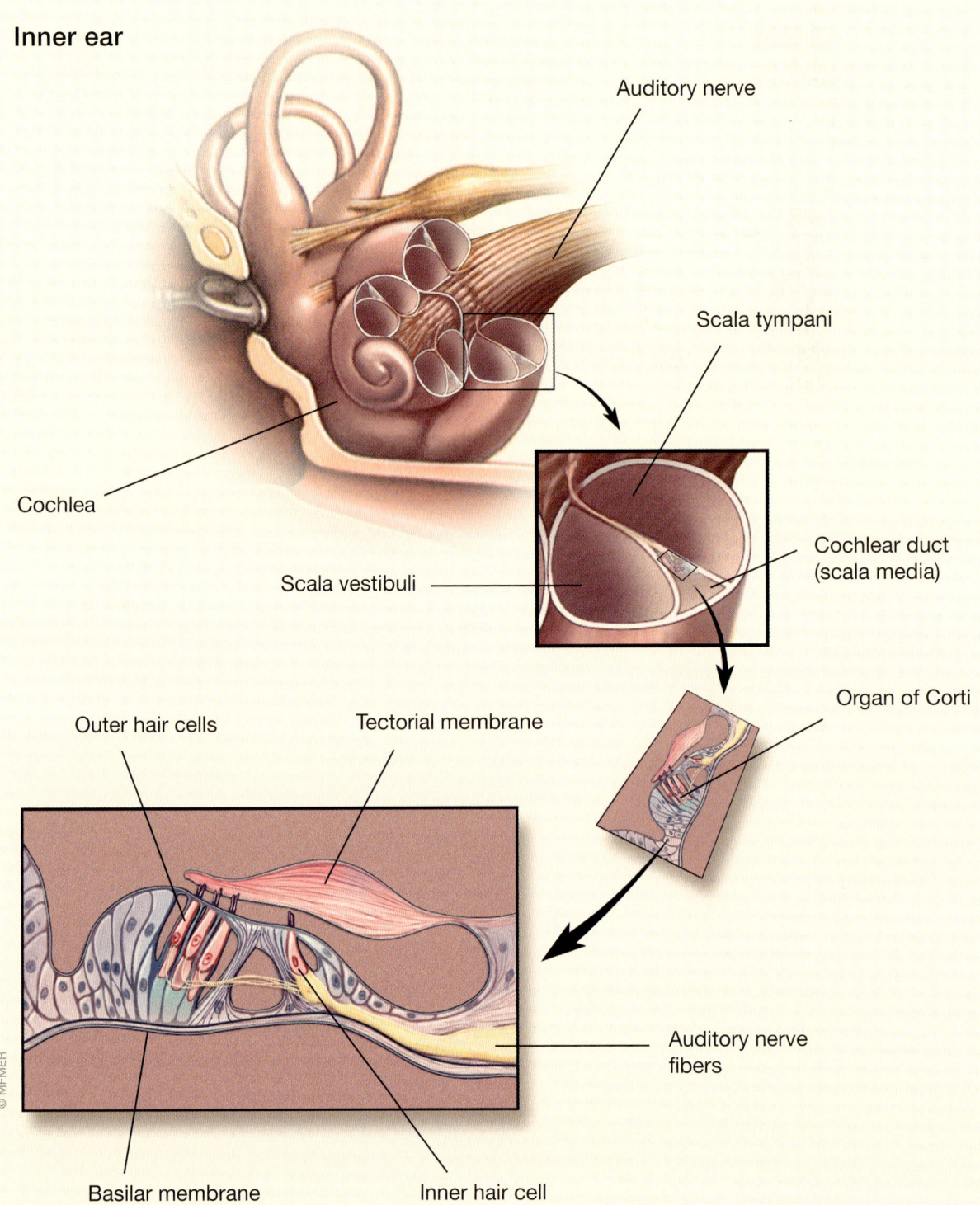

16   Chapter 1: How you hear

membrane. In response to sound, inner hair cells trigger nerve impulses that are transmitted to the brain along the auditory nerve.

The inner ear also contains a structure called the vestibular labyrinth, which assists your sense of balance. It consists of three semicircular tubes that, similar to the cochlea, are filled with fluid and contain hair cells that are sensitive to fluid movement. These cells track every motion of your body to help keep you aware of where your head is in relation to the ground. Chapter 10 describes in greater detail the vestibular labyrinth and symptoms associated with it, such as dizziness and vertigo.

Characteristics of sound

The ear is a series of delicate, complex structures that enables you to collect and make sense of sound. But what is sound exactly?

Sound occurs whenever a substance — or, rather, the molecules that make up the substance — vibrates. And when a substance vibrates, it displaces all the molecules around it, in much the same way that a rock thrown into a pond causes the water to ripple in every direction. The vibration moves from molecule to molecule in the form of a sound wave.

We hear sound waves that travel through air, such as the clap of an audience's applause at the end of a performance or the hum of pistons and belts in a running car engine.

Sounds also travel through fluid, such as when you hear the splashes of nearby swimmers when you're underwater at the pool. Sounds travel through solid matter such as bone or steel, as well. The thump you hear when you bump your head against an object is partially a result of vibrations traveling through your skull as well as through air.

When a sound wave travels through the air to your outer ear and reaches your eardrum, it triggers a chain reaction through the ossicles, cochlea, auditory nerve and brain that allows you to hear the sound.

As you know, one sound can be vastly different from another. Think of the low-pitched rumble of a diesel truck and the high-pitched whine of a lightweight motorbike. Both sounds come from a combustion engine. But there's no mistaking one sound for the other. The differences between sounds arise mainly from three qualities — frequency, intensity and timbre. The first two qualities can be measured, and the third is subjective.

Frequency

The frequency of sound, a quality also known as pitch, is how often a sound wave fluctuates within a given period of time. This is usually measured in cycles per second, or hertz (Hz). The more fluctuations per second, the higher the frequency.

Sound frequencies audible to humans range from around 20 Hz, a very low pitch, to 20,000 Hz, a very high pitch. Common sounds in human speech cover a broad range from near 250 Hz (a low-pitched vowel sound such as *ooo*) to 4,000 to 6,000 Hz (a high-pitched consonant sound such as *ss* or *ff*).

Intensity

The intensity of sound is measured by its loudness (amplitude). This quality is associated with the level of disturbance of the sound wave. It's measured in decibels (dB).

For example, a hushed whisper might be measured at 30 decibels sound pressure level (dB SPL), whereas a gunshot might register at 140 to 170 dB SPL. Noise at this intensity is too loud for the human ear to tolerate, especially when you're exposed to it for a prolonged time. These sounds can cause permanent damage if the ears aren't protected with earplugs or a hearing protective device (earmuffs).

A subjective description of sound intensity is its loudness. For example, noises can be too soft, comfortably loud, too loud or painfully loud.

Timbre

Perhaps the most subjective aspect of sound is its timbre (TAM-bur), which describes the quality of sound. Timbre allows you to distinguish between sounds of the same frequency and intensity, such as the same note played by different musical instruments or the same consonant or vowel spoken by different voices.

The tone of a piccolo or flute, for example, vibrates within a restricted range of frequencies — it would be represented by a relatively smooth, rolling waveform.

Properties of a sound wave

Amplitude measures how loud a sound is. The number of wave cycles per second measures frequency.

A.

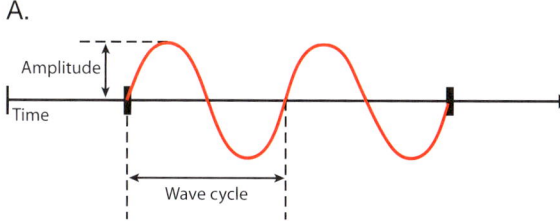

Sound wave A has a frequency of 2 hertz (Hz) — or two wavelength cycles in one second.

B.

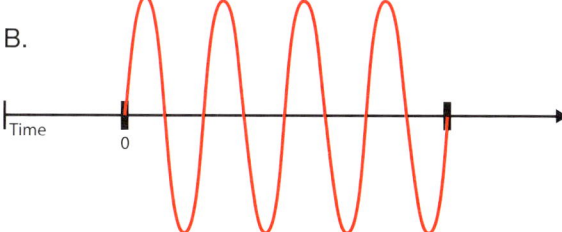

Sound wave B has a higher frequency and amplitude than does sound wave A, making sound wave B higher pitched and louder.

C.

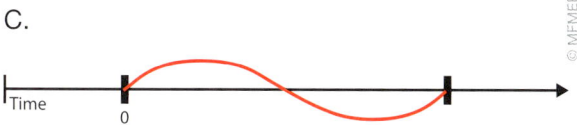

Sound wave C has a lower frequency and amplitude than does sound wave A, making sound wave C lower pitched and softer — in fact, barely audible.

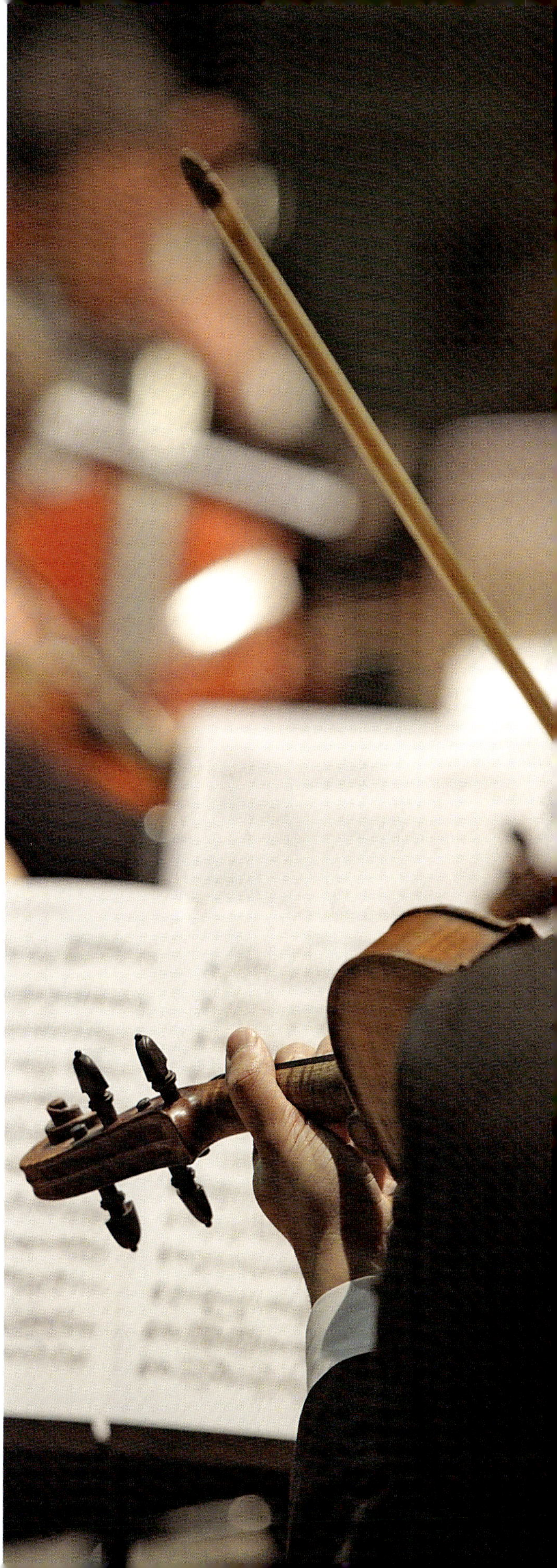

The timbre of a saxophone or piano is more complex — the result of multiple vibrations at many different frequencies — and represented by a jagged waveform. The dissonant ping that results from dropping a wooden pencil on a hard floor is another example of a complex sound.

Sound pathways

Sound is created by molecular vibrations moving through matter, and hearing is the perception of that sound. When you hear a sound, you perceive its qualities of frequency, intensity and timbre practically at once. The journey of a sound wave through the ear and to your brain may be almost instantaneous, but it is nonetheless complex.

It begins as the outer ear (pinna) gathers in sound waves and directs them toward your eardrum. Many mammals, such as cats and dogs, have the ability to rotate their outer ears toward the source of a sound. Humans don't have this ability.

Instead, sound waves reach your outer ears from different directions at different angles and at slightly different times and intensities, producing slightly different patterns depending on where the source of a sound is in relation to your head. This helps your brain to locate the source.

Binaural hearing

Hearing with two ears is called binaural hearing — as opposed to monaural hearing with one ear. The use of both ears is critical to helping you locate the source of a sound. A sound occurring on your left will reach your left ear first and register as louder in this ear than in your right. When your brain compares information from both ears, it can distinguish whether the sound has originated from the left or the right.

With the help of auditory information arriving from both ears, your brain is often able to pick out the sounds you want to hear and somewhat suppress the background noise. An example of this function is your ability to hold a conversation with someone at a crowded, noisy party.

Into the middle ear

After a sound wave travels through the ear canal, it strikes the taut membrane of the eardrum, causing the eardrum

Sound pressure level and hearing level

Decibels are common units of measure that can indicate two different types of sound intensity. Measuring the force of a sound wave in the environment or the amount of pressure it exerts on your eardrum is referred to as sound pressure level. The reference level of 0 decibels sound pressure level (dB SPL) is about the weakest sound that can be heard with the best human ears. The intensity of normal speech is generally around 60 dB SPL.

Decibel units can also establish how well your hearing compares with the average for a large group of young people with normal hearing. This measure is expressed in decibels hearing level (dB HL). A person with a hearing threshold — the faintest level at which he or she can perceive sound — between 0 and 25 dB HL is considered to have normal or near-normal hearing. Someone who has trouble understanding conversations may barely hear sounds at 40 dB HL but not lower and is considered to have moderate hearing loss. A person who can hear only a loud, nearby voice may have a hearing threshold of 70 dB HL and is considered to have severe hearing loss.

In subsequent chapters, sound intensity expressed in terms of dB will represent a measure of sound pressure level. When referring to a measure of hearing level, it will be expressed as dB HL.

to vibrate. These vibrations cause the ossicles that bridge the space between the eardrum and the oval window to vibrate also. The ossicles move together like a tiny lever system.

Because the surface of the eardrum is much larger than the oval window, the vibrations are delivered with greater force to the inner ear. Amplifying the sound increases the energy, which is necessary for the vibrations to travel through the fluid of the inner ear. Fluid offers more resistance than does air and thus requires a greater force to push through it.

If a sound is too loud, muscles in the middle ear constrict to reduce the effects of the sound and protect the inner ear. This is called an acoustic reflex. However, a noise such as a nearby gunshot can cause immediate, permanent damage to the ear. That's because of a slight delay between the auditory nerve's response to a sudden sound and the middle ear muscle's protective contraction. This brief delay leaves the inner ear vulnerable to damage from impact noise.

Into the inner ear

The vibration of the stirrup against the oval window transmits the pattern of the sound wave to the inner ear and the fluid in the upper and lower chambers of the cochlea. The wave sets in motion the hair cells embedded in the basilar membrane (see page 16).

Each frequency of a sound wave affects a specific section of the basilar membrane. This stimulates a response in the hair cells exactly at that location. If the sound you hear has a very high frequency, the basilar membrane resonates near the base of the cochlea. If the sound wave has a low frequency, the basilar membrane resonates closer to the tip of the cochlea.

This motion displaces the cilia on the hair cells, resulting in a chemical reaction within the hair cells. This chemical reaction triggers electrical impulses in the auditory nerve. The louder or more intense the sound, the more impulses that are sent off.

Traveling to the brain

From the auditory nerve, electrical impulses travel along twin neurological circuits in the brain containing several information-processing stations. These stations start analyzing the signals to determine their origin. For example, the stations for the left ear compare what they've learned with stations for the right ear. This activity also filters background noise. See a visualization of the sound pathways on page 24.

The neurological circuits end in the special regions of the brain called auditory cortex areas, which further interpret, analyze and process sound. There is an auditory cortex area on each side of the brain within the temporal lobes. Arrival of the impulses in the auditory cortex areas signals the grand finale of the hearing process.

Scientists are still trying to understand how the brain interprets the impulses and identifies them as distinct sounds. At lower frequencies the electrical impulses follow the same pattern as the sound waves. But at high frequencies, this pattern varies.

Speech and language — how the brain gives meaning to sound — is associated closely with your ability to hear. We know that the knowledge and recognition of specific sounds in a person's memory starts at a young age. For example, at about 3 months, babies can differentiate their parents' voices from other voices.

Types of hearing loss

With such a complex auditory system, many small changes or slight damage to the ear can affect some or most of your hearing. Scientists have identified three types of hearing loss: conductive, sensorineural and mixed.

Conductive hearing loss

The ear canal and the middle ear conduct sound waves to the sensory receptors of your inner ear. If something blocks this pathway, the sound waves are disrupted. The result is a reduced perception of sound.

This can occur, for example, from an excessive buildup of wax in the ear canal. Normally, your ear canal cleanses itself, but in some cases buildup occurs and may require professional removal.

Other problems that can cause conductive hearing loss include foreign objects lodged in the ear, middle ear infections, head trauma and abnormal bone growth in the region of the ear. See Chapter 3 for more information about conductive hearing loss.

Sensorineural hearing loss

Damage to the structures of the inner ear, such as the hair cells in the cochlea or the nerve fibers leading from the cochlea to the brain, can cause sensorineural (sen-suh-ree-NOOR-ul) hearing loss. Such damage is most often associated with the general wear and tear of aging, known as presbycusis (pres-bih-KU-sis), or with too much exposure to loud noise.

Initial sensorineural damage is typically found at the base of the cochlea,

In the ear Sound waves that have traveled through the ear canal cause the eardrum and ossicles of the middle ear to vibrate. These vibrations trigger a chemical reaction in the cochlea of the inner ear, sending electrical impulses along the auditory nerve and into the brain.

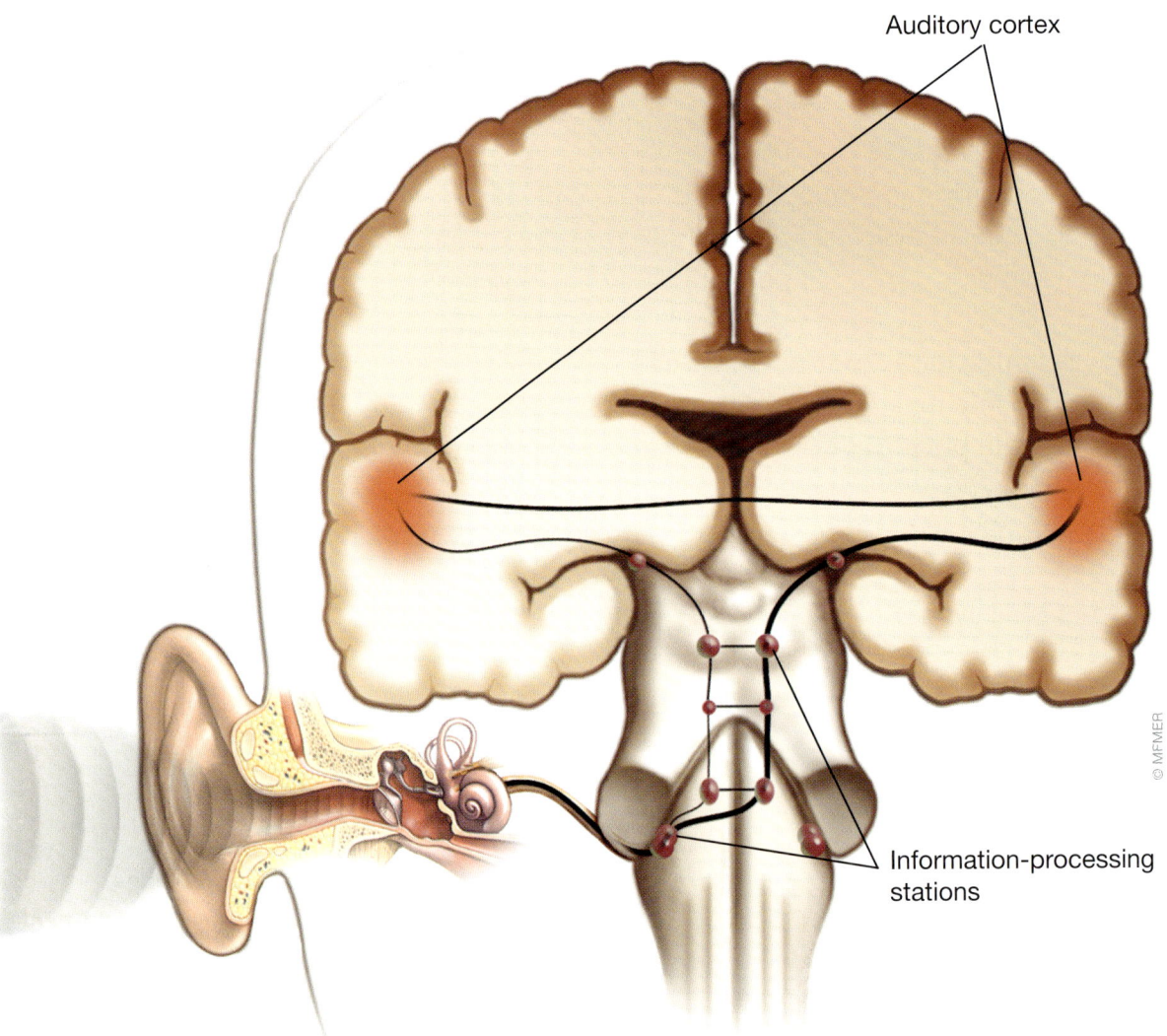

In the brain Electrical impulses from the auditory nerve pass through and cross between several information-processing stations on their way to the auditory cortex areas in the temporal lobes. There, the brain sorts, processes, analyzes, compares and files information about sounds, helping you to make sense of what you hear.

24   Chapter 1: How you hear

where the basilar membrane responds to high frequencies. That's why people with sensorineural hearing loss often have trouble perceiving high-frequency sounds, such as certain consonants used in speech.

For example, someone with high-frequency hearing loss may be unable to distinguish the word *tell* from *sell* or *miff* from *myth*.

Other potential damage to the inner ear may result from high fever or chronic illness, certain powerful medications that can hurt the ear, trauma to the head, and genetic disorders. As well, the auditory nerve can be damaged by abnormal growths, such as tumors, and other causes. See Chapter 4 for more information about sensorineural hearing loss.

Mixed hearing loss

Some individuals may have a combination of conductive and sensorineural hearing loss. For example, someone with age-related sensorineural hearing loss may also develop a middle ear infection. The conductive hearing loss caused by the infection can usually be eliminated with medical treatment. However, the sensorineural damage is likely untreatable.

Compensating for hearing loss

Hearing loss too often bears the brunt of jokes and comedic skits. Frequently, it's associated with inattention, lower intelligence or just plain "getting old." Some people convince themselves that they don't need to hear everything out there anyway and simply resign themselves to their condition.

Losing some of your hearing can be an obstacle at best. At some times, it can be and dangerous. You may mostly think credit hearing for helping you to understand what others are saying. But is also cues you to where you are and alerts you to potential danger. Overall, hearing helps you stay connected to the world.

Many people avoid admitting to hearing loss for fear of being stereotyped as someone who consistently misunderstands conversations and talks to others by shouting. They may compensate for their diminished hearing and try to mask it by:

- Blaming others for mumbling or speaking too softly
- Limiting or withdrawing from social activities

Recognize signs of hearing loss

Look for early signs of hearing loss. The questions below, based on a list from the National Institute on Deafness and Other Communication Disorders, may help you decide whether to see a physician or audiologist for a hearing evaluation. Keep in mind, these general questions may not address everything about your specific situation.

- Do you have a problem with hearing on the telephone?
- Do you have to strain to understand conversations?
- Do you have trouble following a conversation when two or more people are talking at the same time?
- Do you have trouble hearing in a situation with a noisy background?
- Do people say that you turn the TV volume up too high?
- Do you find yourself asking people to repeat themselves?
- Do many people you talk to seem to mumble or not speak clearly?
- Do people get annoyed because you misunderstand what they say?
- Do you respond inappropriately to what people say?
- Do you have trouble understanding the speech of people who may have higher pitched voices or are soft-spoken — often women and children?

If you answered yes to three or more of these questions, you may think about requesting a hearing evaluation. In addition, ask someone who knows you well to consider these questions with you in mind. He or she might notice signs of hearing loss in you long before you do and prompt you to get help.

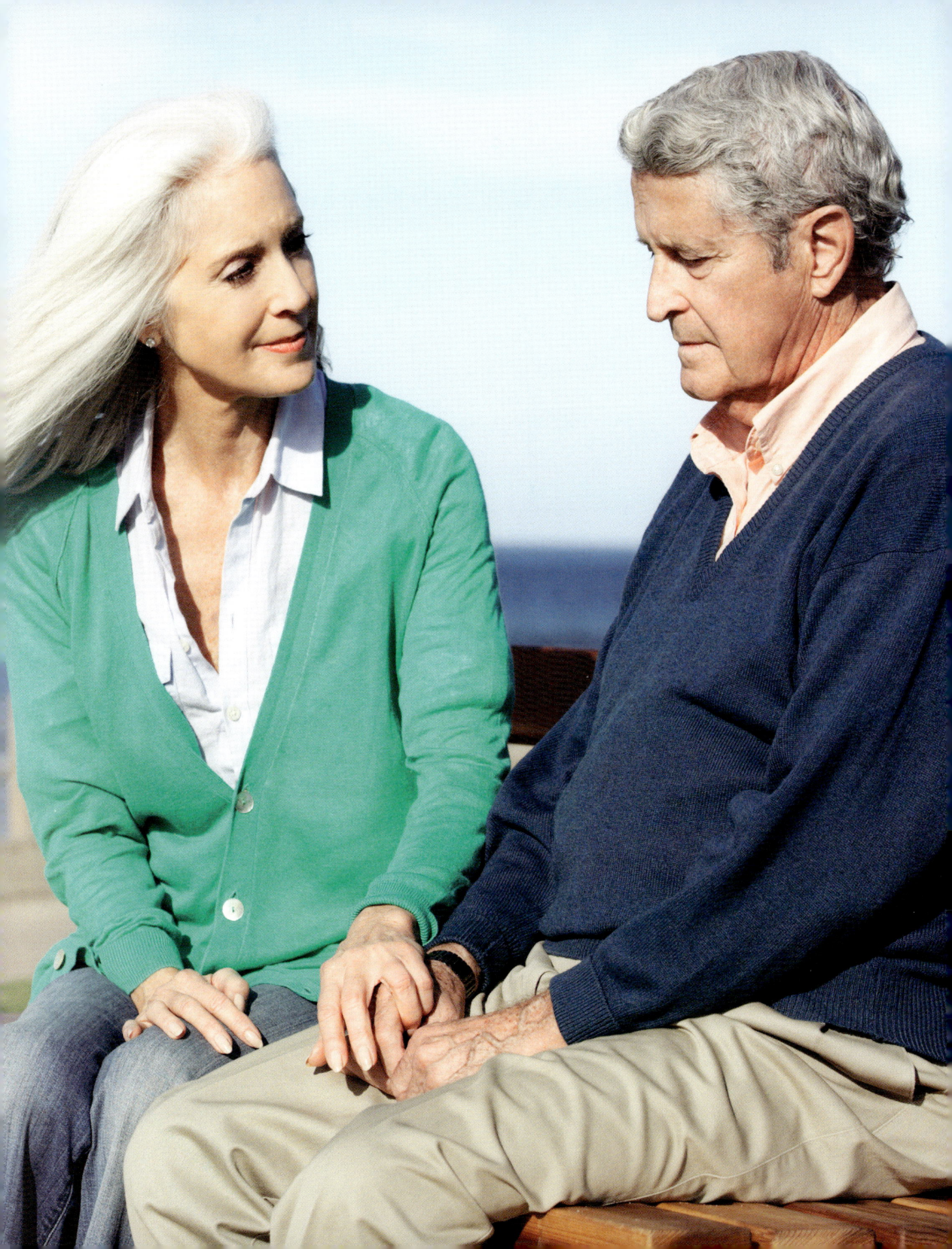

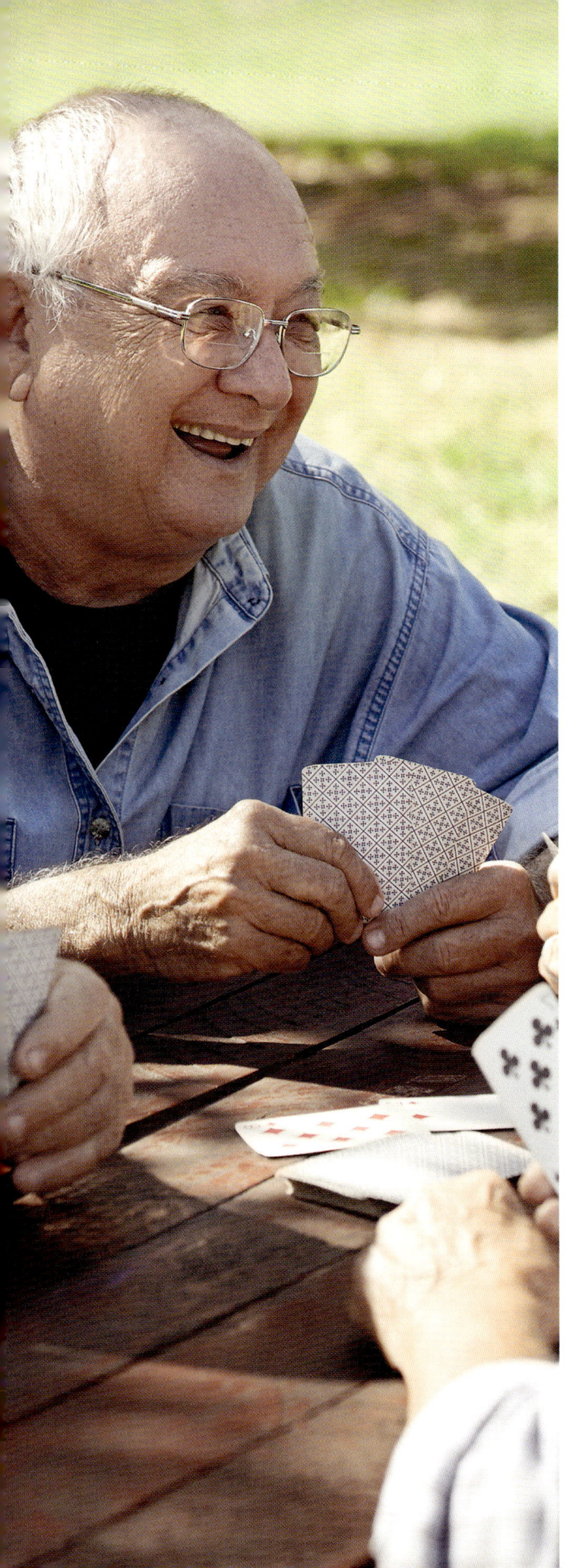

- Turning up the volume on the television or radio
- Smiling and nodding without understanding

If you regularly engage in the actions listed above, you might consider seeking the help of an audiologist to evaluate your hearing.

To deny a real hearing deficit because you don't want others to recognize it is like refusing to look at your shirt in order to detract attention from a stain. Many people will see through your efforts and notice the problem anyway. Addressing a hearing problem can put you on the path to becoming a more active participant in life and a more engaged companion and friend.

Chapter 2

Getting a hearing exam

Perhaps you've noticed lately that you have trouble hearing certain letter sounds when someone is talking to you. While attending a lecture recently, you had difficulty distinguishing the speaker's voice from the background noise. Or you've been having trouble following the typical daily conversation at the dinner table. Because you're unsure of what's being said, you've become more reluctant to join in conversations.

If these situations are becoming all too familiar, you may be experiencing some degree of hearing loss. While you may be tempted to just accept or ignore the problem, consider seeking help. A hearing exam may help identify the cause and lead to treatment that enables you to both hear better and feel more socially engaged and confident.

If you want to get your hearing or your child's hearing checked, whom do you see? You might want to start by talking with your primary doctor or your child's pediatrician. Your doctor can do a preliminary hearing exam and provide explanations for many of your concerns. He or she can also refer you to a hearing specialist (audiologist) if necessary.

In this chapter, you'll get a closer look at each of the specialty areas that may be involved in the diagnosis and treatment of hearing loss. You'll also find out when a hearing exam may be necessary, what's involved in the exam and what the results mean. Knowing what tests to expect and why they're performed can help you get the most out of the hearing exam and put you on your way toward a solution.

Who provides ear care?

Your family doctor may ask about your hearing at medical visits and encourage you to get tested if there are any concerns. In addition, it's wise to talk to your doctor whenever you are routinely exposed to loud noise, notice signs of hearing loss or notice a ringing in the ear (tinnitus).

Always consult your doctor before buying a hearing aid. Sometimes hearing loss results from wax impaction, infection, tumor or other problems that call for medication or surgery, not a hearing aid. Your doctor can guide you to the most appropriate treatment.

There are different kinds of hearing specialists, primarily otolaryngologists, neurotologists and audiologists. Because hearing loss may result from a variety of causes, hearing specialists often work closely with specialists in other fields to make a diagnosis and determine the best course of treatment.

Otolaryngologists

Your primary doctor may refer you to an otolaryngologist (o-toe-lar-ing-GOL-uh-jist) for a thorough hearing examination. Otolaryngologists are medical doctors trained to diagnose and treat diseases of the ears, sinuses, mouth, throat, voice box (larynx) and other structures in the head and neck region. They may also perform cosmetic and reconstructive surgery of the head and neck. These specialists are also known as otorhinolaryngologists (o-toe-rie-no-lar-ing-GOL-uh-jists) or, simply, ear, nose and throat (ENT) specialists.

An otolaryngologist must have broad specialization in the head and neck areas because different parts of the head — ears, nose and throat — are interconnected. The ears and throat are joined by the eustachian tubes. The nose and the throat are joined by the nasopharynx. So, what happens in one area can easily affect the other areas. An upper respiratory infection of the sinuses, for example, can spread to the ears or throat.

All otolaryngologists have completed medical school and at least five years of residency, or specialty training. They're also certified by the American Board of Otolaryngology. After their residency, some otolaryngologists pursue an additional one- or two-year fellowship for more extensive training

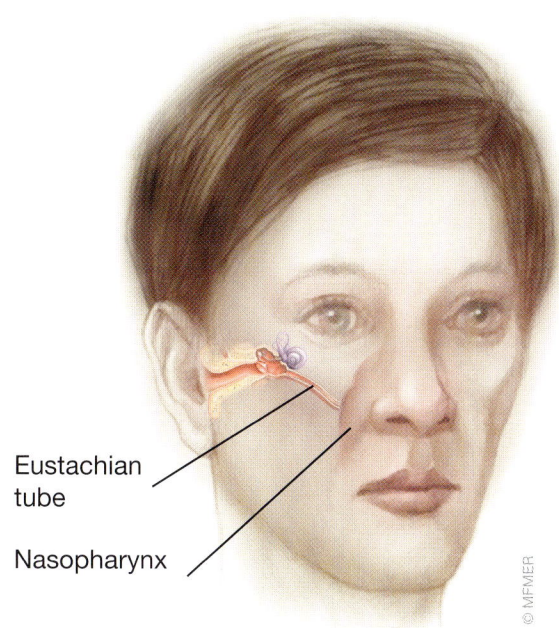

An otolaryngologist must have broad specialization in the head and neck areas because the ears, nose and throat are interconnected.

in a chosen specialty. Some otolaryngologists may choose to focus their practice on ear disorders and refer to themselves as otologists.

Neurotologists

A neurotologist (nooro-TOL-uh-jist) is an otolaryngologist who has completed a specialty fellowship focused on ear disorders. Thus, he or she has the most in-depth training devoted to any physical problems of the ear. If your primary doctor suspects that you have an ear disease, you may be referred directly to a neurotologist.

Some of the conditions that neurotologists treat include ear infections, facial paralysis, dizziness, hearing loss, ringing in the ears (tinnitus), tumors and congenital deformities. If you need surgery for an ear disorder, you'll probably see a neurotologist or an otolaryngologist with special training in ear surgery.

Audiologists

An audiologist (aw-de-OL-uh-jist) is trained to evaluate the perceptual aspects of your hearing. If you complain of hearing loss but your doctor finds no physical signs of disease, you may be referred to an audiologist. The audiologist can assess the type of hearing loss you have and measure its severity. Audiologists also evaluate and fit hearing aids and help with hearing rehabilitation.

Audiologists hold a master's degree or doctoral degree in audiology and must have completed an externship — one year of on-the-job experience — before they're able to practice independently. They may be certified through the American Speech-Language-Hearing Association (ASHA) or by the American

Mayo Clinic on Better Hearing and Balance **31**

Board of Audiology. All states require audiologists to be licensed in the state in which they practice.

Working together

Often, these different specialists work together to diagnose and treat a condition. For example, your neurotologist or otolaryngologist may refer you to an audiologist to have your hearing tested before treating an ear disorder, and again later to see if the treatment is having an effect.

In contrast, an audiologist may be evaluating you and suspect that your hearing loss is due to a medical problem. In that case, you'll likely be referred to an neurotologist or otolaryngologist for treatment. Subsequently, the audiologist may see you again for hearing rehabilitation. The sequence of visits is important because each specialist approaches the problem with different training and from a different perspective.

In addition, audiologists may monitor the hearing of individuals who are undergoing treatment for an illness such as cancer or an infectious disease. Some chemotherapy and antibiotic drugs can damage a person's hearing, so the oncologist or infectious disease specialist will work closely with an audiologist to monitor the person's hearing and, if possible, keep the prescribed drug dosage low enough to avoid auditory damage.

Schedule for hearing exams

Everyone should have their hearing tested, from newborns to older adults. An exam can be performed on request if you're concerned about hearing loss or when situations occur that increase your risk of hearing loss. Sometimes the exam is mandated by law.

Children

The screening of newborns is now a common practice in most hospitals in the United States. In fact, in most states testing is mandatory. That's because hearing loss affects 12,000 children born in the U.S. each year, making it the most common birth defect. Failure to identify the impairment early enough can lead to delayed speech and language development, social-emotional or behavioral problems, and delays in academic development.

Children with unidentified hearing loss often don't do as well in school as their peers do. They're also more likely to be held back a grade or drop out. Because hearing loss isn't readily noticeable, adults may attribute a child's perceived inattention to other causes, such as being distracted or unmotivated. Early treatment can help prevent many of the problems related to hearing loss and provide the child with the necessary tools to be successful at school.

Some types of hearing loss in children don't develop until months or years after birth, so periodic screening is recommended. See page 34 for the recommended screening schedules.

In addition, babies considered to be at high risk of hearing loss should be screened regularly. This group includes infants with a medical history of:

- Severe oxygen deprivation at birth (birth asphyxia)
- Exposure in the womb to an infection such as German measles (rubella) or syphilis
- Exposure to herpes during passage through the birth canal
- Bacterial meningitis infection
- Severe jaundice
- Head trauma
- Chronic ear infection
- Nervous system disorder associated with hearing loss
- Family history of hearing loss during childhood
- Cytomegalovirus infection
- Treatment with chemotherapy

Adults

Screening for adults is not done on a regular schedule. Generally, it's performed at their request. ASHA recommends that adults get their hearing checked at least every 10 years through age 50 and every three years after that.

Hearing loss increases with age — less than 20 percent of individuals between 45 and 64 years of age have some degree of hearing loss. That jumps to more than 30 percent for people ages 65 to 74 and to 50 percent for those age 75 and older.

Employees

Prolonged exposure to loud noise can cause gradual, and often permanent, hearing loss. The Occupational Safety and Health Administration (OSHA) requires that employers monitor their companies for noise levels at 85 decibels (dB) or above, averaged over eight working hours.

Recommended screening schedules

Infants and toddlers
- By 1 month of age: Initial screening, preferably soon after birth.
- By 3 months of age: Further evaluation to confirm hearing loss if indicated by initial screening.
- Before 6 months of age: Appropriate treatment initiated for infants with hearing loss. Ongoing monitoring every six months.
- By age 2 to 2½: Diagnostic assessment for children who pass the initial screening but who have a risk factor for hearing loss. May be needed more frequently for those with higher risk factors or new concerns about hearing.

School-age children
- On first entry into school system
- Annually from kindergarten through third grade
- At seventh grade
- At 11th grade
- On entry to special education
- On repeating a grade
- On entry to a new school system without evidence of previous screening
- When indicated by parent or caregiver, by medical or school concern, or by high risk factors of hearing loss

Adults
- Every 10 years through age 50 and every three years thereafter

Employees
- Before employment
- Before assignment to a hearing-hazardous work area*
- Annually while assigned to a hearing-hazardous work area
- After ending assignment to a hearing-hazardous work area
- At termination of employment

*A hearing-hazardous work area is considered an environment with noise exposure equal to or greater than 85 decibels, if averaged over eight working hours.

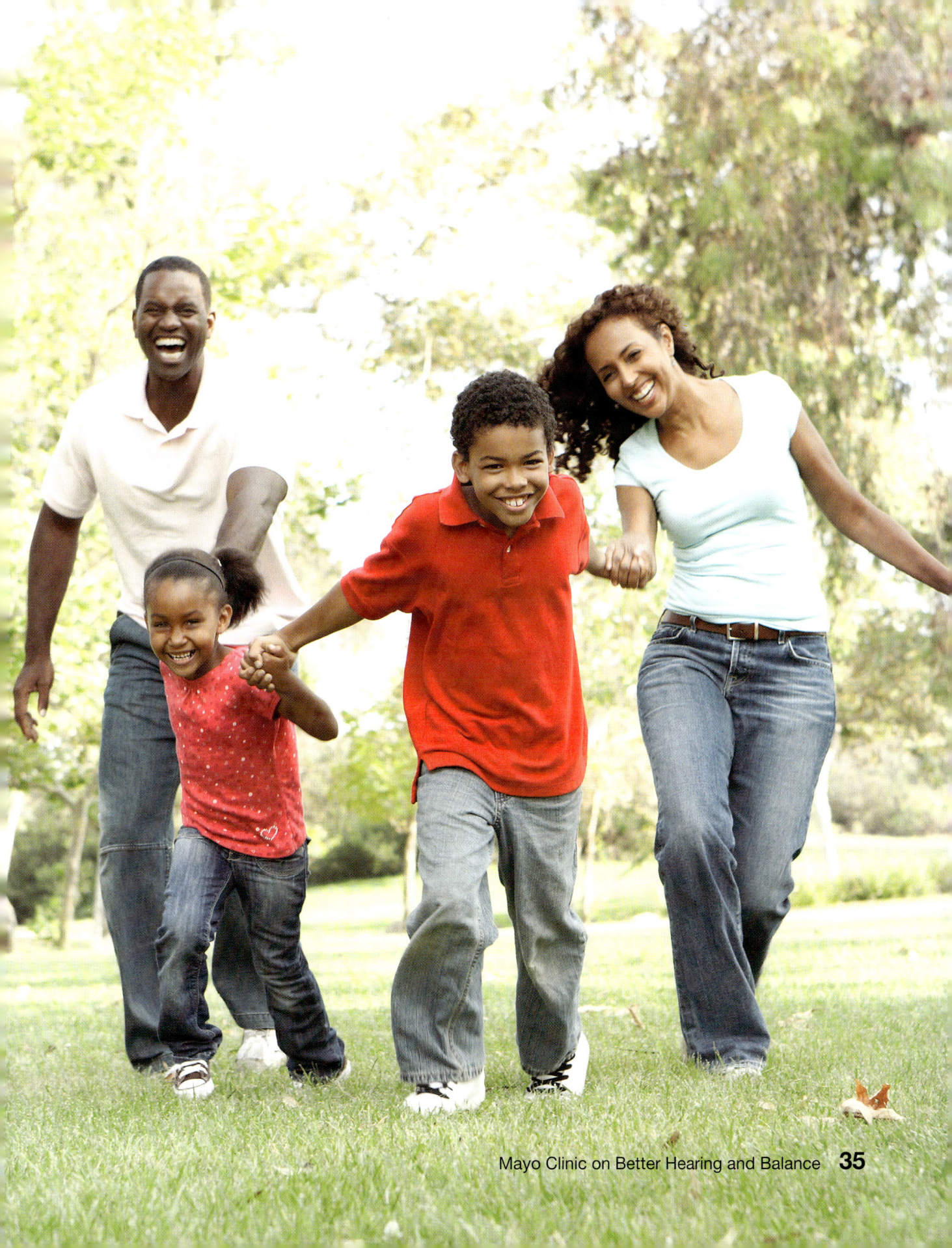

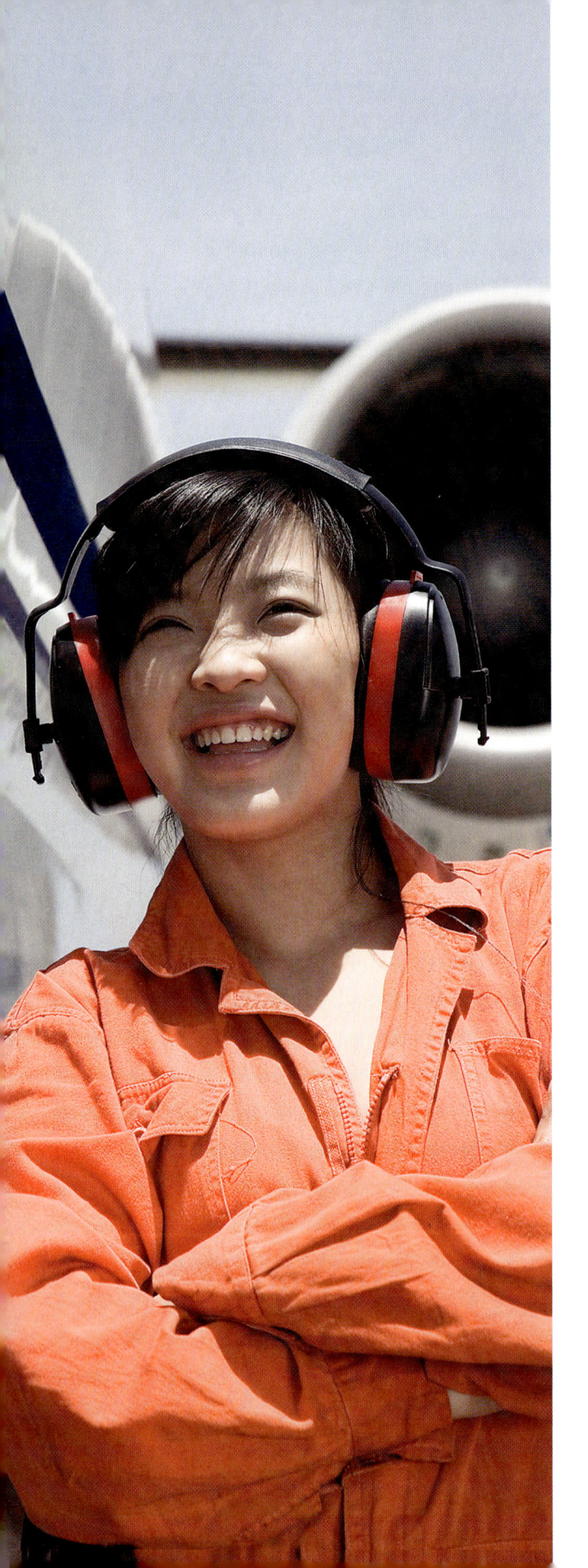

Under such conditions the employer must develop and maintain a hearing conservation program at no cost to the employee. The program would include regular hearing exams, noise monitoring, access to earplugs or protective devices (such as earmuffs), record keeping and employee training regarding hearing protection.

If regular screening indicates hearing loss has occurred, the employee must be informed and wear hearing protectors in work environments with noise levels of 85 dB or more. Hearing protectors are required for all employees when noise levels exceed 90 dB, averaged over eight working hours.

In order for hearing protectors to be effective, it's important that they fit properly and are worn continuously during periods of noise exposure. OSHA requires that a qualified hearing specialist administer the program.

Typical hearing exam

A physician and an audiologist will complete different portions of a hearing examination in order to assess all aspects of your hearing. If there's evidence of hearing loss, they will evaluate the signs and symptoms and check for other medical conditions that may be causing the problem. This will help them determine the severity of your hearing loss and suggest an appropriate course of treatment.

The tests will involve an overall medical evaluation that includes a medical history, physical examination of your ears and laboratory tests. Audiological exams include audiometry, speech reception and word recognition, as well as other tests.

Medical evaluation

The first step in your hearing exam, whether you consult your family doctor or an ear specialist, is to get a full medical evaluation. This helps the doctor determine your overall health status and whether your hearing loss could be the result of an underlying condition. The evaluation generally includes some or all of the following components:

Medical history.
Your examiner will want to fully document the development of your hearing problem. You'll need to be ready for many questions.

- When did you first become aware of the signs and symptoms of hearing loss?
- Is the impairment in one ear or are both ears affected?
- Is the problem getting worse, improving or staying the same?
- Are some sounds more difficult to hear than other sounds, or are all sounds equally hard to distinguish?
- Do you have difficulty recognizing where a sound comes from?
- Are you experiencing signs and symptoms such as ear pain, discharge, infection, dizziness, ringing in the ears and loss of balance?
- Do any members of your family have hearing problems?

Be sure to tell your examiner if you've had long exposure to loud noise, either at work or home. In addition, tell the doctor if you've ever experienced head trauma, ear surgery or chronic illness, or whether you've recently had an upper respiratory infection, such as a cold or pneumonia. Let your examiner know what medications you're taking or have recently taken.

Physical exam
The next part of your exam will be to examine the size, shape and position of your outer ear (pinna) and to inspect it for any swelling, deformity or redness.

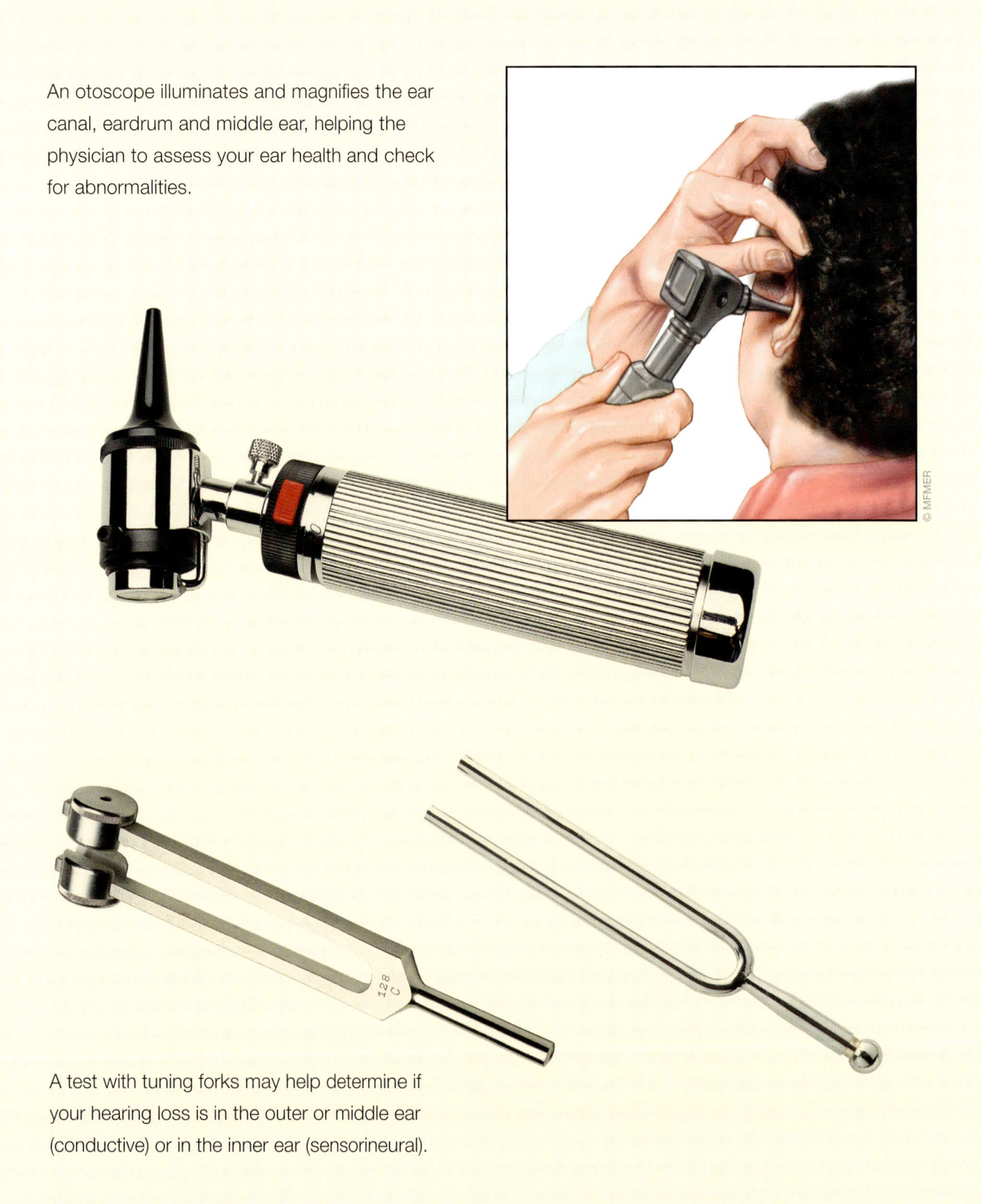

An otoscope illuminates and magnifies the ear canal, eardrum and middle ear, helping the physician to assess your ear health and check for abnormalities.

A test with tuning forks may help determine if your hearing loss is in the outer or middle ear (conductive) or in the inner ear (sensorineural).

38 Chapter 2: Getting a hearing exam

This step may yield information about other problems that may be causing hearing loss.

Your examiner may check your eyes, nasal cavity, mouth and neck for any problems that might be associated with ear damage. A slender, flexible tube with a light at the end is used to check for signs of fluid buildup or infection in the back of your nose and upper throat (nasopharynx) and your eustachian tubes, which connect your ears to your nasopharynx.

Otoscopy

The visual examination of the ear canal, eardrum and middle ear is called an otoscopy — the prefix *oto-* simply refers to "ear." For the test, your physician or audiologist typically uses an instrument called an otoscope, which contains a light and magnifying lens (see page 38). A specially designed microscope called an otomicroscope also may be used to view the ear canal and eardrum.

Generally, an otoscopic examination takes a minute or two and is painless. The examiner may look for wax or fluid buildup, foreign objects, a tumor or skin abnormalities in the ear canal, and any small tears or perforations in the eardrum. He or she also notes whether

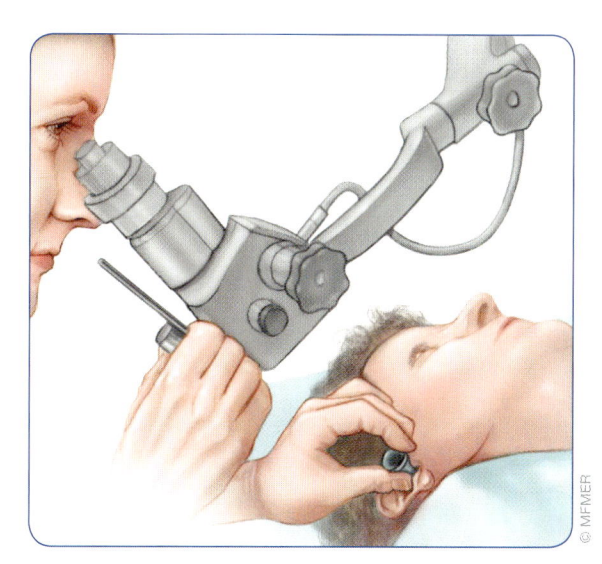

An otomicroscope provides a more detailed look into your ear. The physician gently inserts a small viewing funnel into your ear canal to focus the image.

the eardrum is translucent and has its normal pearly gray color. A bulging eardrum membrane may indicate fluid in the middle ear.

Tuning fork test

A tuning fork looks like a dining fork with only two tines. Made of steel, it sounds a single tone when struck against a solid object — and that tone varies according to the shape and thickness of the tines.

To conduct the test, vibrating forks with different pitches are positioned near your ear to measure your hearing sensitivity to the air conduction of

Mayo Clinic on Better Hearing and Balance

sound waves. The forks are also placed against your skull to measure your sensitivity to the bone conduction of sound waves.

Comparing the results of these tests provides important clues to the cause of your hearing loss. People whose hearing is reduced by air conduction but is normal by bone conduction typically have conductive hearing loss — sound waves have difficulty passing through the ear canal or middle ear. People whose hearing is reduced both by air conduction and bone conduction generally have sensorineural hearing loss due to damage in the inner ear.

Laboratory tests

Your physician may request certain blood tests to confirm or rule out possible infectious or inflammatory diseases that are associated with hearing loss. These include syphilis, German measles (rubella), cytomegalovirus — a gastrointestinal infection — and several autoimmune disorders.

These blood tests are particularly important for pregnant women. One of these diseases in an expectant mother can lead to hearing loss that's present at birth (congenital) in her baby. Blood samples also may be examined for DNA abnormalities.

Imaging tests

If your physician suspects that a tumor, tissue abnormality or damage to the auditory nerve is the cause of your hearing loss, a request may be made for detailed images of the interior of your head. Technology to produce these images includes magnetic resonance imaging (MRI) and computerized tomography (CT) scan.

MRI technology creates detailed images of soft tissues using magnetic fields and radio waves. CT technology produces images of bone structure from a series of X-rays. Both types of imaging can reveal a variety of disorders that would otherwise remain unseen, helping lead to a correct diagnosis. Sophisticated imaging technology also may be used to locate congenital abnormalities and trauma-related damage to the ear.

Audiological exam

The audiological exam is focused on hearing function — how well you hear — rather than on physical signs of disease. Audiologists use various tests to determine your hearing status and degree of hearing loss.

These tests can help distinguish between different types of possible

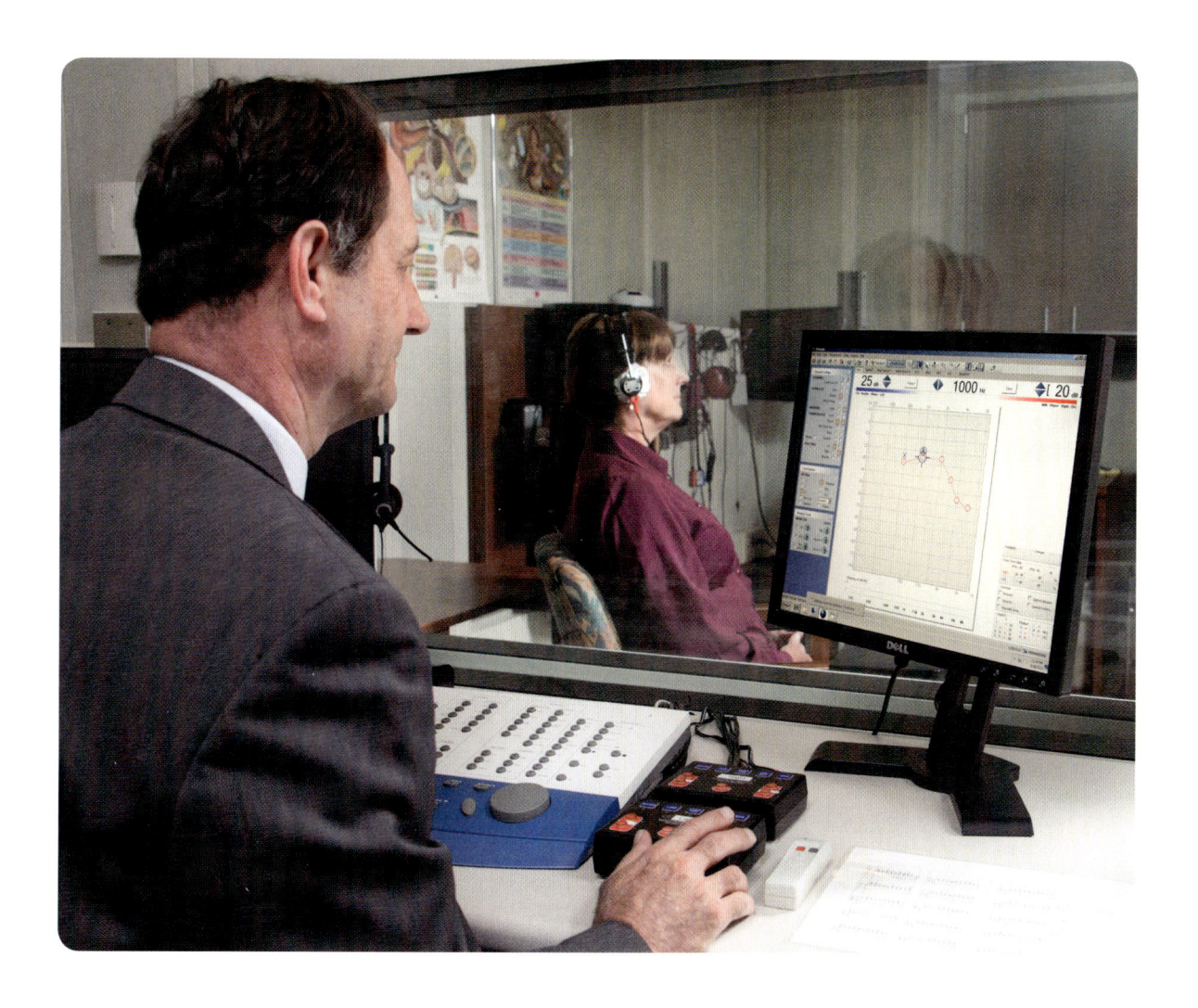

During audiometry, you'll be seated in a sound-treated room (top right in photograph) separate from the audiologist. You'll signal the audiologist whenever you hear a tone played through the earphones. Your hearing thresholds at different pitches will be recorded on an audiogram (graph on the left of screen shot). Also displayed are the results of tympanometry, acoustic reflex and speech recognition tests.

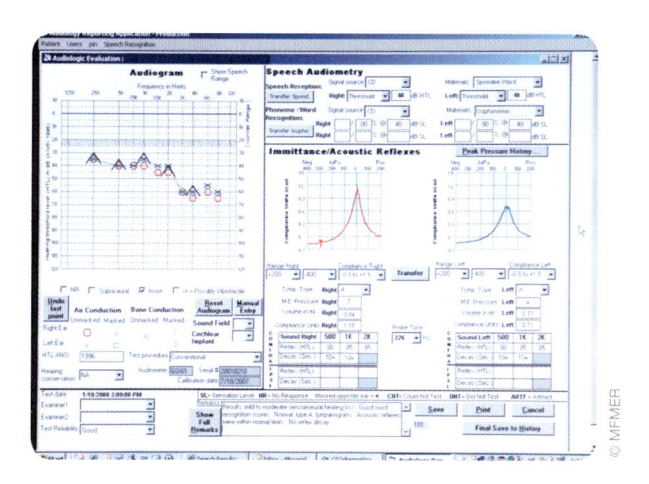

Mayo Clinic on Better Hearing and Balance   **41**

Levels of hearing loss

Decibel (dB) range	Level of hearing loss	Characteristics
16 to 25 dB HL* **	Slight	• Has difficulty hearing faint or distant sounds
26 to 40 dB HL	Mild	• Occasionally misses consonants • Has increasing difficulty in understanding with noisy backgrounds and faraway speakers
41 to 55 dB HL	Moderate	• Can understand normal conversation if face to face and vocabulary is controlled
56 to 70 dB HL	Moderately severe	• May miss most of what's said in a normal conversation • Has difficulty listening in a group setting
71 to 90 dB HL	Severe	• May not be able to hear speech unless very loud • Needs amplification to be able to converse normally
91 dB HL and above	Profound	• May not be able to hear speech at all • Relies on visual cues such as lip reading or sign language

* dB HL = decibels hearing level
** Most clinics consider 0 to 25 dB HL to be the range of normal hearing sensitivity.

Adapted from American Speech-Language-Hearing Association, 2013

hearing loss, reveal whether the impairment is in one or both ears, and determine whether the hearing loss involves one, two or more frequencies. Repeat testing can gauge whether the impairment is getting worse.

Audiometry

This testing measures your ability to hear pure tones, such as a middle C and higher notes, through air and through bone. The previously described tuning fork test is a rudimentary form of the audiometric test.

To check your hearing by way of air conduction, the examiner places earphones over your ears or small, soft tips into your ear canals. Certain tones are introduced through the earphones to one ear at a time.

By varying the frequency and intensity of the tones, the examiner determines the faintest sounds you can hear — your hearing thresholds. You'll be directed to signal, usually by raising a hand or pressing a button, whenever you hear a tone. Your responses are recorded on a type of graph called an audiogram.

Checking your hearing for sounds conducted through the bones of your skull can help locate problems in the outer and middle ear. To do this the examiner places a special vibrating device either behind your ear or on your forehead. The vibrations travel through your skull, thus bypassing any blockage that may be present in the outer or middle ear.

If test results show that you hear sound when it's conducted through skull bone better than through the ear canal and middle ear, then sound isn't getting through the outer ear and middle ear properly. It's likely that you have some form of conductive hearing loss. If results show that your hearing is no better via bone conduction than through air conduction, it's likely to be a sensorineural problem with the inner ear.

Speech reception test

For this test, the audiologist plays a recording of, or speaks, familiar two-syllable words, such as *pancake* or *baseball*, while you listen through headphones. Each syllable of a spoken word is pronounced with equal emphasis.

As you hear a word, you repeat it or point to a picture of it. The intensity of the words gradually softens. The faintest level of speech you can understand at least half the time is called your speech reception threshold, or speech recognition threshold (SRT).

If your SRT is normal — typically in a range between 0 and 25 decibels hearing level (dB HL) — you should not have difficulty hearing and should be able to understand conversational speech in a quiet environment.

If your SRT is 26 dB HL or higher, you're experiencing progressively more severe levels of hearing loss. An SRT greater than 91 dB HL indicates profound hearing loss. Generally, there's a strong correlation between the SRT and your pure tone audiometry test results.

Word recognition test

This test, also known as a speech discrimination test, determines how well you can understand speech at a comfortable volume — typically set at about 40 dB above your SRT level. (Remember that the SRT is a threshold at which sounds below that point are not understandable by you.)

For the test, you must identify a series of familiar single-syllable words such as *come*, *thin*, *sack* and *knees*. When you hear the words, either from a recording or spoken, at a constant, steady volume, you repeat each word or point to a picture of it. Occasionally, background noise is added to see how distraction might affect your understanding.

Your score reflects the percentage of words you've identified correctly. A score between 90 and 100 percent means you should have little difficulty understanding conversation. Scores between 70 and 89 percent indicate occasional difficulty, 40 to 69 percent indicates marked difficulty, and less than 40 percent indicates extreme difficulty in understanding speech.

Word recognition performed with and without a hearing aid may indicate how helpful the device can be to you, and can help guide your decision about whether or not to use one.

Other tests

In addition to the medical evaluation and audiological exam, your doctor or audiologist may wish to test other aspects of your hearing. These tests can help to refine the diagnosis or determine which treatment options would be most beneficial to you. The additional tests include:

Tympanometry
This test is used to check the function of your eardrum and middle ear. Tympanometry (tim-puh-NOM-uh-tree) helps detect conditions such as a perforated eardrum, fluid in the middle ear and reduced air pressure in the middle ear resulting in a retraction of the eardrum.

To conduct the test, your examiner places a soft probe in your ear canal. As small, varying amounts of air pressure are directed toward your ear, the device measures the corresponding movements of your eardrum. The results are charted on a graph called a tympanogram.

Normal response produces a line rising to a sharp peak in the middle of the tympanogram. But if fluid is in the middle ear, the eardrum doesn't move easily and the graph's line doesn't peak. The graph can also reveal whether the air pressure in the middle ear is less than or greater than outside atmospheric pressure.

Acoustic reflex test
An acoustic reflex test measures the level at which the muscle in your middle ear contracts in response to sounds that are too loud. The acoustic reflex is described on page 22.

During the test you hear sounds at varying levels of intensity. The level at which the reflex contraction occurs, or the absence of reflex, helps evaluate your hearing loss and locate problems along the auditory pathway.

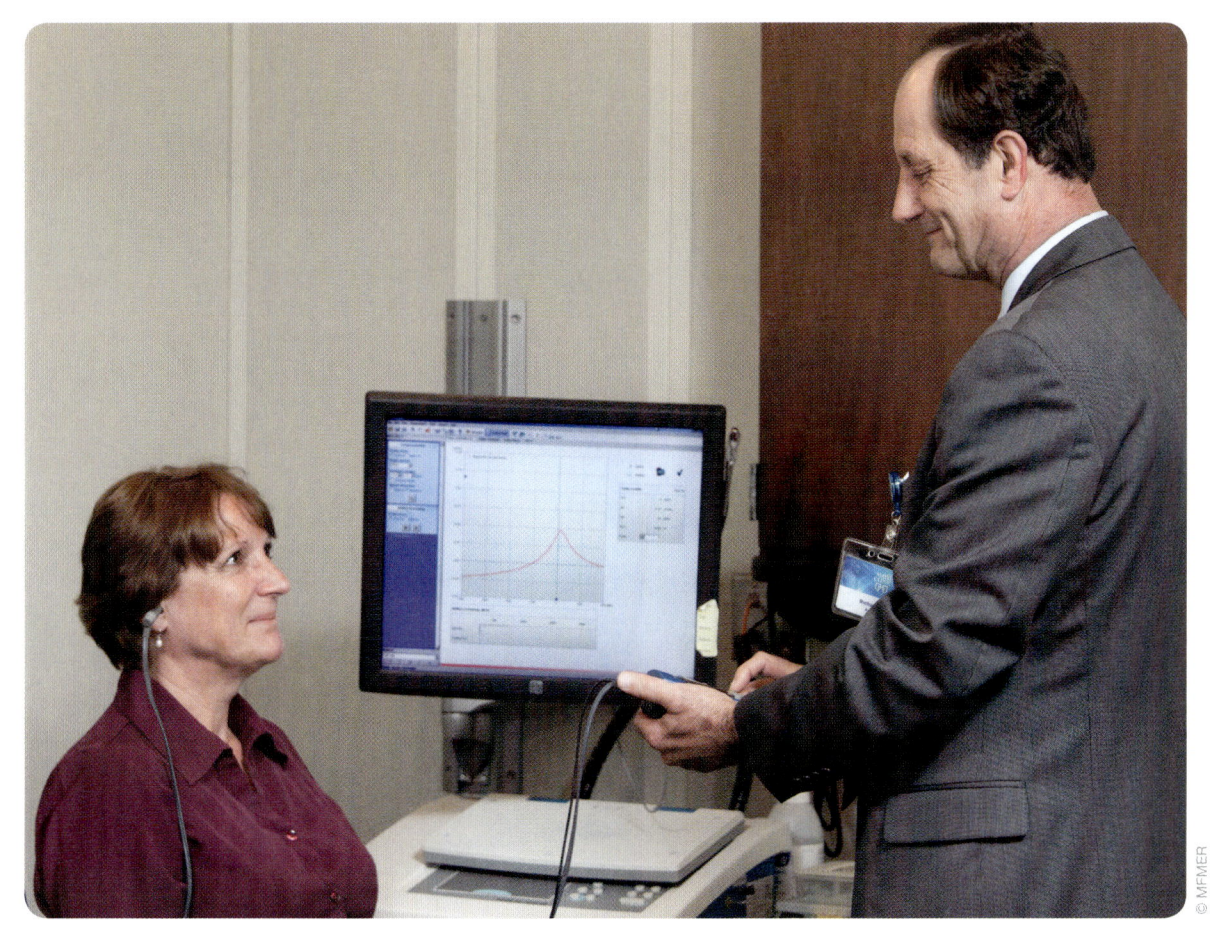

Your doctor or audiologist may use tympanometry to record the response of your eardrum to varying amounts of air pressure. The tympanogram can indicate conductive problems such as a perforated eardrum or fluid buildup in the middle ear.

Auditory brainstem response test

This test measures the electrical nerve impulses sent from the inner ear to the brain when sounds are introduced to the ear. Electrodes are placed in the ear canal or around the ear as well as on your head. Earphones introduce a series of short clicking sounds to your ear. A computer connected to the electrodes records neurological activity as the auditory nerve transmits the impulses to the brain.

Because this test doesn't require a voluntary response, such as a hand signal, from the person being tested, it's often used to screen hearing in newborns and infants. This test can be

Mayo Clinic on Better Hearing and Balance **45**

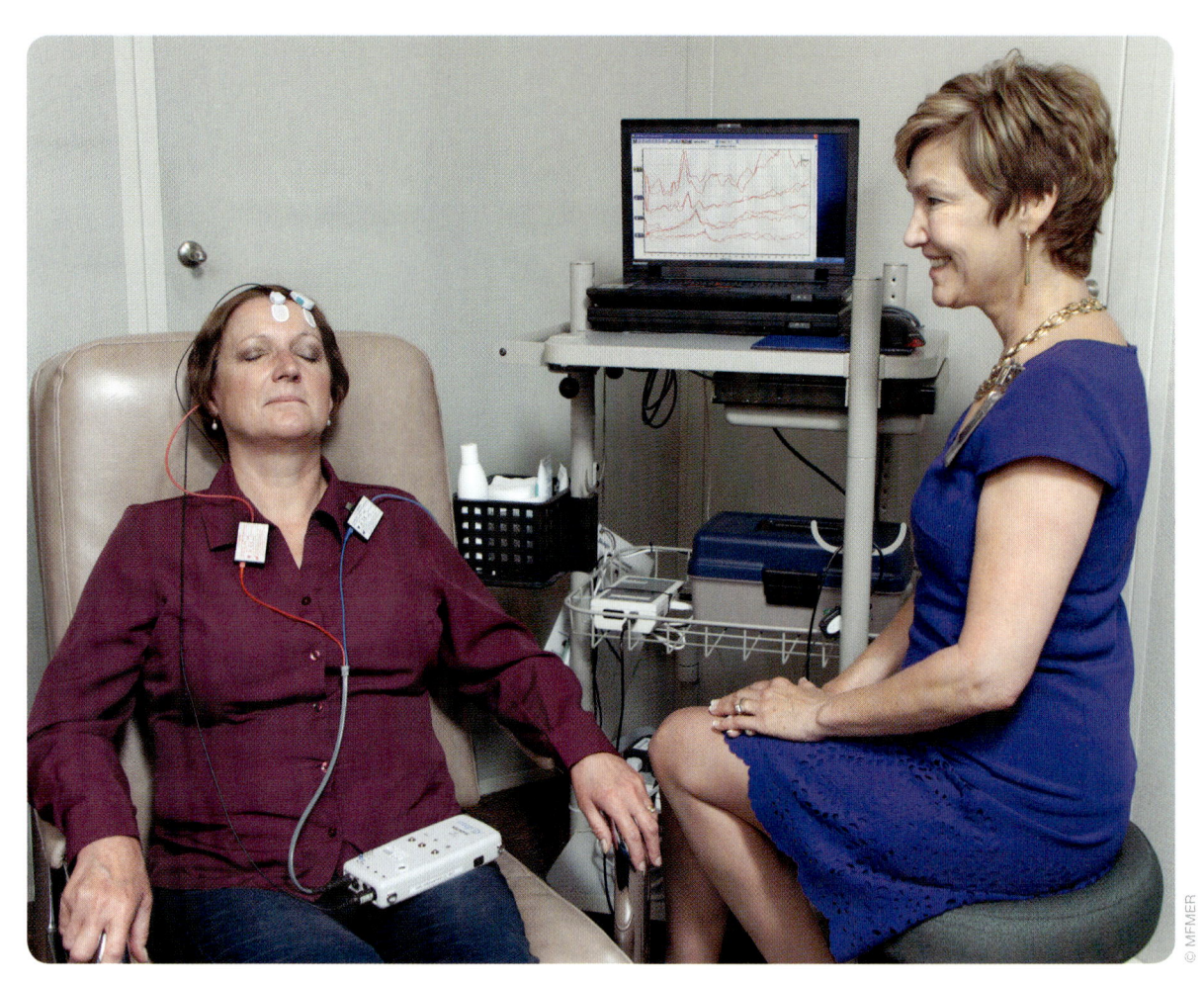

With an auditory brainstem response test, electrodes attached to your ears and head measure how the auditory nerve receives electrical impulses from the inner ear and transmits them to the brain.

used to assess other problems with the auditory nerve.

Otoacoustic emissions test

This test measures an interesting phenomenon that occurs in hair cells of your inner ear. These cells respond to the movement of fluid in the cochlea. The resulting vibrations of the hair cells produce inaudible sounds called otoacoustic emissions. These emissions can be measured by placing a probe equipped with a microphone into the ear canal.

This test is useful because people with normal hearing produce otoacoustic emissions, but people with hearing loss

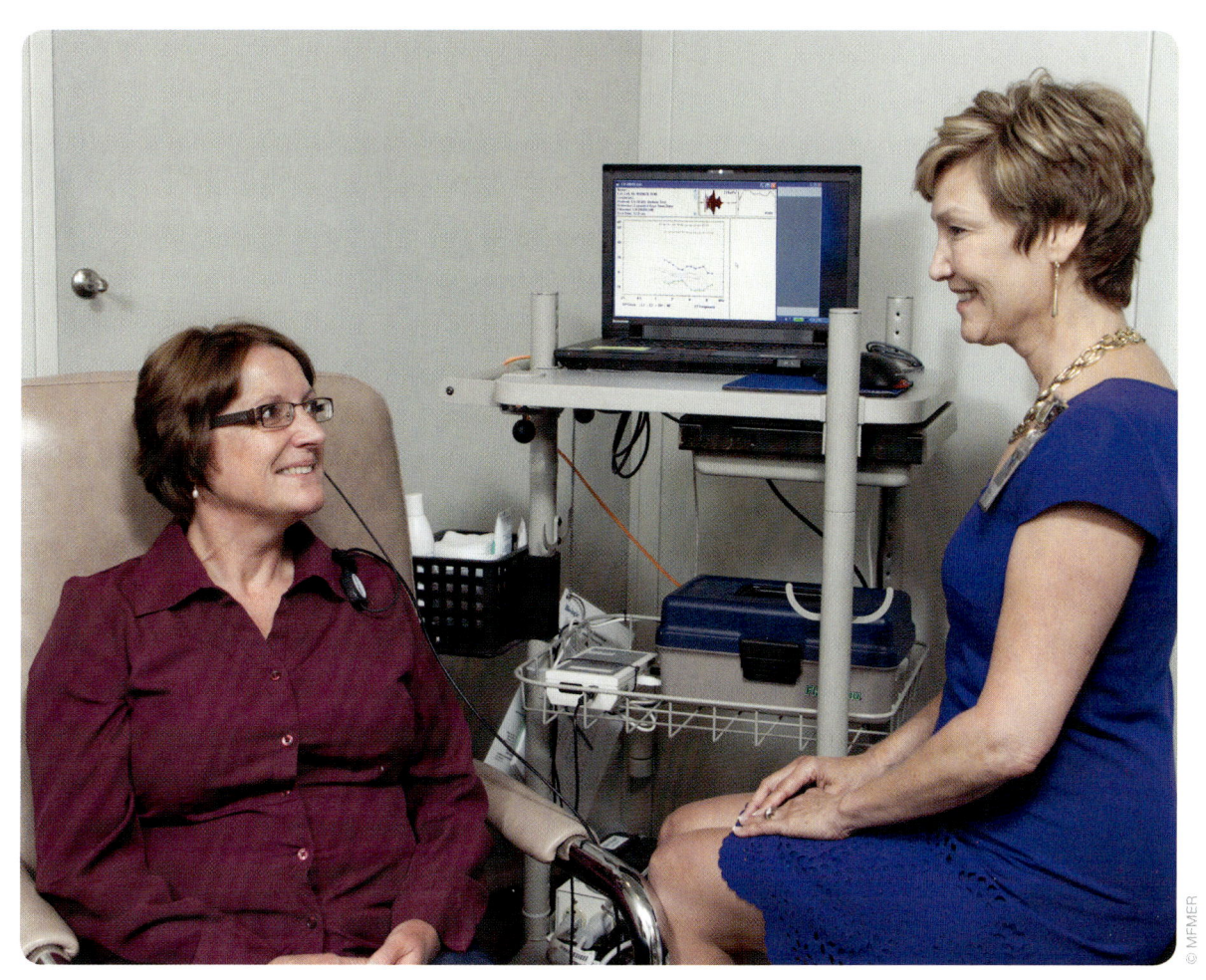

During otoacoustic emissions testing, a probe with a small microphone is placed in your ear canal to check for inaudible sounds called otoacoustic emissions. These emissions are produced in people with normal hearing but not in people with hearing loss.

caused by damaged hair cells don't produce them. Test results help the examiner assess the degree of loss.

The otoacoustic emissions test is also used to screen hearing in newborns and infants because it doesn't require a voluntary response.

Hearing tests for children

As mentioned in the previous section, there are objective tests that can be used for children of all ages — including newborns — because they require no voluntary response. However, there also are several age-related behavioral

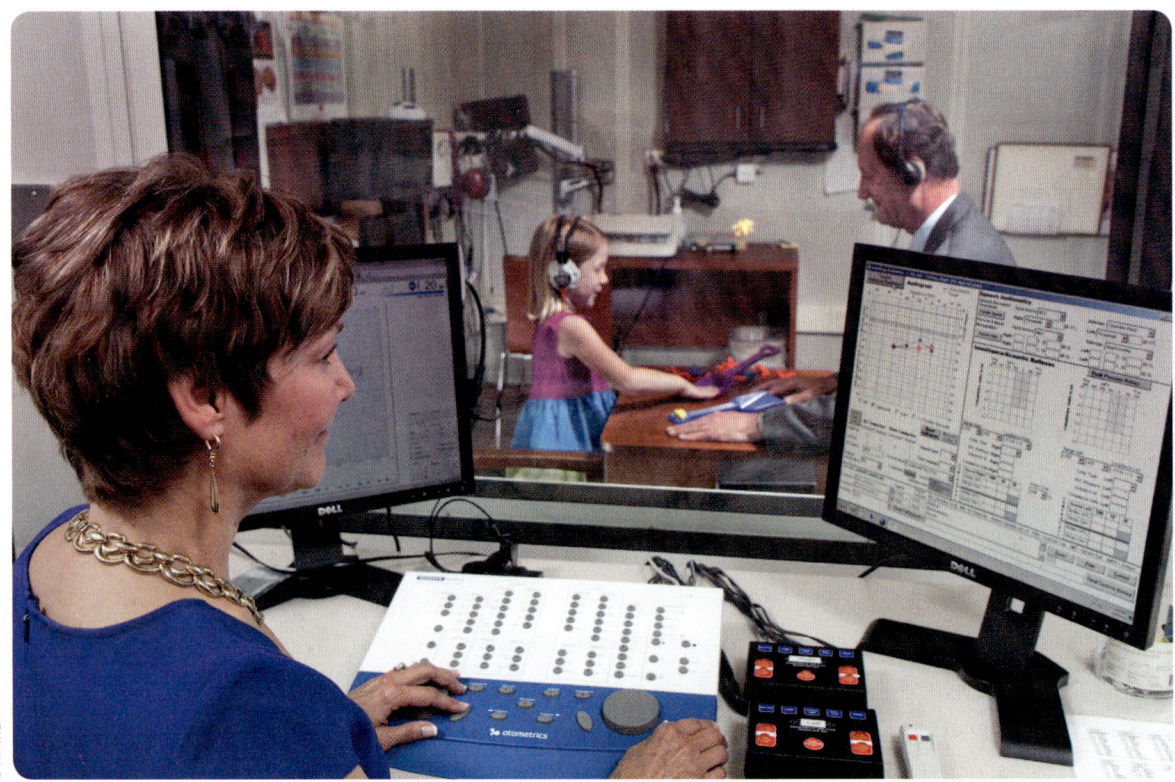

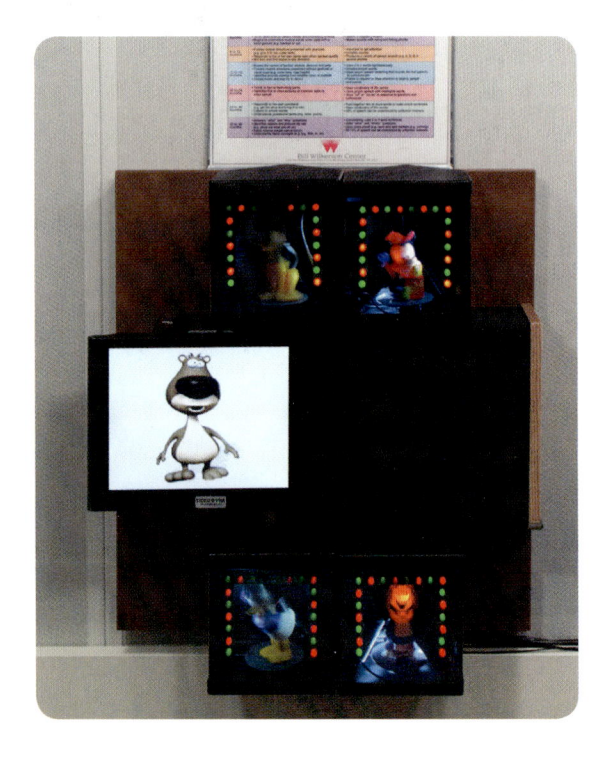

Conditioned play audiometry (above) tries to engage a child's response through play. As simple as they may seem, these play activities can reliably enable the audiologist to determine approximate hearing levels, often for each ear.

Visual reinforcement audiometry (left) incorporates special animated lights and toys to serve as "reinforcers" to a child's eye shifting or head turning to various types of sounds.

48   Chapter 2: Getting a hearing exam

methods that audiologists can use for testing. Results are typically obtained by presenting various sounds through a combination of small earphones, bone conduction devices or sound field speakers.

Behavioral observation audiometry

This type of testing is typically used for the youngest children, from newborns up to 6 months old. It involves careful observation of changes in the child's behavior — such as eye widening, startling motions or changes in sucking behaviors — following the presentation of various sounds. For children in this age group, responses typically aren't as sensitive as they would be in older children, so they're typically used in conjunction with objective tests.

Visual reinforcement audiometry

This testing is commonly used for children of about 6 months to 2½ years old. It incorporates special animated lights and toys to serve as "reinforcers" to a child's eye shifting or head turning to various types of sound. Typical sounds used may include the tester's voice or several low- and high-frequency signals.

Conditioned play audiometry

This testing is often used for children ages 2½ to 5 years old and tries to engage a child's response through play. Some of the more popular techniques include having the child toss small blocks or toy figures into a bucket or pound the end of a small shovel loaded with plastic toys each time a sound is detected. As simple as they may seem, these play activities can reliably enable the audiologist to determine approximate hearing levels, often for each ear.

Understanding your audiogram

Your physician or audiologist may use any or all of the tests described in the previous section to compile a detailed assessment of your hearing. But the test that's relied on most is pure tone audiometry. The resulting graph, the audiogram, is a baseline indicator of your hearing. The graph reveals the softest sounds you can hear at different pitches.

At first glance an audiogram may seem baffling. To understand what the lines and numbers represent, it's helpful to look at each component of the graph separately.

The audiogram portrays sound in terms of two of its most important

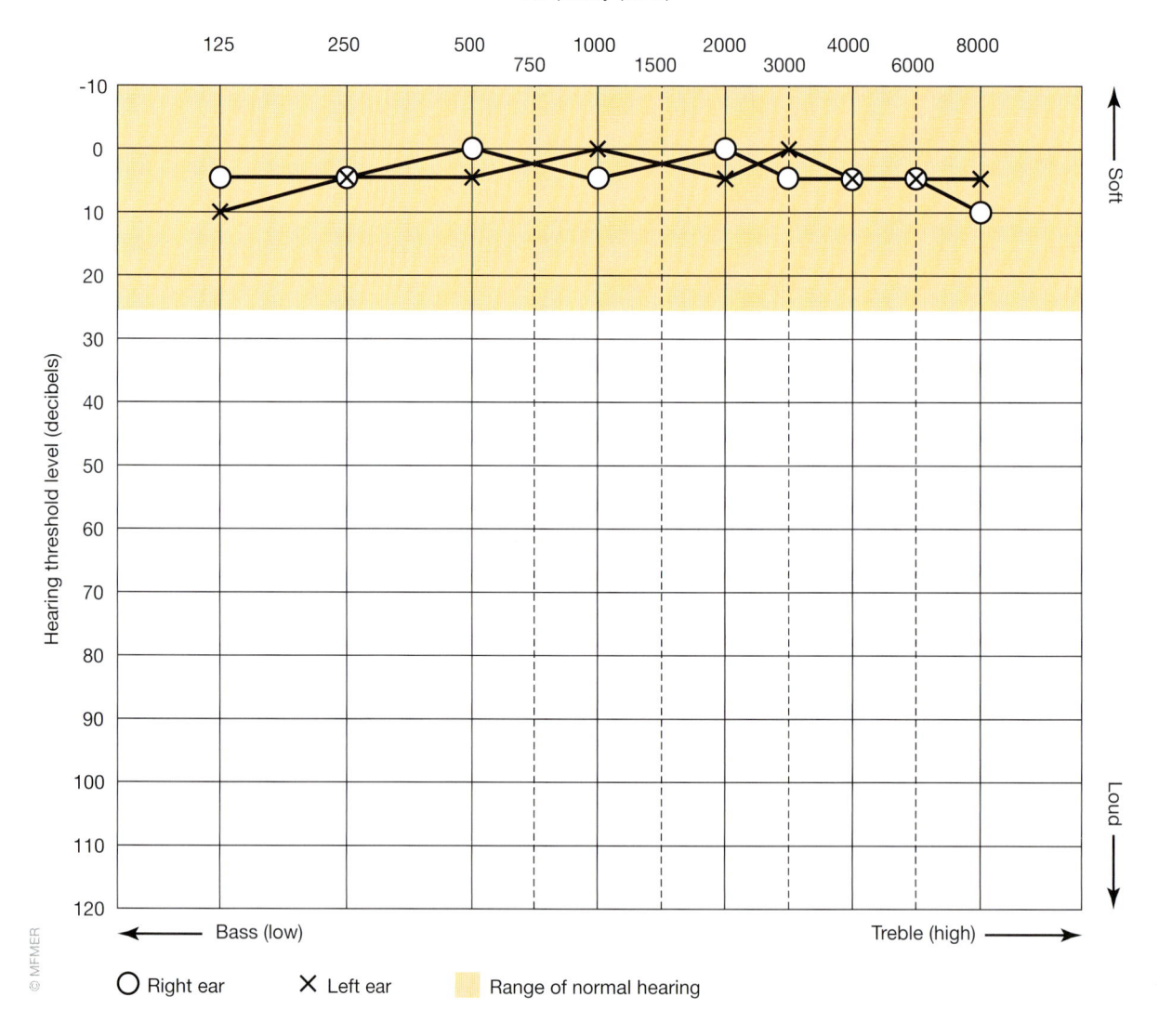

This audiogram shows normal hearing in both the right ear and the left ear. Hearing in the right ear is plotted with O's and in the left ear with X's. If your hearing is normal, all your X's and O's will typically fall in the range between minus 10 and 25 decibels hearing level (dB HL) — the shaded area on the audiogram. As hearing loss develops, the X's and O's fall lower and lower on the graph, and below the shaded area.

50 Chapter 2: Getting a hearing exam

qualities: pitch (frequency) measured in hertz (Hz), and loudness (intensity) measured in decibels (dB).

The vertical lines represent the range of frequencies, which moves from a low (bass) pitch on the left (125 Hz) to a high (treble) pitch on the right (8,000 Hz). The frequencies most common in human speech are between 500 Hz and 4,000 Hz. Some speech sounds have a very low pitch, such as *vv* in vacuum or *mm* in morning. Speech sounds such as *ff* in food and *th* in thanks have a high pitch.

The horizontal lines on the audiogram represent how loud the sound is. These levels range from minus 10 dB HL at the top of the graph (soft) to 120 dB HL at the bottom (loud). Zero dB HL represents very faint sounds that someone with normal hearing can generally hear.

Every point on an audiogram represents a different sound, determined by its pitch at a given intensity. When you take an audiometric test, your response to the different sounds you hear are recorded on the graph. At each frequency, the faintest tone that you can hear in your right ear is recorded as an O and the faintest tone you can hear in your left ear is recorded as an X. The resulting lines of O's and X's on the graph represent hearing thresholds

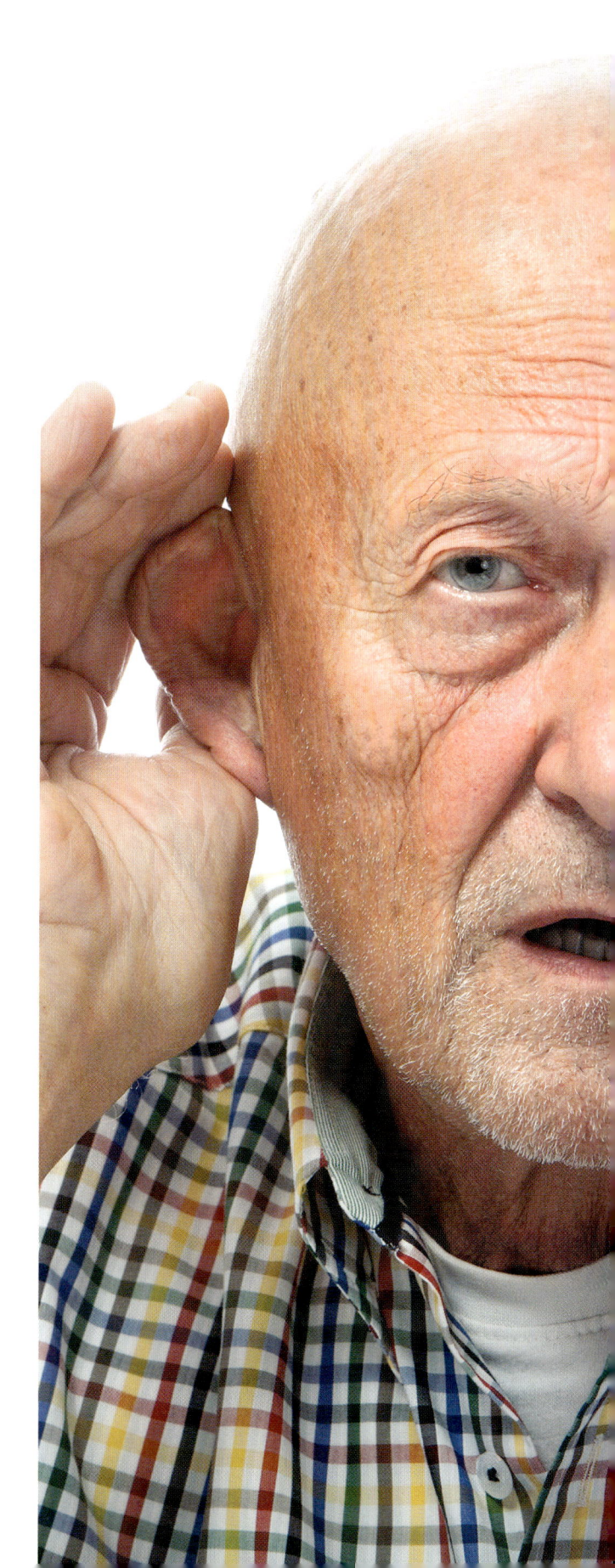

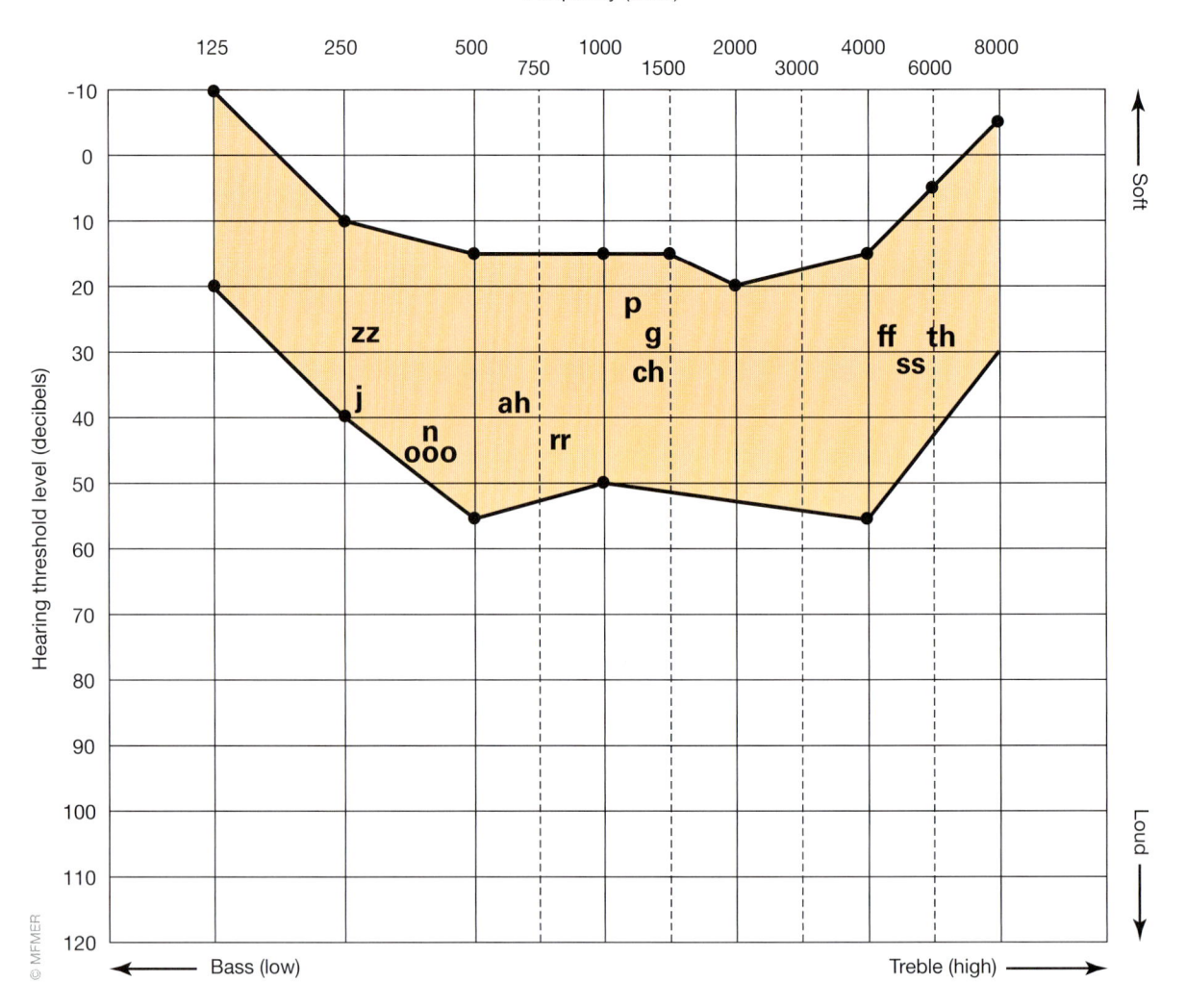

The shaded portion of this audiogram indicates the speech spectrum. This shows the irregular concave arc where the sounds of normal human speech lie. Softer, high-pitched sounds such as *ff*, *th* and *ss* appear on the right-hand side of the audiogram. Louder, low-pitched sounds such as *zz*, *j* and *n* appear on the left-hand side.

52 Chapter 2: Getting a hearing exam

for your ears — any softer sounds are inaudible to you.

Some people may have symmetrical hearing loss, which means the thresholds are approximately at the same level in both ears. Others may have asymmetrical hearing loss, which means one ear has a higher threshold than the other does. Hearing loss may vary according to frequency. For example, someone may have normal hearing at low and middle frequencies in both ears. But he or she may have moderate to severe loss at high frequencies in the left ear and only mild loss at high frequencies in the right ear.

The speech spectrum

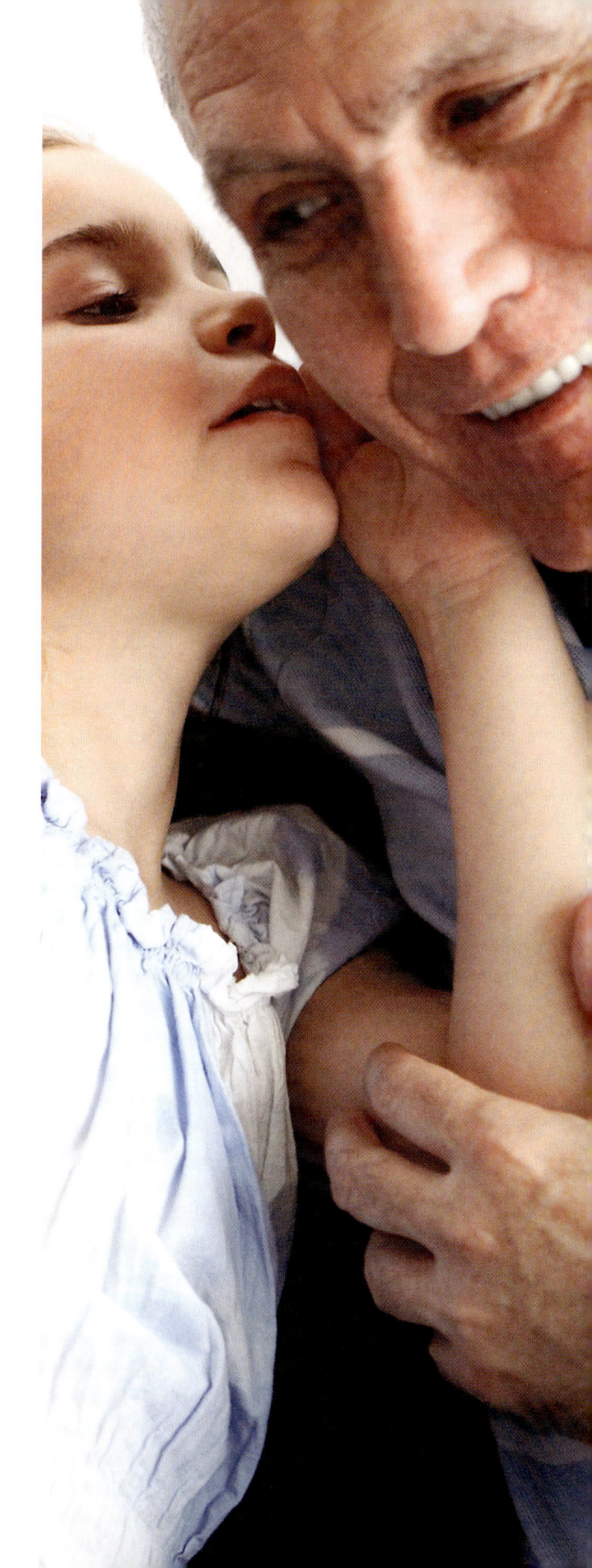

If the audiogram represented all of the sounds that make up human speech at a normal conversational level, it would show up as a concave-shaped — or banana-shaped — area just above the middle of the graph. This area, shown on page 52, is known as the speech spectrum. Soft, high-pitched sounds such as *ss*, *ff* and *th* would be in the right-hand portion of the spectrum. Loud, low-pitched sounds such as *zz*, *j* and *n* would appear in the left-hand portion. Sounds such as *ch* and *g* fall somewhere in between.

If the graph showed the speech spectrum superimposed over your audiometric test results, you would have a visual representation of which portions of conversational speech are audible to you and which are inaudible. The inaudible sounds could be heard only if the decibel level were increased and the sounds made louder.

Hearing loss is generally greater in the high frequencies where many of the consonant sounds occur. Often, this results in a person saying they can hear speech but not understand it.

Sometimes you don't think about getting your hearing checked until you notice that something is obviously wrong or another person calls a hearing problem to your attention. Hearing loss may be tough to admit to and is often viewed as a sign of old age.

But protecting your hearing can have an immediate and positive physical, social and emotional impact on your life. Treatment may help eliminate feelings of isolation and frustration and allow you to participate more actively in the world around you. A decision to take action today and schedule a hearing exam can determine how well you'll be hearing in the weeks, months and years ahead.

Chapter 3

Problems of the outer ear and middle ear

A primary function of both the outer ear and the middle ear is to direct (conduct) sound waves to the sensitive auditory structures of the inner ear. This function allows strong, clear signals to be processed by the brain into sounds that you can make sense of and recognize.

Conductive hearing loss occurs when something interferes with the passage of sound waves through the outer ear and middle ear. Very often in these situations, the function of the inner ear remains normal.

When you have conductive hearing loss, all sounds that you hear, no matter the frequency (pitch) or intensity (loudness), seem muffled. What are soft or faint sounds to someone with normal hearing become inaudible to you.

A number of problems can obstruct the sound waves on their passage to the inner ear. Common causes of conductive hearing loss include too much earwax, ruptured eardrum or infection that causes a fluid buildup in your middle ear. The development of cysts and benign tumors also can be a cause.

Often, conductive hearing loss can be reversed with proper treatment. Sometimes simple self-care measures are enough. Other problems may require medication or surgery. The good news is that problems of the outer ear and middle ear generally don't cause permanent damage.

This chapter describes many of the common causes of conductive hearing loss and guidelines for preventing and treating these conditions.

Outer ear problems

Problems in your outer ear are more often a discomfort and annoyance than a serious medical condition. With proper self-care and, if necessary, treatment from a doctor, outer ear problems usually can be resolved and your hearing restored to its normal level. The most common outer ear problems include earwax blockage, a foreign object lodged in the ear and swimmer's ear.

Earwax blockage

The skin lining the outer portion of your ear canal contains glands that produce a waxy substance called cerumen, more commonly known as earwax. This wax is part of your body's normal defense against harm. Earwax has natural oils that help keep the skin of the ear canal soft and protect the skin from water. It traps dust and other foreign particles that collect in the outer ear to keep them from injuring the delicate eardrum (tympanic membrane). Wax also helps inhibit the growth of bacteria.

Normally, earwax is carried to the outer edge of the ear canal by a conveyor belt growth pattern of ear canal skin and either falls out or is wiped away when you clean your outer ear. At times you may produce more wax than your ear can expel, causing the wax to accumulate in your ear canal.

Generally, an excess amount of earwax doesn't lead to hearing loss because it doesn't completely block the passageway. But many people insert objects such as cotton swabs, hairpins, keys and fingers into the ear canal, presumably to clean it. These actions push the wax farther into the passageway and impact it. Impacted earwax, as it builds, can reduce your hearing by blocking sound vibrations in your ear canal.

Blockage can make your ear feel full or plugged. Rarely, it can cause noise such as ringing, buzzing or roaring in your ears (tinnitus).

Treatment
To remove excess wax from your ears, you may consult a doctor or try the following self-care method:

- Soften the earwax with a few drops of baby oil, mineral oil or olive oil from an eyedropper twice a day for several days.
- When the wax is softened, fill a bowl with water heated to body temperature — if the water is colder

Frequency (hertz)

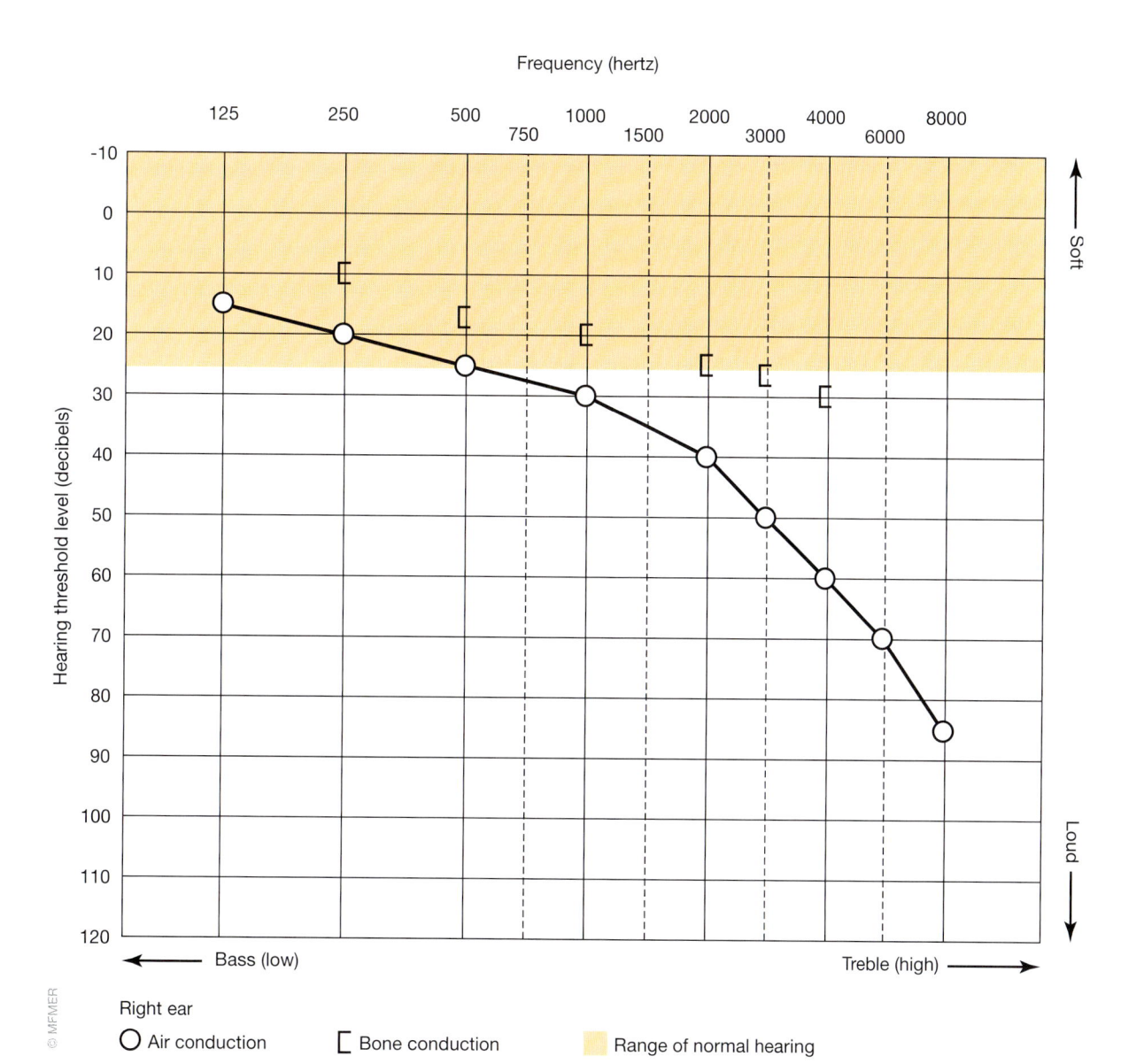

Right ear
- ○ Air conduction
- [Bone conduction
- ▨ Range of normal hearing

This audiogram shows a typical pattern of hearing loss due to earwax blockage in the right ear. Results show increasing difficulty in hearing sounds at higher frequencies. You would need sounds at 6,000 hertz to be at least 70 decibels hearing level (dB HL) in order to hear them.

Mayo Clinic on Better Hearing and Balance **57**

or hotter than body temperature, application may make you feel dizzy during the procedure.
- With your head upright, grasp the top of your ear and pull upward. With your other hand, squirt water gently into your ear canal with a 3-ounce rubber-bulb syringe. Lower your head to the side and allow the water to drain into the bowl.
- You may need to repeat the previous step several times before the excess wax falls out.
- Dry your ear carefully with a towel or hand-held hair dryer. Insert a few drops of an alcohol-vinegar preparation (half rubbing alcohol, half white vinegar) with an eyedropper to help dry your ear.

Earwax removers sold in stores (Debrox, Murine Earwax Removal Drops, others) also can be effective. One note of caution: If you've previously ruptured an eardrum or had ear surgery, don't flush your ears unless your doctor approves. Such action could lead to pain or infection.

Mayo Clinic experts don't recommend ear candling — a technique that involves placing a lit, hollow, cone-shaped candle into the ear canal. Research shows that this technique is ineffective at removing earwax. In fact, it can actually push earwax deeper into the canal. It can also lead to various injuries, such as burns.

If after self-care you still have excess wax in your ears, seek the help of your doctor. He or she may repeat the washing of your ears or use special instruments to either scoop or suction out the impacted earwax.

Foreign object in the ear

Occasionally, an object such as a piece of cotton thread from a swab, a bit of paper, an earplug or even an insect can become stuck in your ear. You may notice this when your ear begins to tickle, hurt or feel plugged.

Most foreign objects lodge in the ear canal and don't cause lasting hearing problems. But if an object is pushed too far into your ear, it may rupture your eardrum and potentially damage your middle ear, which can have more-serious consequences.

Treatment
Here's advice for occasions when a foreign object becomes lodged in your ear:

- Don't attempt to remove the foreign object by probing with a cotton swab, matchstick or any other tool.

To do so is to risk pushing the object farther into the ear, making it harder to extract and possibly causing more-serious damage.
- You may be able to dislodge the object by tilting your head toward the affected side and shaking it gently in the direction of the ground.
- If the object is clearly visible to an observer, is pliable and can be grasped easily with tweezers, he or she may be able to gently remove it.
- If the object isn't accessible, contact your doctor or a hospital emergency room. The doctor will need to remove the object with tiny forceps or suction or by flooding the ear with fluid. He or she can check to see if any damage has occurred.
- If an insect is lodged in the ear and is still alive, tilt the affected ear upward. Insects instinctively crawl up, rather than down, in order to free themselves.
- If the insect doesn't exit the ear on its own, place a few drops of warm — not hot — baby oil, mineral oil or olive oil into the ear. You can ease the entry of the oil by gently pulling the top of the ear back and upward. The insect should suffocate and float out in the oil bath.
- Don't use oil to remove objects other than an insect. Also, don't apply oil if any of the signs or symptoms of a perforated eardrum are present, such as pain, bleeding or discharge from the ear.

Swimmer's ear

Swimmer's ear (acute otitis externa) is an infection of the ear canal. Usually, it's the result of persistent moisture in the ear — for example, frequent swimming — often in combination with a mild injury to the skin of the ear canal.

This condition can result from scraping the ear canal to clean out wax. This creates ideal circumstances for bacteria and fungi to invade the ear canal and

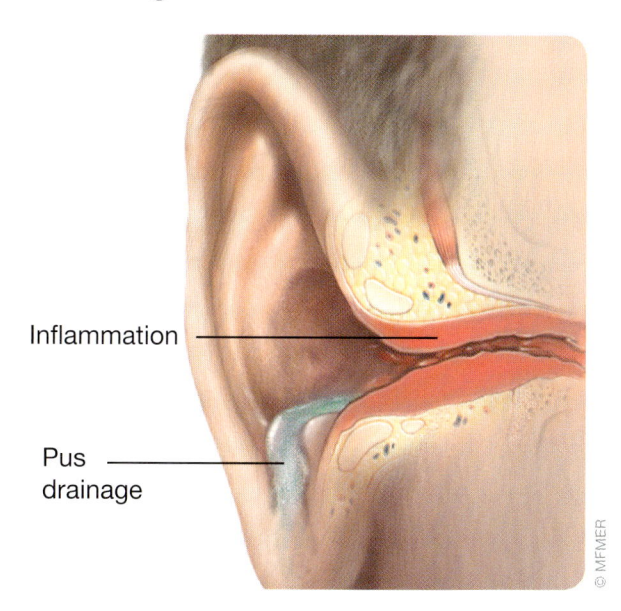

Inflammation

Pus drainage

With swimmer's ear, a small cut allows bacteria and fungi to invade the ear canal and cause an infection.

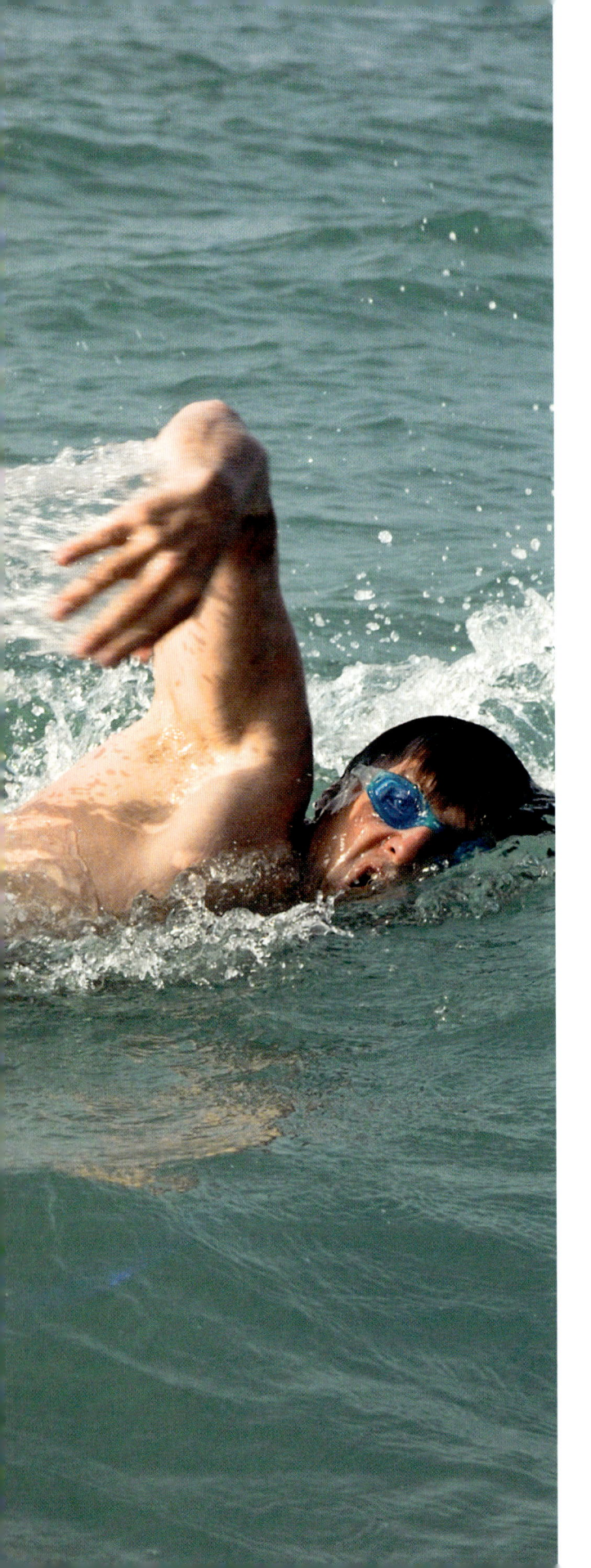

cause infection. Hair spray and hair dyes also may cause infection or allergic reaction. Swimmer's ear is most common in children and young adults.

Pain or itching in the ear, a swollen ear canal, and the drainage of pus are signs and symptoms of an outer ear infection. Temporary hearing loss may occur if the swelling or pus blocks the ear canal.

Treatment

If the pain is mild and you don't have ear drainage or hearing loss, follow the self-care tips below. Otherwise, seek medical attention.

- Place a warm — not hot — heating pad over your ear. But don't lie on the heating pad.
- Consider taking a pain reliever such as ibuprofen (Advil, Motrin IB, others) or acetaminophen (Tylenol, others), if needed.
- Keep water, fluids and other substances out of your ear canal while it's healing.
- Place a few drops of an alcohol-vinegar preparation (half rubbing alcohol, half white vinegar) in your ear after showering or swimming. The alcohol helps keep the skin of your ear canal dry, and the vinegar helps prevent bacterial and fungal growth from occurring.

If the ear pain doesn't subside after a day or two, or if you have additional concerns, see your doctor. After cleaning your ear, the doctor may prescribe eardrops containing a corticosteroid to relieve itching and decrease inflammation, and antibiotics to control infection. More-severe infections may be treated with oral antibiotics.

Particularly among people with diabetes or a weakened immune system, swimmer's ear may lead to infection of the bones and cartilage at the base of the skull (necrotizing otitis externa). This is often accompanied by increasingly severe pain. Such a complication can be life-threatening and usually requires prolonged antibiotic therapy under the care of a team of specialists.

If you're a frequent swimmer, you also may want to consider preventive measures. Over-the-counter ear-water drying drops (Auro-Dri, Swim-Ear, others) are available for use after you swim. These are easy to use.

Benign tumors

Benign tumors, or exostoses may develop in the ear canal, caused by an overgrowth of bone. The tumors can grow large enough to block the ear canal and trap wax and water. Ear infection also may develop.

This condition is known as surfer's ear because it develops in many individuals who participate in surfing. That's because the growths are associated with prolonged exposure to water and wind. Furthermore, the colder the water temperature, the higher the risk — cold-water surfers are more likely to develop exostoses than are warm-water surfers.

Treatment

The exostoses are slow growing and often present no problem. Should they block the ear canal, they can be surgically removed. This is an outpatient procedure, but recovery may require several weeks, during which time the ear canal is kept dry. Antibiotics can take care of infection, although treatment in a partially blocked canal is more difficult than in an open canal.

Eardrum problems

Your eardrum (tympanic membrane) is a resilient structure but subject to constant strain. Two common problems are rupture of the eardrum membrane and barotrauma. Both conditions prevent the eardrum from vibrating properly, which disrupts the relay of sound waves into the middle ear. This results in mild to moderate hearing loss, which is usually temporary.

Ruptured eardrum

Your eardrum is a thin, elastic membrane that plays the crucial role of gatekeeper for the sound waves traveling from your outer ear to your middle ear. Occasionally, the eardrum may be torn or perforated as a result of an ear infection or from ear trauma.

Ear infection
Fluid buildup in the middle ear caused by infection can exert strong pressure on the eardrum, forcing it to rupture. Pain associated with the buildup usually improves once the eardrum has ruptured — because fluid draining out of the ear relieves the pressure. But chronic ear infections can gradually wear down the eardrum membrane, even if there is no pressure buildup, causing a hole.

Trauma to the ear
The eardrum can be ruptured by a sharp blow to the head or by a sudden increase in outside air pressure, such as

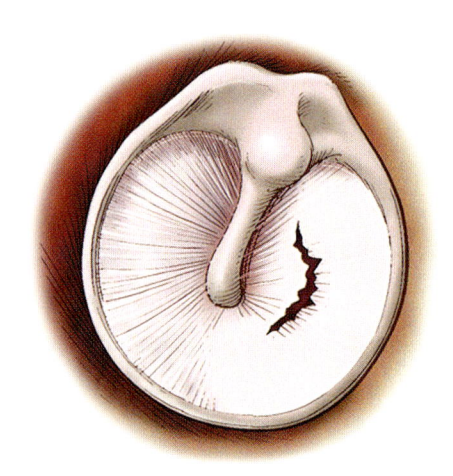

Although a ruptured eardrum usually will heal itself, the risk of infection and hearing loss still exists. It's important to see your doctor if you think your eardrum may be damaged.

from an explosion, slap across the ear or diving accident. The eardrum also can be punctured if you push an object such as a cotton swab or paper clip too deeply into the ear canal.

Signs and symptoms of a ruptured eardrum include earache, partial hearing loss, noise such as ringing, buzzing or roaring in your ears (tinnitus) and slight bleeding or discharge from the ear. In some cases, the three tiny bones (ossicles) in the middle ear may be damaged, resulting in more-severe hearing loss and, possibly, dizziness.

Treatment
Often, a ruptured eardrum heals by itself without complications and with

little or no permanent hearing loss. Some ruptures cause recurring infection.

If you think you may have a ruptured eardrum, contact your doctor immediately. The following self-care tips may ease ear pain and promote healing:

- Take aspirin or other pain relievers, if needed.
- Place a warm — not hot — heating pad over your ear.
- Keep your ear dry.
- Before showering, place a cotton ball coated with petroleum jelly into the ear canal to keep water out.

Your doctor may prescribe an antibiotic to make sure the infection is out of your ear and to help prevent it from recurring. He or she may also place a thin paper patch over your eardrum to seal the opening while it heals. If your eardrum hasn't healed within several months, you may require a surgical procedure to repair the tear.

Barotrauma

Barotrauma (bar-o-TRAW-muh), also called airplane ear, results from a sharp difference between the air pressure in your middle ear and the outside pressure in your environment.

Normally, the narrow channel that connects your ear to your nose and upper throat (eustachian tube) allows air to flow in and out of your middle ear. This air movement helps equalize pressure on both sides of the eardrum. You may notice clicks or popping sounds in your ears when you swallow or yawn to equalize the pressure.

Barotrauma occurs when you experience a sudden, drastic change in outside air pressure or water pressure, such as a rapid descent during an airplane landing or a rapid ascent during a deep-sea dive.

The rapid change in outside pressure — or restricted airflow in the eustachian tube — can create a situation where air pressure in your middle ear is less than the outside pressure. This imbalance causes the air-filled parts of your ear to compress and your eardrum to bow inward (retract). The distortion of your eardrum interferes with the passage of sound waves, so your hearing will be slightly reduced.

Your participation in activities that may involve rapid changes in outside pressure can require you to open your mouth or swallow frequently to equalize the pressure in your ears. Signs and symptoms of barotrauma include pain in one or both ears, slight hearing loss, and a feeling that both ears are plugged.

A more serious problem occurs if the pressure change is extreme or if your eustachian tube is completely blocked. Small blood vessels in your middle ear may rupture, filling your ear with blood and resulting in hearing loss.

Treatment

Although barotrauma may cause discomfort, it usually doesn't result in permanent hearing loss. The pain usually disappears within a few hours after the pressure has equalized, and your hearing returns to normal.

If you must fly while you have a cold or nose congestion, try a nonprescription decongestant nasal spray (Afrin, Neo-Synephrine, others) 20 to 60 minutes before the flight. This helps keep your eustachian tubes clear. However, don't use a decongestant if you have a heart condition or blood pressure problems without first obtaining your doctor's approval.

During the flight, suck on candy or chew gum to encourage swallowing. A method used by pilots is to pinch the nostrils shut, inhale and swallow, or to close the nostrils and try to blow air out the ears. The pop in your ears is a sign that air has gone through the eustachian tube to your middle ear.

If symptoms persist, consult your doctor. If the eustachian tube remains obstructed or unable to perform its function, it may become necessary to make a small incision in your eardrum. This helps equalize air pressure and allows fluid to be removed from your middle ear — a procedure known as myringotomy (mir-ing-GOT-o-me).

Middle ear problems

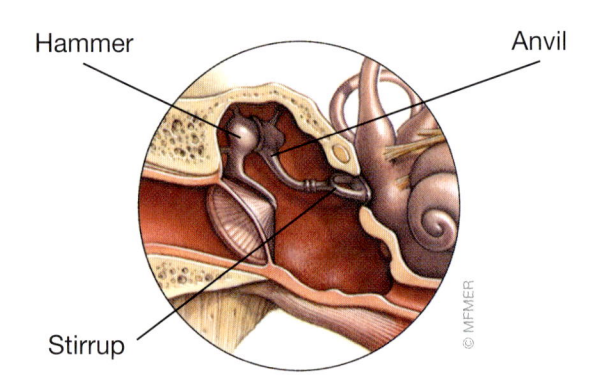

Infections, cysts, tumors and abnormal bone growth can affect your middle ear. These problems cause hearing loss when they disturb the eardrum or the tiny bones in the middle ear: the hammer (malleus), anvil (incus) and stirrup (stapes). Often, normal hearing can be restored with medical or surgical treatment. However, if the problem is left untreated and allowed to expand into the inner ear, permanent hearing loss may result.

Middle ear infection

An infection of the middle ear is known as otitis media. The condition is associated with colds and other upper respiratory infections, which can block the eustachian tube. The blocked tube prevents proper ventilation of the ear, causing swelling, inflammation and buildup of fluid in the middle ear.

In addition, bacteria from the nose, mouth or throat may travel through the lining of the eustachian tube and infect the trapped fluid in the middle ear, which causes a thick mucus or pus to form. Infected fluid usually causes ear pain. It may also obstruct proper movement of the eardrum and ossicles, causing conductive hearing loss.

Rarely, pressure from an infection may tear or rupture the eardrum. When this happens, the tear usually heals quickly, without lasting problems. Acute otitis media is a single, severe episode that typically lasts no more than two weeks.

The signs and symptoms of otitis media include:

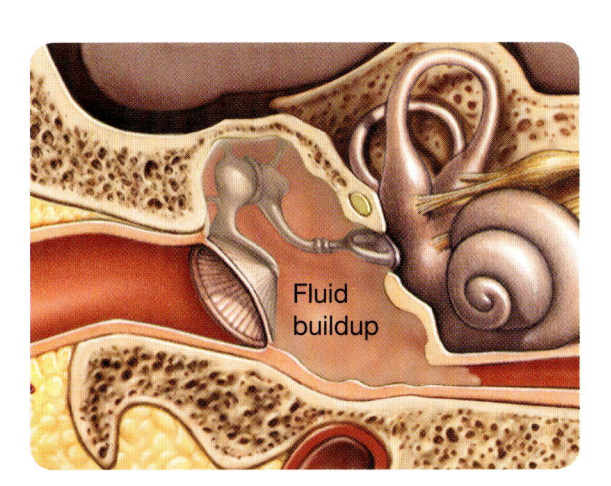

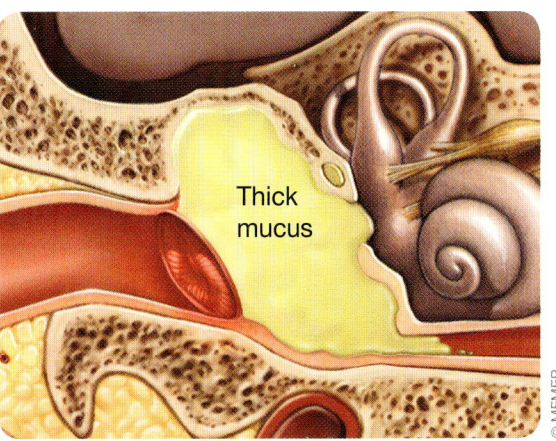

(Left) Otitis media may occur when the eustachian tube becomes blocked due to a cold or other respiratory infection. Fluid may build up in the normally air-filled middle ear. (Right) Bacteria from the nose and throat may infect the trapped fluid, forming a thick mucus or pus that obstructs movement of the eardrum and ossicles.

- Severe pain or pressure in the ear
- Fever above 101° F
- Disrupted sleep
- Sensation of a plugged ear

Other signs and symptoms associated with otitis media are dizziness, imbalance, nausea, vomiting and drainage from the ear.

Although otitis media may occur at any age, it's most common in young children. In fact, 3 out of 4 children will have at least one ear infection by their third birthday. This is partly due to the shape of a child's eustachian tube, which is shorter and more horizontal than an adult's is. A horizontal orientation means fluid is less likely to drain and more likely to accumulate in the ear.

The trapped fluid is an ideal breeding ground for bacteria or viruses that cause infection. At times, the fluid remains trapped, even after the infection is gone. This may cause recurring infections (see "Chronic ear infection").

Treatment

The pain, fever or drainage that's often associated with a middle ear infection will likely cause you to see a doctor. An examination of your ear may reveal a discolored, bulging or indented eardrum. Tympanometry, which measures movement of the eardrum, may indicate reduced pressure in the middle ear or diminished mobility of the eardrum membrane. Your doctor may take a sample of the draining fluid to identify the organism that's causing the infection.

Studies have found that most ear infections heal on their own without medical treatment. You and your doctor may decide to hold off on using antibiotics and follow a course of watchful waiting. If fluid in the ear isn't infected or if the infection is viral rather than bacterial, the antibiotics provide no benefits — and research shows that viruses cause most ear infections.

To ease ear pain, use over-the-counter pain relievers such as ibuprofen (Advil, Motrin IB, others) or acetaminophen (Tylenol, others). Applying a cold pack or cold wet washcloth to the outer ear for 20 minutes can help while the medicine takes effect. If you prefer, a warm compress may be used instead of a cold pack. Taking an antihistamine or decongestant may improve nasal breathing and help increase airflow through the eustachian tube.

In follow-up visits, you and your doctor will check to see if the ear infection gets better or worse and watch for signs and symptoms of more severe illness. These signs include severe pain, high fever, stiff neck, dehydration, difficulty breathing and extreme irritability.

If the acute symptoms last more than 48 to 72 hours, an antibiotic may be prescribed to fight the infection. Unless the exact organism causing the infection is identified, your doctor will probably prescribe an antibiotic that's effective against a range of bacteria. If the infection doesn't respond to one kind of antibiotic, your doctor may prescribe a different one.

After the infection is cleared up, fluid in the middle ear usually disappears within three to six weeks. Once you begin taking an antibiotic, it's important to complete the full prescription, even if your symptoms improve before you finish. This ensures that all of the bacteria are killed.

Chronic ear infection

Chronic otitis media is a recurring or persistent middle ear infection. Sometimes, a low-level infection continues even after you've been treated for acute

Acute ear infection: Key points

Keep in mind the following points regarding acute ear infections:

- Ear pain and possible ear infections do not typically require urgent medical attention.
- Most ear infections are not serious and will heal on their own without the use of antibiotics.
- Ear pain can be successfully controlled with pain relievers and other pain management strategies.
- Doctors most often recommend antibiotics for ear infections when ear pain lasts more than 48 to 72 hours or if you signs of a more severe illness appear.
- If you're beginning to experience signs or symptoms of a more severe illness, seek immediate medical care.

otitis media. Other times, the acute infection clears up but the ear is left more vulnerable to future infections. Persistent inflammation of the adenoid tissue behind your nasal passages also may cause swelling and block the eustachian tube.

The signs and symptoms of chronic ear infection may appear milder than do those of acute infection. In fact, a chronic condition may not be noticed until after the infection is established. But a chronic infection can be more harmful than an acute one because it can cause permanent ear damage and hearing loss.

When the eustachian tube is frequently blocked, tissues of the middle ear gradually begin to thicken and become inflamed. Mucus trapped in the middle ear also thickens. The blocked tube may create a vacuum in the middle ear that, over time, can deform or rupture the eardrum.

As these changes come about, the structures of the middle and inner ear begin to deteriorate, causing permanent damage and hearing impairment. Infection also can spread to the bone behind the ear — a projection of bone called the mastoid process — and even to the brain.

Seek medical attention if pus is seeping from your ear canal, if your ear continually hurts or if you experience hearing loss. Your doctor can refer you to an audiologist to determine the type and severity of hearing loss.

The doctor may also try to identify the source of infection. A computerized tomography (CT) scan may be taken, albeit rarely, to check if infection has spread to the mastoid process.

Treatment

Your doctor may prescribe an antihistamine or decongestant if nasal congestion from a cold or allergy is contributing to the infection. This will help open the eustachian tube, improve nasal breathing, and increase airflow to and from the middle ear. However, some studies cast doubt on how effective these drugs are with chronic ear infections.

Some doctors may recommend taking low-dose antibiotics to prevent recurrent middle ear infections. Hower, antibiotics have not been shown to prevent these infections. Additionally, because widespread, prolonged use of antibiotics has contributed to the growth of drug-resistant bacteria, doctors don't agree on whether antibiotics should be used preventively.

If the middle ear remains filled with fluid for more than three months and the eardrum is not ruptured, a small surgical incision in your eardrum may be necessary to relieve pressure and help drain fluid. Hearing often improves immediately after the procedure.

Typically, it takes less than 10 minutes to make the tiny incision, suction out the fluid, and insert a metal or plastic tube into the hole. This ventilation tube keeps the drainage pathway open. Without the tube, the incision would heal in about a week — sometimes before all of the fluid has drained out. Some tubes are intended to stay in place for up to a year and then fall out on their own. Other tubes stay in longer and may need to be surgically removed.

If significant damage has occurred to the eardrum and ossicles, surgery may be needed to remove infected tissue and repair these structures. This procedure is known as tympanomastoidectomy (tim-puh-no-mas-toid-EK-tuh-me).

The entire procedure may be done all at once, or an initial surgery may be undertaken only to eliminate the infection. Later surgery is performed to reconstruct the middle ear structures. Chronic ear infections often require multiple surgeries.

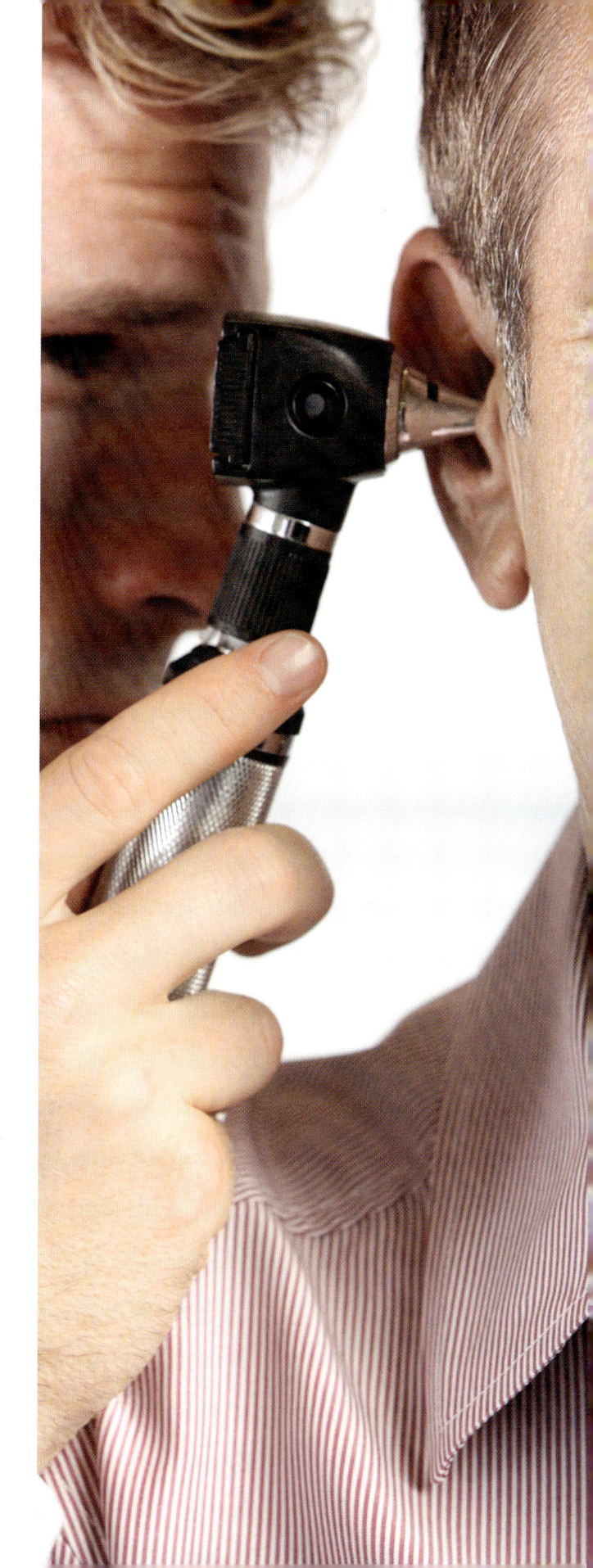

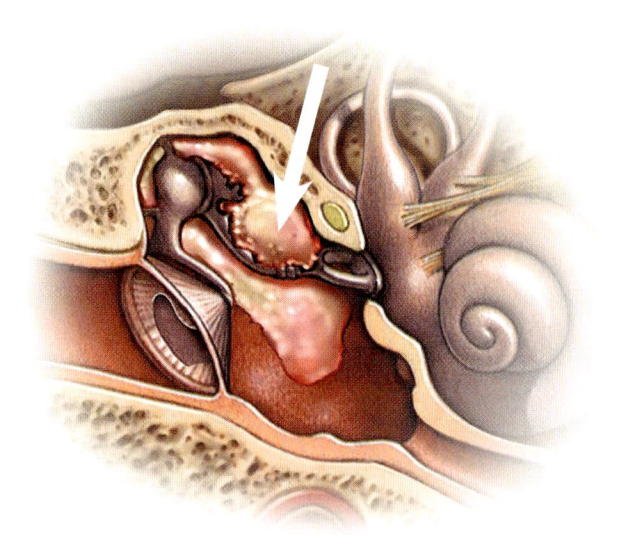

An untreated cholesteatoma (see arrow) has eroded bones in the middle ear and ruptured the eardrum. Surgical removal of the cyst may require patching the eardrum and replacing the ossicles with a prosthesis.

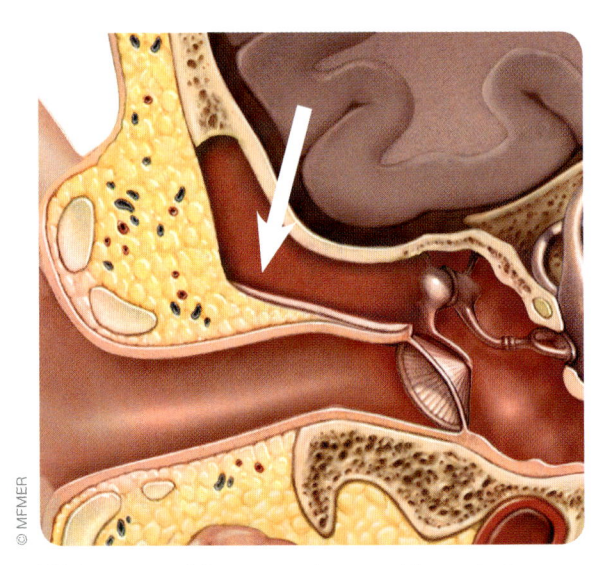

With a mastoidectomy, damaged bone in the mastoid caused by a cholesteatoma is removed to stop the disease process (see arrow).

Cholesteatoma

Cholesteatoma (koe-luh-ste-uh-TOE-muh) is a cyst commonly found in the middle ear or the mastoid process. It can occur when skin from the ear canal grows into the middle ear through a hole or tear in the eardrum. It may also happen when a blocked eustachian tube creates a vacuum in the middle ear, bending your eardrum inward to form a pocket. Old skin cells that are caught in the eardrum pocket develop into a cyst-like cholesteatoma.

Occasionally during fetal development, skin cells become trapped behind the eardrum so that a baby is born with congenital cholesteatoma. Unlike the adult form, this type of cholesteatoma may grow quickly.

Signs and symptoms of cholesteatoma include pus drainage from your ear, hearing loss, ear pain or numbness, headache, dizziness, and weakness of the facial muscles.

A cholesteatoma isn't cancerous and won't spread to other locations. The degree of hearing loss you may experience from a cholesteatoma will depend on the size and location of the cyst. Frequently, it impedes or erodes the delicate bones of the middle ear (ossicles), causing significant conductive hearing loss.

If left untreated, a cholesteatoma may also affect the cochlea and vestibular labyrinth of the inner ear — resulting in permanent hearing loss and problems with balance. A cholesteatoma may damage the facial nerve and, rarely, cause an infection of the central nervous system (meningitis).

Treatment

A cholesteatoma can only be treated surgically. A large or more advanced cholesteatoma may require a series of operations to correct damage to the bones of your middle ear and possibly to rebuild them. If all of the cyst isn't removed, it will grow back, possibly requiring later surgery.

In severe cases when the cholesteatoma is large or located in an area of the ear that's difficult to access, the surgeon may perform a procedure called a canal wall down mastoidectomy (mastoid-EK-tuh-me) to remove damaged portions of the mastoid bone. This leaves a cavity that must be cleaned out periodically, but doesn't effectively restore lost hearing. Subsequent surgery may be undertaken to reconstruct the ossicular chain in the middle ear, if it has been damaged.

Other cysts and tumors

Abnormal growths may develop in the middle ear and surrounding tissues, such as the temporal bone of the skull — although these types of growths are less common.

Most middle ear tumors are noncancerous (benign), although some, such as squamous cell carcinoma, are cancerous (malignant) and capable of spreading to other parts of the body. Benign tumors usually grow slowly, whereas malignant tumors tend to grow at a faster rate.

The sensation of a plugged ear may indicate a tumor. Other warning signs include hearing loss, noise such as ringing, buzzing or roaring in your ears (tinnitus), drainage from the ear, facial paralysis, dizziness, and loss of balance.

Consult your doctor if you experience any of these symptoms. A CT scan or MRI can help determine if a tumor is present. Your doctor may take sample tissue from the tumor (biopsy) to determine whether it's malignant.

The more common tumors include:

- **Glomus tympanicum and glomus jugulare.** Both types of tumor are masses of cells that interfere with the function of the ossicles. Often a glomus tumor will cause a pulsing sound in your ear that accompanies each heartbeat. Most glomus tumors are benign, although rarely they can spread to the lymph nodes in your neck and become a more serious problem.

- **Squamous cell carcinoma.** Malignant tumors of the ear are rare, but of those that occur, squamous cell carcinoma (SKWAY-mus sel kahr-sih-NO-muh) is the most common. This type of tumor develops in the skin cells of your outer ear and ear canal and spreads into your middle ear and mastoid. Though what causes the tumor is unclear, it has been associated with chronic inflammation. Ear pain, periodic draining of fluid from the ear and extended periods of bleeding from the ear are signs and symptoms of squamous cell carcinoma. This cancer is usually fatal if left untreated.

Treatment

Tumors of the ear may be treated with surgery, radiation or both. Sometimes, the tumors may also be monitored with watchful waiting, especially in older adults. With this approach, regular MRI or CT scans are taken to check the tumor for growth.

When surgery is performed to remove a tumor, it's a delicate, complex procedure. Surgery may involve removing some or all parts of the ear, depending on the nature and size of the tumor. This can result in permanent loss of hearing. It can also cause a loss of function in the nerves leading to your face and throat, which can affect your voice and swallowing ability.

Radiation therapy may be used as a primary treatment or in combination with surgery to improve the chances of controlling the tumor. With any malignant tumor, treatment must be prompt and aggressive. Radiation therapy is often used after surgery to destroy all remaining cancerous cells.

Otosclerosis

Otosclerosis (o-toe-skluh-ROE-sis) develops when an abnormal growth of spongy bone forms at the entrance to the inner ear (oval window). Due to this growth, the stirrup, one of the tiny bones in the middle ear, becomes fixed to the oval window, losing its ability to vibrate. The immobile stirrup disrupts the sound pathway.

For a small number of people with otosclerosis, hearing loss can be profound, especially when tissue in the cochlea of the inner ear also becomes involved. Other signs and symptoms of otosclerosis include dizziness, balance problems and tinnitus.

Otosclerosis is a frequent cause of conductive hearing loss in young adults. It's more common in women than in men and affects whites more often than individuals of other races. Signs and symptoms of the condition usually appear between the ages of 15 and 45. The disease develops gradually and can affect one or both ears.

An increasing body of evidence suggests that genetic defects may predispose a person to the disease — among all the individuals who have otosclerosis, approximately 60 percent of this population will have a family history of the disease.

Treatment

Because otosclerosis typically results in mild to moderate hearing loss and doesn't progress far beyond that, hearing aids can successfully overcome most hearing loss due to the condition.

Another treatment option is surgery through the ear canal to replace the fixed stirrup with a tiny wire or other prosthesis. This procedure is known as a stapedotomy (stay-puh-DOT-uh-me). The prosthesis allows sound vibrations to again pass from the eardrum to the inner ear. Hearing improvement is usually permanent, although it may not be noticeable until about three to six weeks after surgery.

In rare cases, a person undergoing the procedure loses all hearing in the affected ear. Other potential complications: The prosthesis may eventually

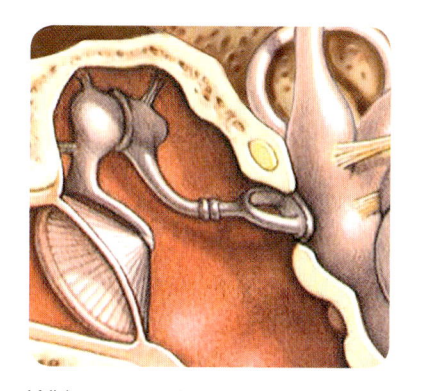

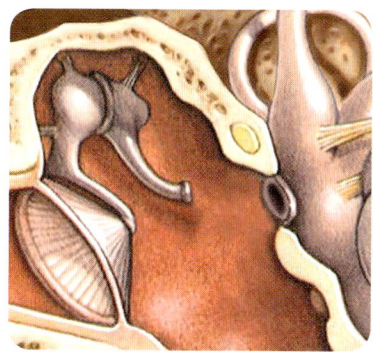

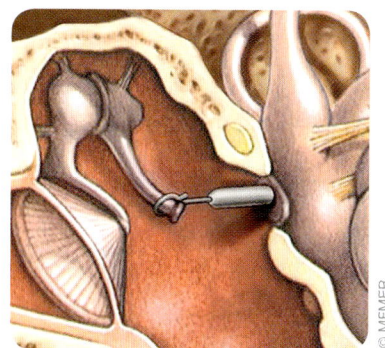

With a stapedotomy, a malfunctioning stirrup (stapes) is partly or completely removed and replaced with a tiny wire or other prosthesis that resumes the sound pathway to the inner ear.

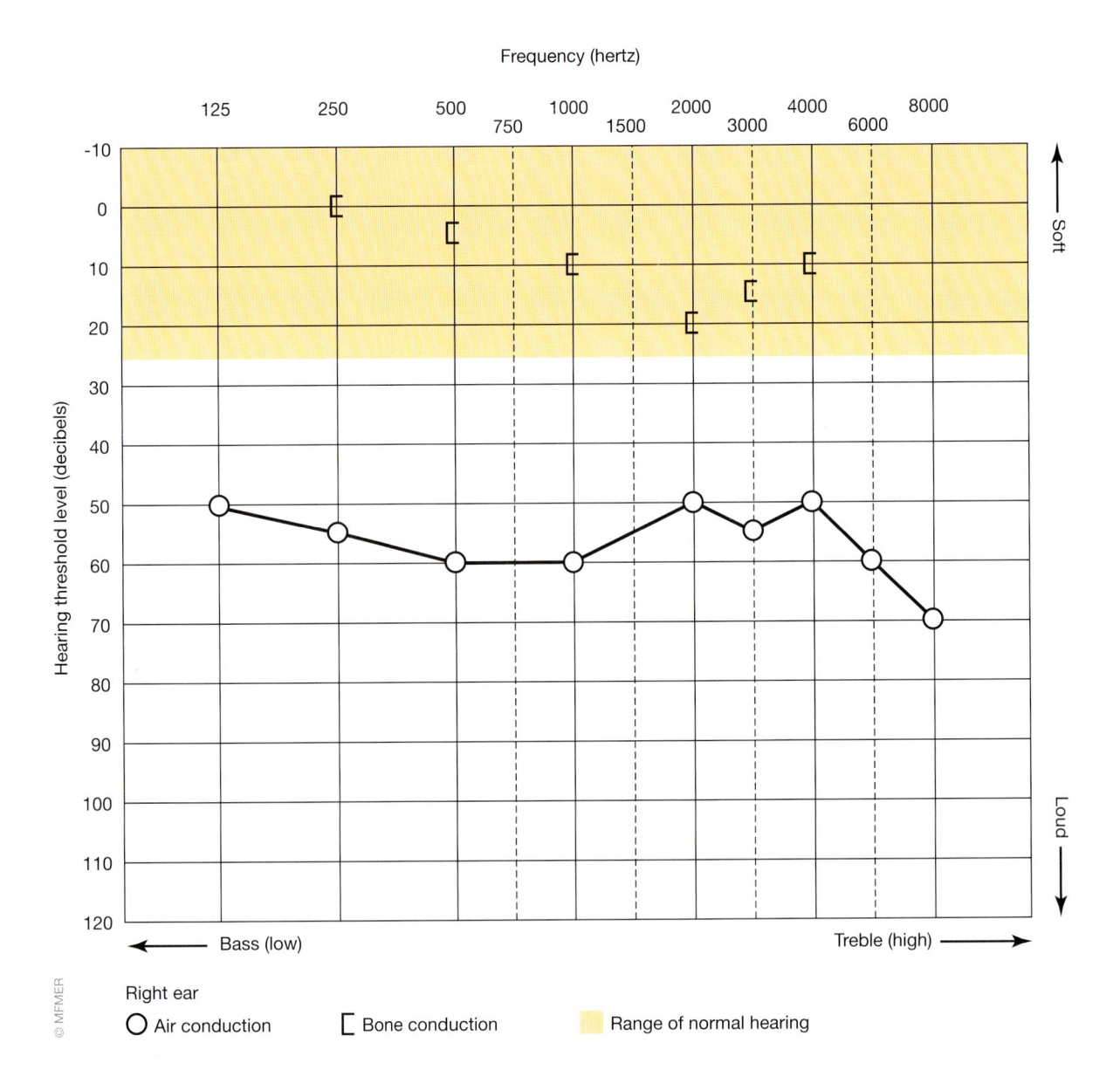

This is a typical audiogram of hearing loss due to otosclerosis in the right ear. Because the stirrup can no longer vibrate and transmit sound waves to the inner ear, air conduction for all frequencies is far below what is generally considered normal. Bone conduction remains good.

Chapter 3: Problems of the outer ear and middle ear

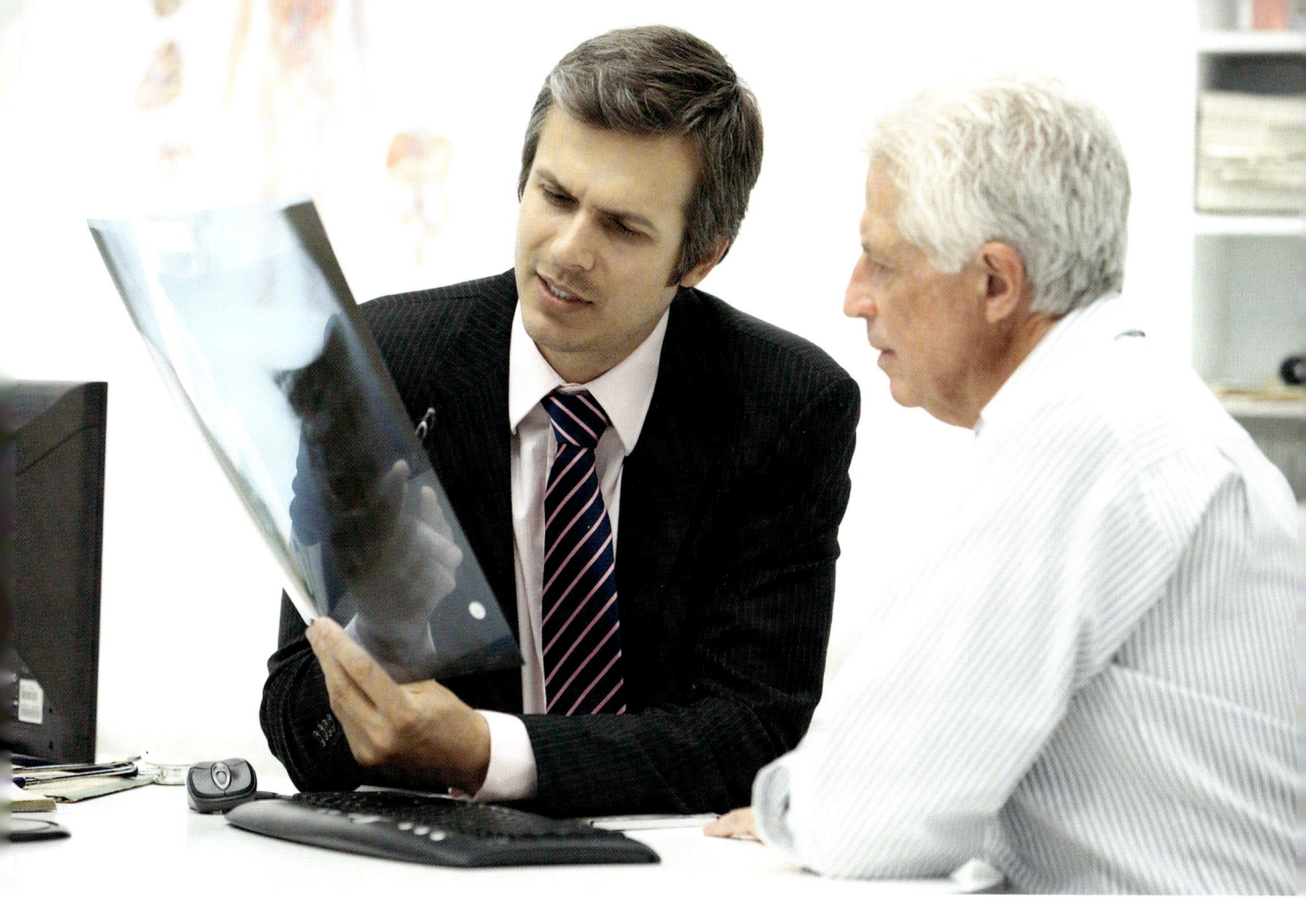

become displaced, a growth of spongy bone may recur over the oval window, or the anvil (incus) — to which the prosthesis is attached — may erode. If the disease progresses after surgery, the function of the prosthesis may be reduced over time.

If you have otosclerosis, you may be told to take tablets of sodium fluoride to help preserve hearing. But the value of this treatment is controversial. Advocates of this treatment note that fluoride may help harden the spongy bone, preventing progressive changes in the inner ear and the resulting hearing loss. However, fluoride is already present in most public water supplies in the U.S., so additional fluoride treatment is usually not necessary.

Ossicular chain disruption

A traumatic head injury can result in the displacement or breakage (fracture) of the small bones of the middle ear. These bones — the hammer, anvil and stirrup — are referred to collectively as the ossicular chain.

The most common site of displacement from a trauma is at the joint where the anvil connects to the stirrup. Often, the anvil itself is partially broken. The disruption of the ossicular chain causes a breakdown in the sound pathway from the eardrum to the inner ear, resulting in significant hearing loss.

Treatment

Obviously, a complete medical examination should follow any serious head trauma. Tests can help determine the nature of any hearing loss and the degree of its severity. If you still have hearing loss six months after the trauma, your doctor may propose surgery or recommend that you talk to an audiologist about a hearing aid to remedy the loss.

Surgery involves a procedure called ossiculoplasty (os-IH-coo-low-plas-tee), which attempts to rebuild the displaced ossicles or to replace them either with a prosthesis or with small pieces of bone or cartilage. Because the ossicles are tiny, the operation is a delicate one, and you may not recover all of your hearing.

If head trauma has damaged the cochlea, resulting in hearing loss in the inner ear (sensorineural hearing loss), a hearing aid may be your best option. This is because surgery can't be used to correct cochlear damage.

Although complications are rare, some risks that accompany all types of ear surgery are:

- Total deafness in the affected ear
- Tinnitus
- Dizziness and loss of balance
- Damage to the facial nerve, resulting in changes to your sense of taste or facial paralysis on the affected side

Your ear doctor will discuss such risks with you before any decision is made regarding surgery.

Chapter 4

Problems of the inner ear

The word *sensorineural* refers to the response of your nerve cells to stimuli from the external environment and from the internal functions of your body. With regard to hearing, the term is associated with the cochlea — the primary structure of the inner ear — and the auditory nerve.

The organ of Corti, located inside the cochlea, contains rows of ultrasensitive receptors known as hair cells, which respond to incoming auditory stimuli. These hair cells convert sound waves into electrical impulses that are carried by the auditory nerve to centers in the brain (see page 16).

Sensorineural (sen-suh-ree-NOOR-ul) hearing loss involves damage to the cochlea, the auditory nerve or both. For example, when hair cells in the organ of Corti are damaged due to trauma or simply to the wear and tear of age, the electrical impulses aren't transmitted as efficiently, resulting in hearing loss.

A common form of sensorineural hearing loss is presbycusis (pres-bih-KU-sis). As you get older, the hair cells gradually wear out, causing you to lose some sensitivity to sound. Some adults lose very little hearing as they age; others lose considerably more due to hair cell loss.

How much hearing loss you experience depends on various genetic and environmental factors, including:

- **Cumulative noise.** A lifetime of hearing the sounds of power tools, machinery, firearms, appliances and motor vehicles can gradually affect your ability to hear.

- **Sudden intense noise.** A single loud report from a nearby explosion or gunshot is another cause of sensorineural hearing loss.
- **Medications.** Certain drugs that are harmful to hearing are referred to as ototoxic (o-toe-TOK-sik).

Other causes of sensorineural hearing loss may be disease, physical trauma and genetic disorders.

Typically, sensorineural damage is permanent and irreversible. But with the use of hearing aids and other assistive devices and techniques, it's possible to communicate effectively despite a sensorineural hearing impairment.

Presbycusis

Presbycusis refers to age-related hearing loss. It's known that hearing tends to decrease as people age. An estimated one-third of Americans ages 65 to 74 have hearing loss, as do close to one-half of Americans age 75 and older, according to the National Institutes of Health.

There's a lot of variation in how people age, but in general you can expect the physical and mental changes to cause your senses to become a little less sharp and for sensory details to be a little harder to distinguish. In your ears, for example, you may lose hair cells in the cochlea — leading to sensorineural hearing loss. In addition, your brain may not be as quick to interpret incoming signals from the auditory nerve into recognizable sounds.

At first, you may notice that you're losing your sensitivity to sounds that have a high frequency (pitch). That's because the initial damage to hair cells often occurs where high-frequency sounds are processed. When this happens, you may be unable to hear or distinguish between certain sounds of speech, such as *ss*, *ff* and *th*.

At the same time, your ability to hear sounds with a low frequency usually remains intact. Some sounds, such as a booming bass instrument or a passing truck, may even seem too loud.

Presbycusis is sometimes accompanied by ringing or buzzing in your ears, which is a condition known as tinnitus (TIN-ih-tus). More about tinnitus can be found in Chapter 5. Presbycusis also makes it hard to hold a conversation in public spaces, such as a busy store or restaurant, where there's often commotion and background noise.

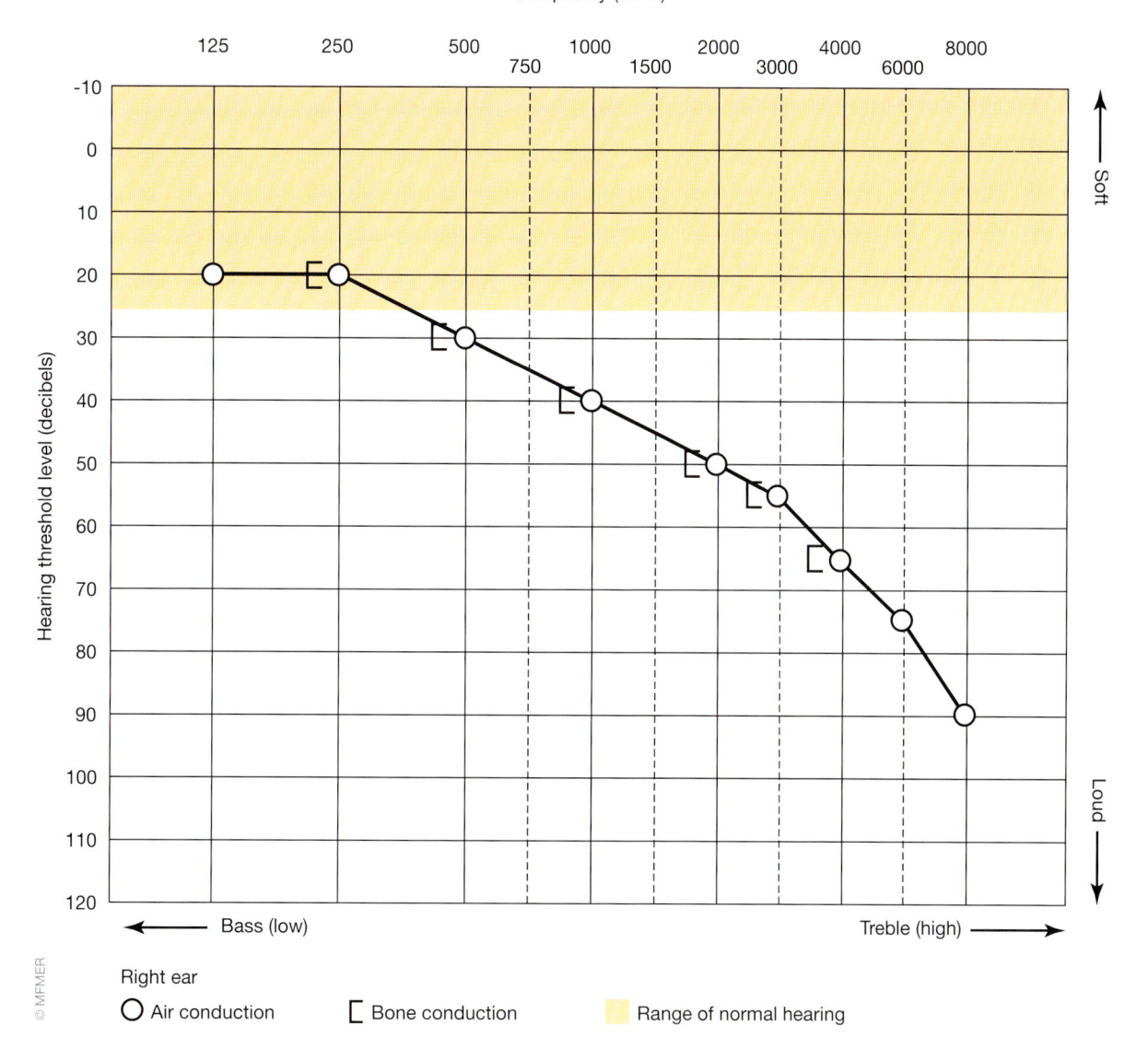

Audiogram of the right ear showing a typical pattern of hearing loss due to presbycusis. Often as you age, your sensitivity to low-frequency sounds remains relatively intact but you'll have increasing difficulty hearing high-frequency sounds. Certain high-frequency sounds, such as doorbells or bird songs, may become inaudible.

Mayo Clinic on Better Hearing and Balance **79**

Not being able to hear everything spoken in a conversation is the equivalent of reading a book from which random pages have been removed or trying to recognize a song based on just the throbbing bass line from a radio playing at your neighbor's house. It's usually a frustrating, if not annoying, experience.

Presbycusis tends to run in families, which suggests that genetics are involved. Its onset may be earlier in some families than in others.

Just as you adjust to other changes that may accompany aging, such as vision loss and high blood pressure, you can also compensate for presbycusis. In particular, hearing aids can make high-frequency sounds audible without amplifying the low-frequency sounds that you already hear.

Noise-induced hearing loss

Every day we're surrounded by noise — the bustle of traffic, the hums and grinds of machinery, people conversing, music and chatter from the radio, airplanes flying overhead.

Typically we think nothing of these familiar sounds. Most of the time they aren't loud enough to interfere in our routines or hurt our ears. But sometimes a noise is too loud for our ears, and some sounds may cause permanent damage.

There are two ways that noise exposure can damage hearing:

- **Single explosion of noise.** Sudden unprotected exposure to a sound measuring 140 decibels (dB) or above, such as a rifle gunshot or firecracker blast, can cause immediate hearing loss. The sounds of artillery and explosions are more dangerous. In fact, noise-induced hearing loss is a common injury in the military.
- **Prolonged exposure to loud noise.** Long-term exposure to noise levels above 85 dB can damage your hearing. This may happen at work or during recreational activities. Noise sources include power tools, lawn equipment, tractors, motorcycles and snowmobiles, and sound equipment such as personal listening devices set to high volume.

Noise-induced hearing loss can occur in one or both ears. You may begin noticing that familiar sounds seem muffled

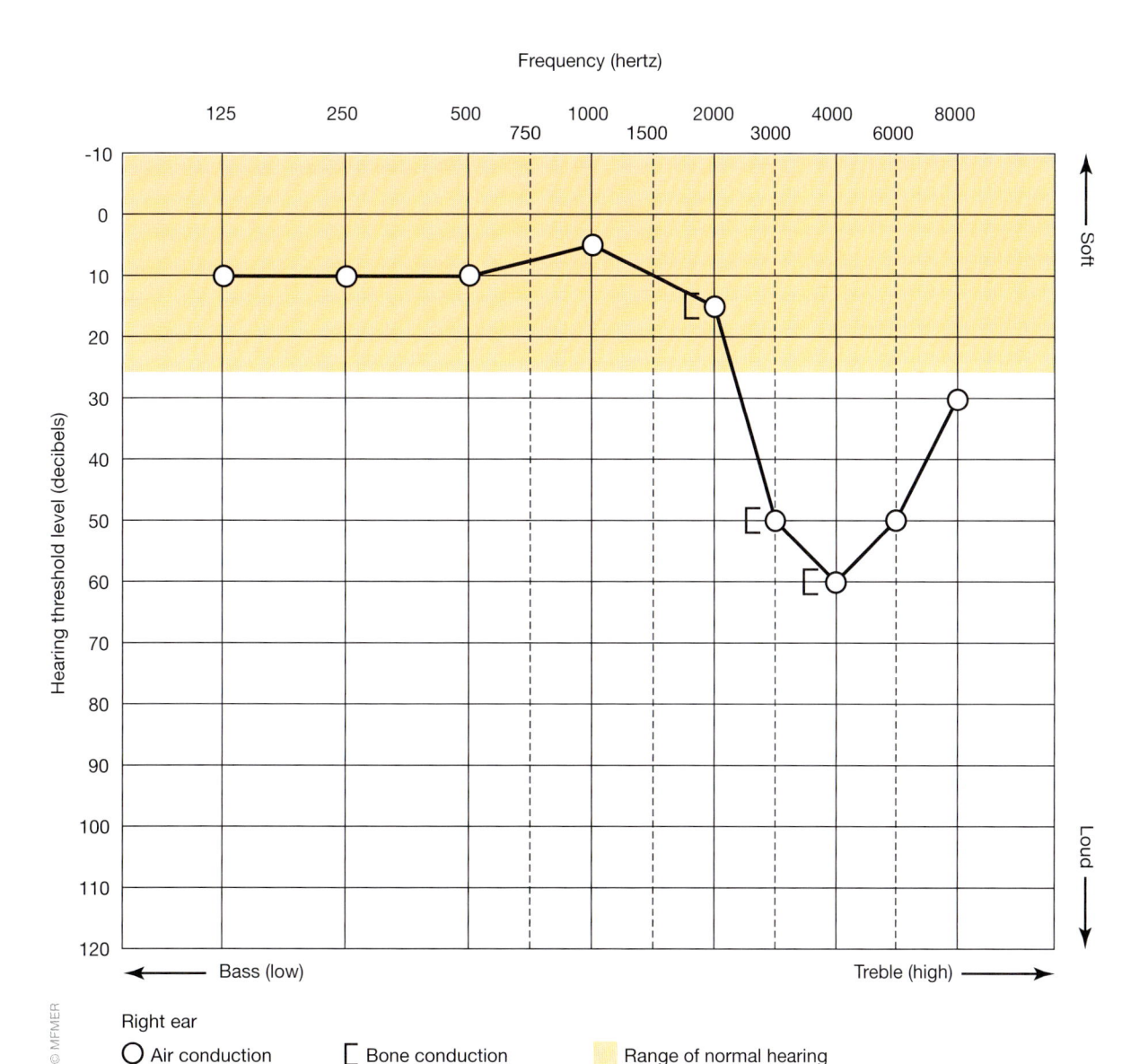

Audiogram of the right ear showing a typical pattern of hearing loss due to noise. Hearing sounds at low frequencies may remain in the normal range, while the ability to hear high frequencies takes a characteristic dip, usually greatest at 4,000 hertz.

Mayo Clinic on Better Hearing and Balance **81**

Hold down the noise

Most of us are aware of the dangers of work-related noise. But we easily overlook the racket at home. Here are steps you can take to hold down the noise level around your house:

- Turn down the volume on your television or home sound system.
- Wear snug-fitting headphones that block background noise on personal listening devices so that you don't have to turn up the volume so much.
- Choose quieter appliances.
- Place pads under noisy appliances.
- Don't run multiple appliances at the same time.
- Install carpeting to absorb sound.
- Seal windows and doors to block the noise of traffic.
- Wear earplugs or earmuffs when using power equipment.
- Rest your ears. Alternate noisy activities with quiet ones.

Hearing loss that results from many recreational activities is becoming more common. Don't forget to wear ear protectors when riding a snowmobile or motorcycle, using firearms, or listening to extremely loud music.

---

or distorted. This may be accompanied by the ringing or buzzing sensation in your ears known as tinnitus, which may or may not subside.

After a sudden exposure to loud noise, you may experience these symptoms immediately. However, with prolonged exposure, the hearing loss may be so gradual that you're not aware of a problem until it's pointed out to you or you have a hearing test.

If your hearing loss is temporary, it's called a temporary threshold shift. With this condition, normal hearing usually returns within 16 hours of being exposed to noise. But sometimes, hearing loss from your exposure to loud noise may be permanent.

Approximately 15 percent of Americans between ages 20 and 69 have some degree of high-frequency hearing loss due to exposure to loud sounds or noise at work or in leisure activities. Although noise-induced hearing loss usually can't be restored, there are ways in which it can be prevented:

- Avoid exposure to the loud noise.
- Take breaks from prolonged exposure.
- Move farther away from its source.
- Wear hearing protectors when involved in loud activities.

So how loud is too loud? Here's a good rule of thumb: If you have to shout in order to be heard by someone an arm's length away, you're being exposed to too much noise.

Hearing protectors are effective when they can be worn for the entire time that you're exposed to loud noise. Earplugs are small inserts that fit snugly inside the ear canal. Earmuffs fit over

Approximate sound levels of noise

Sound level (decibels)	Noise
30	Whisper
40	Refrigerator hum
50	Rainfall
60	Normal conversation, sewing machine
70	Washing machine
85	Heavy city traffic
95	Motorcycle, power lawn mower, MRI
100	Snowmobile, hand drill, blow dryer, subway train
105	Personal listening device at maximum volume
110	Chain saw, rock concert
120	Ambulance siren
130	Jet engine at takeoff
150	Firecracker
165	12-gauge shotgun blast
180	Rocket launch

Adapted from National Institute on Deafness and Other Communication Disorders, 2011, National Institute for Occupational Safety and Health, 2011, and American Tinnitus Association, 2013

Personal listening devices

The greatly improved sound quality, small size and convenience of personal listening devices has translated into more time listening to music. Unfortunately, many users listen for too long at too high a volume. This can cause noise-induced hearing loss, which may not be noticeable until significant damage has occurred.

Personal listening devices typically produce sound levels ranging between 55 and 105 decibels (dB). Listening to sounds of 80 dB or less isn't likely to cause damage. Keeping the volume at a level where you can still comfortably carry on a conversation means you won't need to limit the amount of time that you listen. Using snugly fit or sound-isolating earphones may help block background noise, allowing you to listen at lower decibel levels.

While you can't easily measure the decibel level of your music, a simple guideline for safe use is the 80/90 rule. This guideline says that it's OK to use a music player at 80 percent of maximum volume for up to 90 minutes a day. If you choose to listen for longer, the volume should be reduced. This guideline assumes that there are no additional high-level noise exposures within that 24-hour period.

Some other ways to tell if the volume is set too high:

- You can't hear conversations going on around you.
- You find yourself shouting when you talk to people nearby.
- After listening, you experience muffled sounds or ringing in your ears.

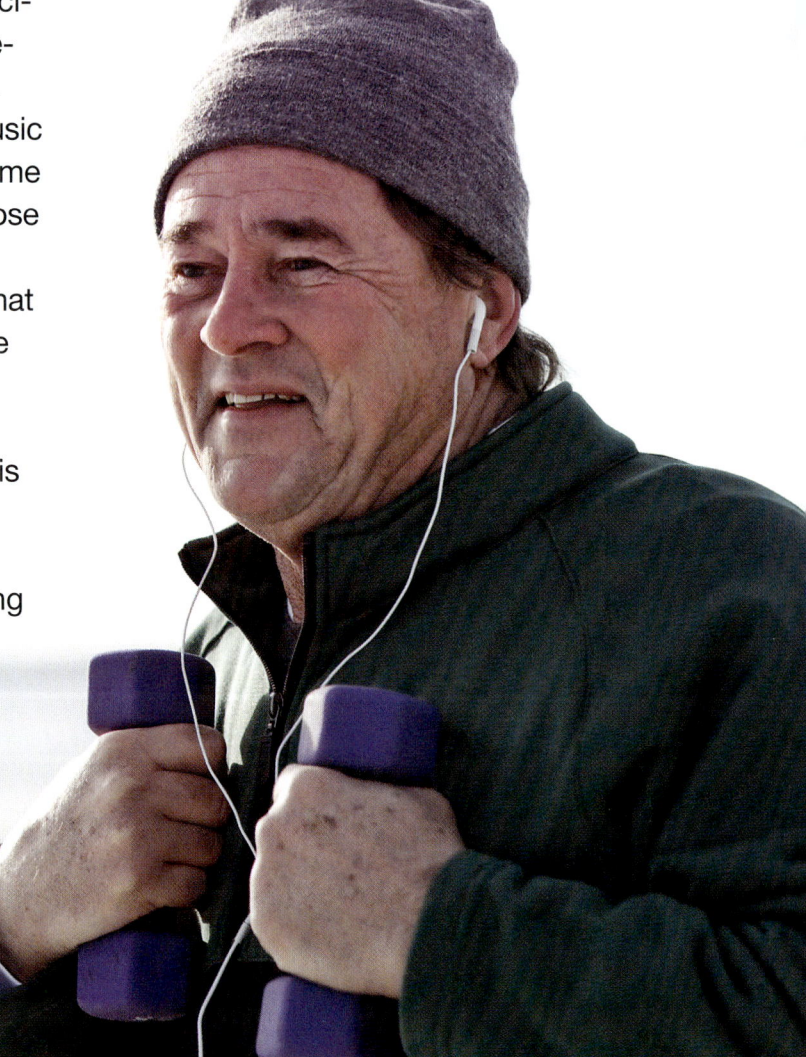

the entire outer ear. Each can reduce the noise by about 15 to 30 dB. When earplugs and earmuffs are worn together, they offer an additional reduction of 5 dB — which is important when noise levels are high.

Whatever type of ear protection you use, make sure it's clean and it fits correctly. Earplugs should maintain an airtight seal in your ear. Earmuffs must contact the skin entirely around your ear. Devices that meet federal standards are available at drugstores, hardware stores, sporting goods stores and with hearing aid dispensers.

In companies that operate at noise levels averaging 85 dB or more over an eight-hour day, employers are required to have a hearing conservation program. These programs include conventional noise measurements, the provision of hearing protectors to employees, an annual hearing test to screen employees, as well as education and training sessions.

See Chapter 2 for information on screening for hearing loss. If testing reveals significant loss in an employee, he or she is required to wear hearing protectors. If noise levels reach 90 dB or above, everyone is required by law to wear hearing protectors.

Sudden deafness

Sometimes hearing can be lost all at once or within only a few days. This condition is known as sudden sensorineural hearing loss (SSNHL).

SSNHL is almost always confined to one ear. You may notice a popping sound when it happens, or you may detect it when you first wake up or try to use the impaired ear. Dizziness or tinnitus also may develop. About 4,000 cases of sudden deafness occur every year in the United States.

If you notice the symptoms, contact your doctor immediately. The condition is often misdiagnosed as a routine ear infection or other dysfunction — however, it can be sorted out with a good examination.

You'll be checked to determine the extent of hearing loss. The less hearing loss that has occurred, the more likely you'll return to normal hearing within a few weeks. Although many individuals regain their former hearing, some may have no recovery or else regain only partial hearing in the affected ear.

Pinpointing the cause of SSNHL can be difficult. If your hearing returns quickly, you may not need medical treatment.

If the cause is known, taking care of the underlying problem may resolve the hearing loss. When the cause isn't obvious, your doctor may consider several possible suspects, including:

- Viral inner ear infection
- Abrupt disruption of blood flow to the cochlea
- Membrane tear within the cochlea
- Acoustic neuroma

Most of the time the cause is unknown. Your doctor may prescribe a corticosteroid such as prednisone or dexamethasone to reduce the inflammation as soon as possible. Sometimes, the corticosteroid is injected directly into the middle ear through the eardrum.

There is emerging evidence that hyperbaric oxygen therapy may aid in recovery from SSNHL if done within three months of the hearing loss. However, the therapy is not widely available and often is not covered by insurance.

Other causes of hearing loss

Factors other than aging and noise exposure may damage the inner ear and auditory nerve. The sensorineural hearing loss that results may be sudden or may worsen gradually.

Viral infections

Before the widespread practice of childhood immunization, the viruses responsible for several illnesses were also major causes of hearing loss. For example, the measles virus usually attacks cells lining the lungs and the back of the throat. And the mumps virus typically affects one of the salivary glands between the ear and the jaw. Either infection may spread to your inner ear and destroy hair cells in the cochlea.

Hearing loss from these once-common illnesses is now rare in the United States because they can be prevented with a vaccine. Children routinely get the measles, mumps, rubella (MMR) vaccine at ages 12 to 15 months and again at 4 to 6 years. You also gain immunity if you've previously had a measles or mumps infection.

Viruses may also travel through your bloodstream to the cochlea, leading to hearing loss. These viral illnesses include influenza, chickenpox, mononucleosis and cytomegalovirus (CMV).

If you're not sure whether you've been immunized or you need a vaccination before traveling to a place where the illnesses are still prevalent, talk to your doctor about vaccination.

Head trauma

A blow to the head can sometimes cause hearing impairment, especially if the part of the skull containing your ear (temporal bone) is fractured. Such a fracture may damage the delicate structure of the cochlea or your auditory nerve. Damage to the nerve interferes with communication to the brain. Occasionally, hearing loss isn't apparent until some time after the trauma.

Normally, your brain rests inside your skull protected by a cushion of spinal fluid. A sharp blow to the head will cause your brain to abruptly shift, which can tear blood vessels, pull nerve fibers and bruise tissue. Pressure waves from the blow can disrupt structures in the cochlea (damage known as a cochlear concussion) and cause sensorineural hearing loss.

If you've experienced a cochlear concussion, your hearing may improve over a six-month period. Another result of head trauma may be bleeding into the cochlear fluids, which also can result in hearing loss.

Meniere's disease

Meniere's (meh-NYAYRZ) disease is characterized by spontaneous episodes of sudden hearing loss, tinnitus, and the feeling of a plugged ear. This is often followed by a sensation of spinning or rotating (vertigo), often accompanied by nausea and vomiting. One attack may last anywhere from 20 minutes to several hours.

The attacks are unpredictable and can occur as often as several times a week or as infrequently as once a year. Typically, dizziness is the worst symptom. Between attacks you may not feel any symptoms at all. Although hearing comes and goes with the attacks, it may gradually worsen. Meniere's disease usually affects only one ear.

No one knows what causes Meniere's disease, but scientists associate the signs and symptoms with fluctuations in the fluid volume of the inner ear. Excess fluid increases pressure on the membranes of the inner ear, which may distort and occasionally rupture them. This development affects your hearing and sense of balance.

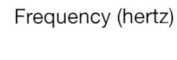

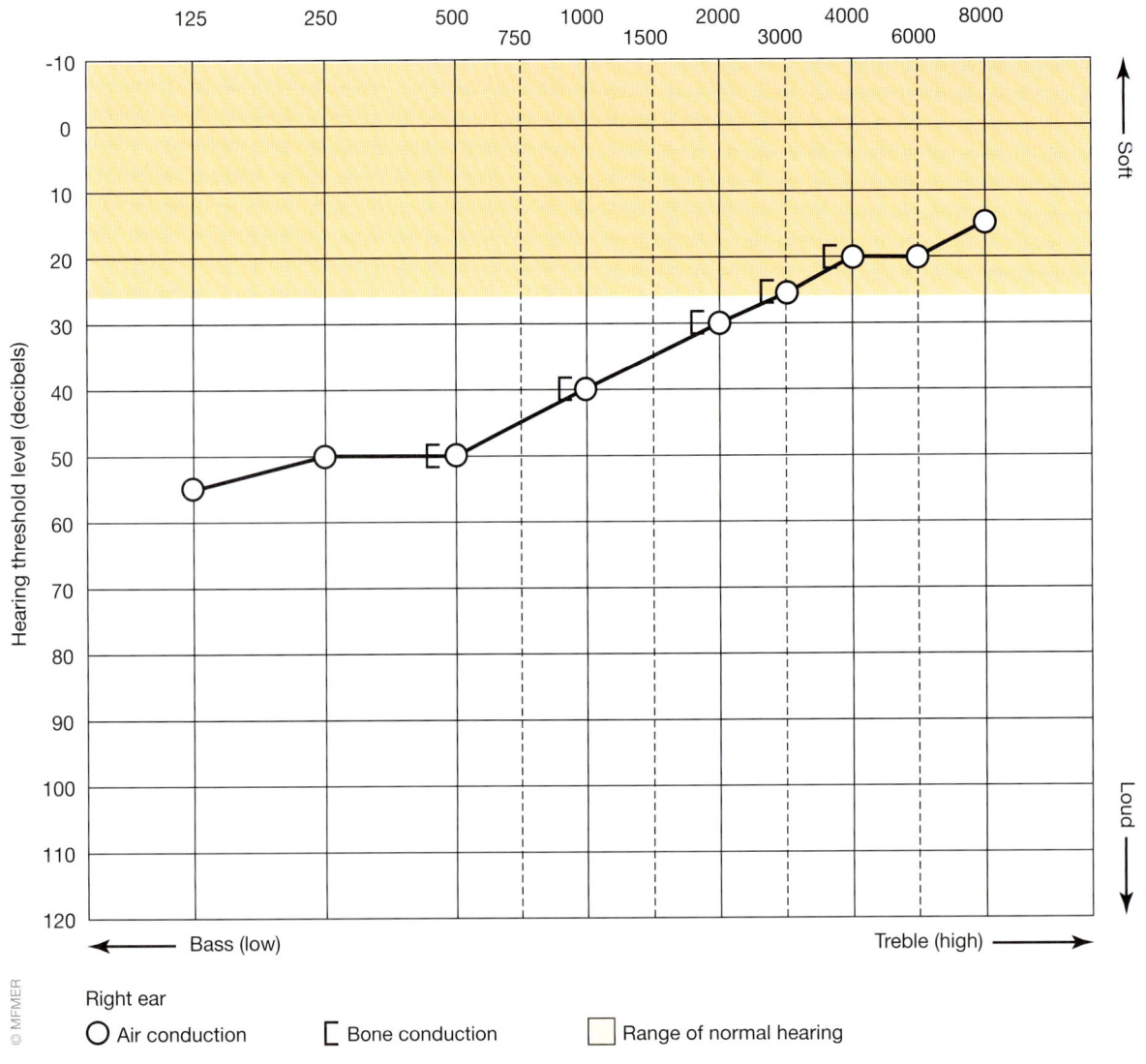

Audiogram of the right ear showing how Meniere's disease typically affects hearing. During attacks, sounds at lower and middle frequencies are more difficult to hear than are sounds at higher frequencies.

Chapter 4: Problems of the inner ear

Treating Meniere's disease usually involves taking medications to manage the symptoms of dizziness and nausea, limiting your intake of caffeine, alcohol and chocolate, and eating a low-salt diet.

Your doctor may also prescribe a diuretic, antihistamine or migraine medication to help reduce fluid retention. Medications such as corticosteroids, which reduce inflammation, or the antibiotic gentamicin, which reduces vestibular activity, may be injected into the middle ear to reduce or eliminate attacks.

If dizziness is severe, inner ear surgery may be an option. For more information on surgery of this kind, see the brief summary on page 224.

Labyrinthitis

Labyrinthitis (lab-uh-rin-THIE-tis) is an inflammation that can affect both the cochlea, which is vital to hearing, and the vestibular labyrinth, which plays a role in balance and eye movement. If the inflammation affects only the vestibular labyrinth, it's known as vestibular neuritis.

The inflammation often follows a viral infection or, more rarely, after a bacterial infection. Bacterial meningitis can cause severe to profound hearing loss. Vaccinations against the pneumococcal and meningococcal organisms responsible for this infection are now routinely recommended for children and many adults.

Labyrinthitis may also occur after a blow to the head, or it may occur with no associated illness or trauma.

Signs and symptoms of labyrinthitis include dizziness, hearing loss, tinnitus, nausea, vomiting and involuntary movements of your eyes. You may lose all of your hearing in the affected ear.

To minimize dizziness, it's helpful to frequently sit still and avoid sudden changes of position. Most of the time, the inflammation goes away on its own after a few weeks.

If the underlying problem is bacterial, your doctor may prescribe antibiotics. Drugs to relieve dizziness and nausea also may be recommended.

If the dizziness persists, physical or occupational therapy may be recommended. Many individuals recover completely from labyrinthitis, but some continue to experience problems with balance and hearing loss.

Acoustic neuroma

An acoustic neuroma is a slow-growing, benign tumor on the balance and hearing nerves leading from your inner ear to your brain. The tumor results from an uncontrolled growth of Schwann cells covering the nerves. It causes hearing loss by applying severe pressure on these nerves and affecting their blood supply. The condition is also known as vestibular schwannoma.

Because an acoustic neuroma affects nerves related to both hearing and balance, hearing loss and tinnitus in one ear are common signs and symptoms of the disorder. As the tumor grows, it can affect other nerves, causing facial numbness and weakness.

Although an acoustic neuroma is generally slow growing, it can become large enough to push against the brain and interfere with life-sustaining functions. Some tumors stop growing or grow slowly enough that they can be safely observed without treatment. Others may be removed with surgery or treated with a specialized, single dose of radiation.

To remove an acoustic neuroma, a surgeon will make a small incision behind or above your ear and remove a segment of your skull in order to get at the tumor. Once the tumor is located and

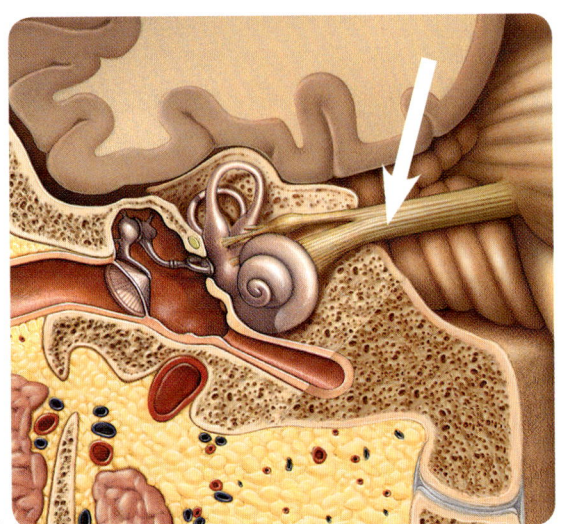

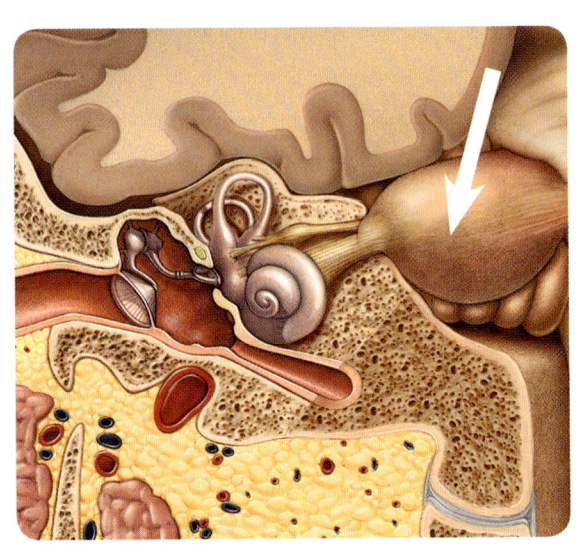

An acoustic neuroma is a tumor on your balance and hearing nerves. The arrow in the left-hand image shows a normal nerve. The arrow in the right-hand image indicates a large tumor that has developed at the base of the bony internal auditory canal.

removed, the bony segment is replaced to cover the opening in the skull and protect the brain.

If the tumor can be removed without injuring the nerves, your hearing may be preserved. In general, the larger the tumor is, the greater are the chances of your hearing, balance and facial nerves being affected.

A noninvasive treatment to stabilize small or medium-sized tumors is stereotactic radiosurgery. This closed-skull procedure involves sophisticated imaging that targets several focused radiation beams on a tumor. The separate beams are too weak to harm tissue they pass through — they only affect tissue at the spot where the beams crisscross.

One of the benefits of this procedure is that the skull isn't opened, eliminating the chances for surgical complications. And recovery time is shorter than with open surgery. A drawback is that it's not 100 percent effective. In some cases, the tumor continues to grow and may require surgical removal.

Reaction to medications

The action of certain medications or chemicals can cause hearing loss, tinnitus and balance problems. Medications can also aggravate an existing hearing problem. These medications are considered ototoxic.

The effects of ototoxic medications can range from mild to severe. Effects generally depends on the dosage strength and on the length of time you take the drugs. Common ototoxic medications are listed on page 93.

Hearing problems caused by some ototoxic drugs will go away after you stop taking the medications. Drugs that are known to cause permanent hearing loss are usually given only when no other option exists for treating a life-threatening disease.

About 200 medications are considered ototoxic. If you and your doctor decide that it's in your best interest to take an ototoxic drug, an audiologist will likely test your hearing before, while and after you take the drug.

While you're taking the ototoxic drug, your physician will closely monitor test results to determine how long you can continue with the regimen or when to alter the dosage.

Signs and symptoms of an ototoxic reaction include:

- Onset of tinnitus
- Worsening of existing tinnitus
- Feeling that one or both ears are plugged
- Loss of hearing or worsening of existing hearing loss
- Dizziness, sometimes accompanied by nausea

Notify your doctor if you have an existing hearing or balance problem or if you experience inner ear problems from certain medications. This may help you avoid unnecessary exposure to ototoxic drugs. If needed, an audiologist can help you plan for a hearing aid and hearing rehabilitation.

Autoimmune inner ear disease

Autoimmune inner ear disease (AIED) occurs when your body's immune system mistakes normal cells in your inner ear for a virus or bacteria and begins attacking them. This produces an inflammatory reaction that can lead to problems with both hearing and balance. AIED is rare, probably accounting for less than 1 percent of all cases of hearing loss.

It's unknown why the immune cells start attacking other normal cells. As with many other disorders, scientists suspect that AIED may have something to do with abnormal genetics.

A characteristic of AIED is hearing loss that progresses rapidly in both ears, occurring over weeks or months. Sometimes, the hearing loss starts in one ear and moves to the other.

Other signs and symptoms include tinnitus, a plugged ear and, in about half the AIED cases, dizziness. Because these signs and symptoms are similar to those of many other ear disorders, diagnosis can be difficult.

In addition, AIED is often associated with other autoimmune disorders of the body, such as:

- Ankylosing spondylitis, a disease that affects your spine
- Sjögren's syndrome, also known as dry eye syndrome
- Cogan's syndrome, which affects your eyes and ears
- Ulcerative colitis, which affects your intestinal tract
- Wegener's granulomatosis, which inflames blood vessels
- Rheumatoid arthritis, which inflames your joints
- Scleroderma, which affects your skin and other connective tissues

Ototoxic medications and chemicals

Listed below are some of the drugs and environmental chemicals that may cause hearing loss. If you're taking one of these medications, it's important not to stop taking it until you've consulted your doctor.

Category	Examples	Effects
Salicylates	• Aspirin • Aspirin-containing products	Ototoxicity only occurs at high doses. Hearing loss is almost always reversible.
Antivirals	• Chloroquine (Aralen) • Quinidine • Quinine (Qualaquin)	Ototoxicity usually occurs at high doses. Hearing improves when use of the drug is stopped.
Loop diuretics	• Bumetanide (Bumex) • Ethacrynic acid (Edecrin) • Furosemide (Lasix) • Torsemide (Demadex)	Ototoxicity is temporary. If these drugs are given with an ototoxic antibiotic, risk of permanent damage may increase.
Aminoglycoside antibiotics	• Amikacin • Gentamicin • Neomycin • Streptomycin • Tobramycin	Risk of ototoxicity usually increases when the antibiotic is administered directly into the bloodstream, which allows the greatest amount of the drug into the body. Damage may be permanent.
Anti-cancer drugs (anti-neoplastics)	• Carboplatin • Cisplatin	Drugs designed to kill cancer cells may also kill inner ear cells. The damage is often permanent and may make you more vulnerable to noise-induced hearing loss.
Environmental chemicals	• Lead • Manganese • N-butyl alcohol • Toluene	Excessive exposure to these chemicals in the workplace may result in permanent hearing loss.

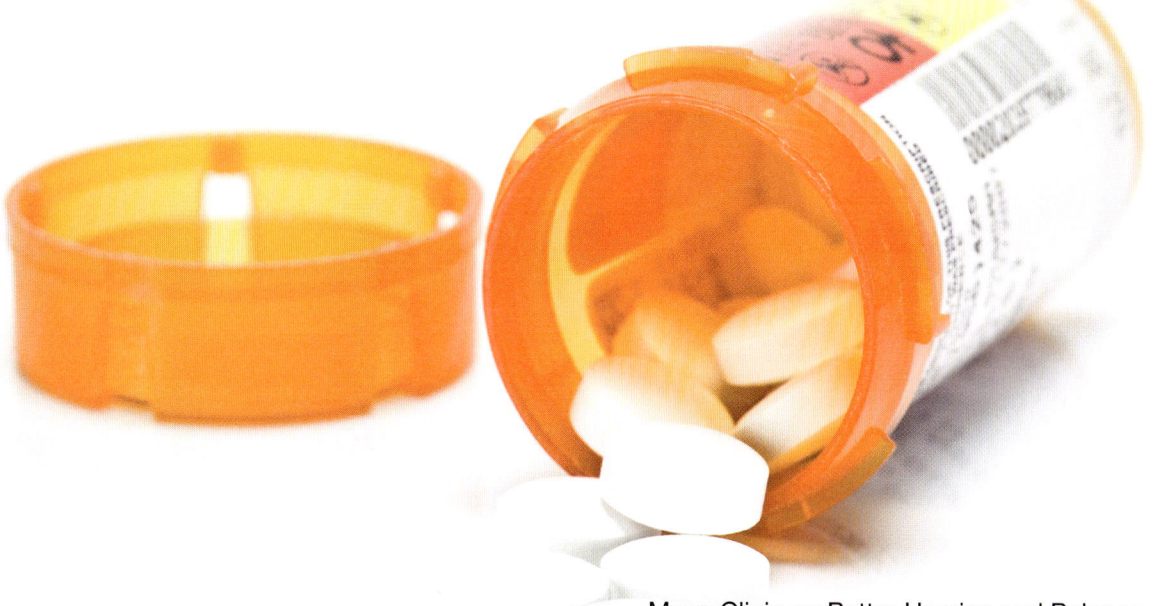

Mayo Clinic on Better Hearing and Balance

- Systemic lupus erythematosus (SLE) and Behçet's syndrome, both of which can affect multiple systems in your body

If you have AIED, your doctor may prescribe oral corticosteroids (prednisone, dexamethasone) to reduce the inflammation. Corticosteroids are the most effective treatment for AIED but have side effects that can limit long-term use. In certain cases, steroids may be injected directly into the ear in an attempt to avoid the side effects.

Several treatment options for AIED that have been used in the past but are less commonly used today include certain immunosuppressive agents such as methotrexate (Rheumatrex) — drugs that suppress your immune cells — and etanercept (Enbrel) — a drug that blocks a protein triggering some of the inflammation.

Congenital hearing problems

A congenital problem means the condition exists at birth. These types of hearing problems may be hereditary in nature. Some may also develop in the womb or from conditions during the birthing process.

Genetic factors may be responsible for more than half of all incidents of congenital hearing loss. A child whose hearing loss is inherited usually has two parents who carry a recessive gene for hearing loss (autosomal recessive hearing loss). This gene isn't expressed in the parents, who therefore have normal hearing, but is expressed in the child who inherits both recessive genes. So far, multiple genes have been identified that cause recessive hearing loss not related to other illnesses.

Often, congenital hearing loss is part of a collection of symptoms (known as a syndrome) caused by a genetic defect. Conditions linked with congenital hearing loss include Pendred's syndrome, Waardenburg's syndrome, Usher's syndrome and Treacher Collins syndrome.

Other factors that may cause hearing loss in an infant include:

- Severe jaundice
- Infection in the mother, such as German measles (rubella), cytomegalovirus, herpes or syphilis
- Premature birth
- Lack of oxygen during or shortly after birth
- Blood incompatibilities between mother and child

- Diabetes in the mother
- Fetal alcohol syndrome
- Inner ear malformations such as Mondini malformation or enlarged vestibular aqueducts

As mentioned in Chapter 2, most newborns will be screened for hearing loss before they leave the hospital. Even with normal results, it's important to continue monitoring your child's hearing as he or she develops — a hearing impairment that goes unnoticed may significantly interfere with speech and language development. Once identified, the impairment may be successfully corrected with hearing aids or cochlear implants.

Research on the horizon

The fact that sensorineural damage to the inner ear so often causes severe or profound permanent hearing loss has challenged scientists to come up with new approaches for treatment. They're testing certain drugs that may reduce the effects of noise exposure on the inner ear. They're also studying drugs that may inhibit the effects of aging on your hearing.

Hair cell regeneration

An exciting area of new research involves hair cell regeneration. Hair cells are the delicate sensory receptors of the inner ear, and damage can result in serious hearing problems.

Until recently, scientists believed the inner ear was incapable of producing new hair cells. Then they discovered that birds have a natural ability to generate new hair cells in response to damage. Furthermore, the new cells restored the birds' hearing. This discovery has led researchers to consider how to regenerate lost or damaged hair cells in humans.

Human hair cells might be regenerated using hormone-like substances called growth factors, which regulate cell growth. Researchers are testing various growth factors to identify ones that might cause the hair cells to develop. In one recent study, researchers demonstrated for the first time that hair cells can be regenerated in an adult mammal's ear by using a drug to stimulate cells to become new hair cells. This resulted in a partial recovery of hearing.

Although progress so far is promising, many challenges remain.

Gene therapy

Scientists have also made important progress in understanding the relationship between genetics and hearing loss. They've discovered that many genes can affect hearing and that genetics and environment likely interact to cause hearing loss. For example, an individual may be genetically predisposed to hearing loss caused by specific environmental factors such as noise exposure, drugs or illness.

With this growing body of knowledge, researchers are investigating gene therapy as a way to treat hearing loss. Gene therapy, also called gene transfer, involves replacing a defective gene with a normal gene, with the hope that a cell will accept and use it.

Gene therapy holds great potential for treating hereditary forms of deafness, preventing hair cell damage and stimulating hair cell regeneration. Research is still at an early stage. There's a long way to go before effective and affordable genetic treatment for hearing impairment is feasible.

Chapter 5

Tinnitus

Tinnitus (TIN-ih-tus, or in some places pronounced as tih-NIE-tus) is the perception of sound in your ear caused by no apparent external source. The sound is characterized as a ringing, buzzing, whistling, chirping, hissing, humming, roaring or clicking, among other descriptions. Some people refer to it as music or the sound of boiling water.

Regardless of how it's described, it's a sound that's not produced in your surroundings. Often the noise seems to originate in your head.

Many people experience brief episodes of tinnitus after being exposed to an extremely loud noise or by taking certain medications. But few people are overly alarmed by such episodes, and the noise usually goes away.

According to the American Tinnitus Association, about 17 percent of people in industrialized countries — 50 million people in the U.S. — experience tinnitus at some time in their lives. And 5 percent have prolonged tinnitus that requires medical evaluation.

The impact of tinnitus on people's lives can range anywhere from annoying to debilitating. At night the ringing or hissing noise may make it difficult for some people to fall asleep. Tinnitus also makes it hard for them to focus on daily tasks and jobs. Frustration with the unexplained sounds can often lead to anxiety, fear and depression.

Tinnitus is a symptom associated with many ear disorders as well as with other diseases, including cardiovascular disease, allergies and anemia.

Unraveling the mystery

Physicians and medical researchers have grappled with a precise definition of tinnitus. It's unclear whether tinnitus is a syndrome — a set of symptoms that accompanies another disorder — or whether it's a disorder in itself.

What mechanisms trigger tinnitus — which might explain how and why the noise occurs — are still unclear. Although descriptions of tinnitus exist as far back as the time of the Pharaohs of ancient Egypt, much about the condition remains a mystery.

Several theories have been proposed regarding the cause of tinnitus. One hypothesis is that it's a phenomenon of the central nervous system, similar to the phantom-like sensations experienced after a limb amputation. A person may feel pain in his or her foot even after the leg has been removed.

Similarly, the central auditory nervous system may be responding to the loss of hair cells in the inner ear by becoming hyperactive. That is, one or more of the auditory-information processing stations in the central auditory nervous system may generate abnormal activity.

In addition to auditory centers, nonauditory areas also may play a role. In some people with tinnitus, there seems to be a link between the auditory system and the limbic system (which is responsible for emotions such as fear and anxiety). There's also evidence that the somatosensory system (which signals the sensation of touch and the movement of body parts such as jaw clenching and certain neck movements) may influence activity in the auditory system. These movements can cause changes in the loudness and pitch of tinnitus.

This evidence is based on positron emission tomography (PET) scans, which reveal the parts of the brain that are used to accomplish specific tasks. Careful study of PET imagery of people with tinnitus suggests that these non-auditory areas can interact with the auditory system for some patients, leading to changes in the perception of tinnitus.

Other researchers think the cause of tinnitus may lie with the activity of chemicals in the auditory nerve, which carries messages between your inner ear and the brain. Tinnitus may also stem from turbulent blood flow through arteries and veins that lie close to the inner ear.

Regardless of their preferred theory, many scientists agree that tinnitus is a

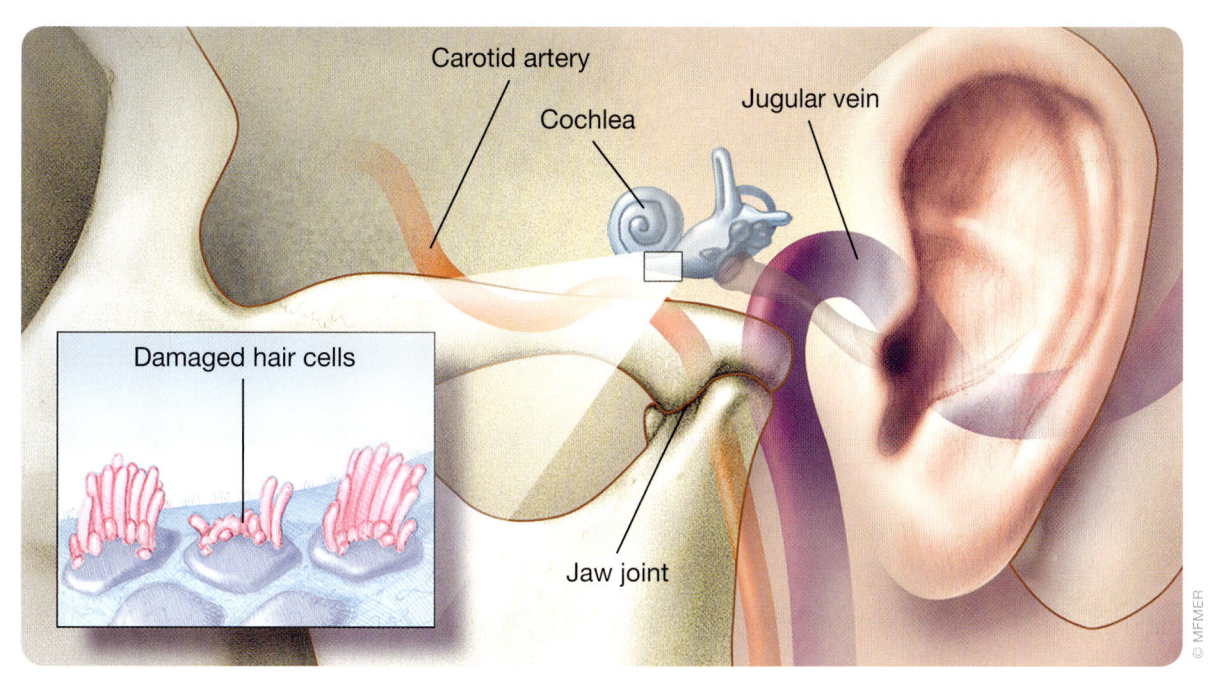

Tinnitus may develop from multiple causes. Some researchers believe that tinnitus results from damage to the hair cells inside your cochlea, leading to hyperactivity in the central auditory nervous system. Turbulent flow through your blood vessels also may produce a sound sensation, since blood vessels such as the carotid artery and the jugular vein lie close to the inner ear. Tinnitus may also result from a misalignment of the jaw joint (temporomandibular joint), head or neck trauma, or a variety of other medical conditions.

complex systemwide problem involving both the auditory and nonauditory segments of the central nervous system.

The good news is that tinnitus is generally not a serious or life-threatening medical concern. In a few cases, tinnitus may be caused by an underlying condition that's treatable.

While tinnitus may not be curable, you can learn various ways to manage it so that its effect on your daily life is minimized. These options often require the assistance of a physician and audiologist along with your active participation.

Types

How people describe tinnitus varies greatly from one person to the next. The only thing they have in common

Mayo Clinic on Better Hearing and Balance **99**

seems to be the existence of an unexplained noise in their head or ears.

For a general framework on which to classify tinnitus, some experts have categorized the condition by two broadly defined types: objective and subjective.

Objective tinnitus

Objective tinnitus, sometimes referred to as pulsatile (PUL-suh-tile) tinnitus, is a sound sensation that can be heard by other people as well as by you. The sounds originate within your body, most commonly from turbulent blood flow in your arteries and veins.

If you have atherosclerosis, for example, a buildup of cholesterol and other fatty deposits causes your blood vessels to lose elasticity. This restricts the vessels from flexing slightly with each heartbeat. Narrower openings require a more forceful blood flow. Your heart works harder — to the point where your ears can detect each heartbeat. Your doctor may hear the sound with the help of a stethoscope.

High blood pressure can make tinnitus more noticeable. So can factors that temporarily increase blood pressure, such as stress, alcohol or caffeine use, and high amounts of sodium in your diet. Repositioning your head usually can cause the sounds to disappear.

The malformation of small blood vessels (capillaries) connecting your arteries and veins also can produce an audible pulse. Other sources of objective tinnitus include muscle spasms, movement of the eustachian tube and spontaneous vibrations of hair cells.

Only a small percentage of all the individuals who have tinnitus have the objective type. Treating the underlying disorder may help reduce or even eliminate the sounds. That's why it's important to describe the tinnitus to your doctor and receive an accurate diagnosis. Be as specific as you can about the noises you hear and under what circumstances they occur.

Subjective tinnitus

Subjective tinnitus involves sounds that only you detect. Scientists aren't sure what causes these sounds. And in order to study the problem, they must depend on how well people describe what they're hearing.

Still, there's a consensus that subjective tinnitus originates within the structures

Hyperacusis

Hyperacusis (hi-pur-uh-KOO-sis) is another condition that's often associated with tinnitus. Hyperacusis involves a heightened aversion to sound. Everyday noise, such as traffic, conversation or a telephone ring, seems uncomfortably loud. Like tinnitus, the cause of hyperacusis is unknown.

Hyperacusis may be even more debilitating than is tinnitus. A person with severe hyperacusis may avoid social situations for fear of painful noise exposure (phonophobia), choosing instead to stay in a secluded environment. Although some form of hyperacusis may occur in people with hearing loss, those reporting hyperacusis usually have normal hearing.

Treatment consists of counseling and participating in a program that gradually increases your tolerance of normal sounds. This may involve a white noise generator — an electronic device that generates a persistent hissing sound, similar to what you may hear when a radio is tuned between stations. Initially the device is tuned to barely audible levels and then gradually increased to higher levels over time.

---

of the inner ear, the central auditory pathways or elsewhere in the brain.

Although the nature of subjective tinnitus remains unclear, several factors are believed to be capable of triggering the condition or making it worse.

Hearing loss

Exposure to loud noise, even for a short time, can damage the hair cells in your cochlea and cause permanent hearing loss. Most people with tinnitus have some form of noise-induced hearing loss. It may be that the damage to hair cells also causes the tinnitus.

Some researchers believe that age-related hearing loss (presbycusis) may also precipitate tinnitus. As the presbycusis muffles sounds from the outside world, existing tinnitus may become more noticeable. Other conditions that can reduce hearing, such as impacted earwax or ear infection, also may increase tinnitus.

Medications

More than 200 prescription drugs are associated with tinnitus. Some of these drugs are ototoxic and may permanently injure the ear. Usually such prescriptions are made only when absolutely necessary.

Other drugs can produce tinnitus as a side effect. Always discuss potential side effects of any prescription medication with your doctor. After you begin taking the drug, inform your doctor if your hearing is reduced or you experience tinnitus. Stopping the drug or adjusting the dosage often eliminates the problem. If you already have tinnitus, be sure to tell your doctor.

Jaw disorders

A misaligned joint connecting your jaw and the temporal bone of your skull may cause clicking or grating noises whenever you move your jaw. Some people claim the noises are present even when no jaw movement occurs, but this is debatable. A dentist who specializes in treating this joint may be able to correct the misalignment and reduce or eliminate the associated noises.

Other factors

Various conditions or lifestyle factors may cause tinnitus:

- Schwannomas (shwah-NO-muhz), which are benign tumors that grow on the fibers of the balance and hearing nerves
- Serious trauma or injury to the head or neck
- Otosclerosis, or a stiffening of the ossicle bones in the middle ear
- Meniere's disease, which causes excess fluid in the inner ear
- Exposure to excessive noise
- Too much sodium in your diet
- Stress, either emotional or physical

Diagnosis

There's little doubt that tinnitus can be troublesome. In many cases, the tinnitus triggers a cycle of growing discomfort: Annoyance leads to increased attention to the noise, which builds greater frustration. Some people find the distraction so severe that they're unable to carry on with their regular daily activities.

Several options are available that may allow you to manage tinnitus and still function in life with a reasonable degree of comfort. First, talk about the condition with your physician or audiologist. He or she can help identify or rule out a treatable cause of your tinnitus. Other specialists may become involved in the diagnosis.

If an underlying condition is causing the tinnitus, treatment of that primary condition may resolve the problem. Measures such as treating an ear infection or removing impacted earwax also may help reduce tinnitus.

If the cause of your tinnitus remains unknown, you and your medical team can decide how best to treat your symptoms. A medical history, physical examination, hearing tests and laboratory tests may provide vital clues.

For a more detailed description of your tinnitus, the doctor may ask:

- Is one ear affected or both? If only one, which one?
- Do you have hearing loss?
- What does the noise sound like? Is it high pitched or low pitched? How loud is it?
- Are the sounds constant, or do they change in loudness or pitch?
- What circumstances make the tinnitus better or worse?
- How does this condition affect your work habits and your ability to sleep and to concentrate?
- How has this condition affected your stress level?

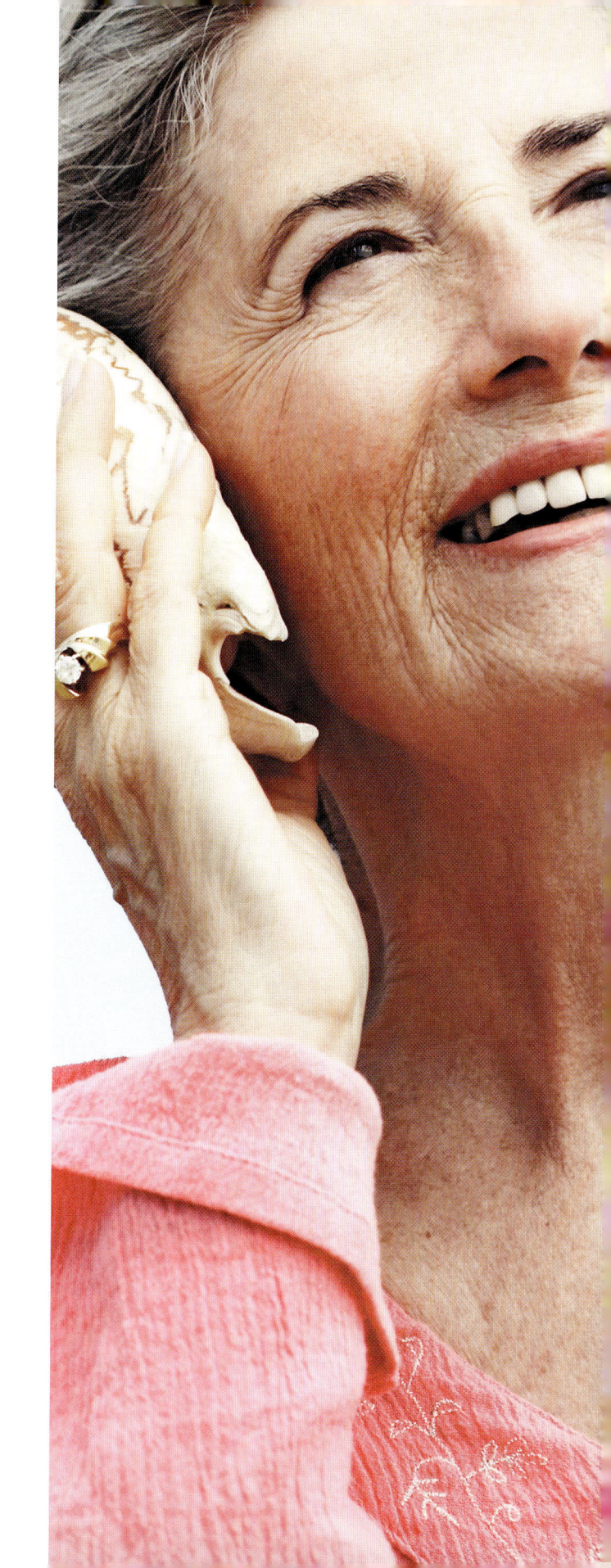

In addition to this assessment, an audiologist may try to determine the specific frequency (pitch) and intensity (loudness) of your tinnitus through audiological tests. This information can help you and your medical team select the best treatment for your situation.

Management

Though many questions remain about tinnitus, effective treatment strategies focus on managing its signs and symptoms. This focus allows you to continue functioning in your daily responsibilities and to lead a more fulfilled life.

You and your medical team may try several management approaches — including counseling and some types of therapy — before deciding which one works best for you. It's often helpful to use multiple strategies.

Hearing aids with maskers

One treatment approach involves wearing hearing aids that can produce a low-level background masking noise that's typically easier to tolerate than tinnitus. You may not have difficulty hearing, but you may benefit from the addition of subtle background noise to cover, or mask, the sounds of tinnitus.

These sounds usually resemble static noise or wind chimes. You may have controls to adjust the loudness, but the frequency is usually programmed by the manufacturer and your audiologist to achieve the best effect.

If you do have hearing loss, then a hearing aid may not only reduce your perception of tinnitus but also improve your ability to hear. Programmed specifically for your hearing loss, hearing aids amplify environmental sounds that could result in making the tinnitus less noticeable. Many people, but not all, who have hearing loss and tinnitus report that their tinnitus diminishes when they wear hearing aids.

Before committing to the purchase of hearing aids, you should confirm that they can provide enough benefit to be worth the investment. Be sure to ask your hearing health care provider about the return policy in case hearing aids are not the best answer for you.

Other masking sources

Tinnitus maskers are devices worn behind or in the ears. They resemble a hearing aid, but instead of amplifying environmental sounds they produce low-level background noise that may be easier to tolerate than tinnitus. Recent models allow the user to adjust the loudness and in some cases select from several types of noise to obtain the most benefit. The frequency is usually programmed by the manufacturer and your audiologist.

Often, tinnitus is most noticeable at night, when the outside world is more quiet. Some people find it helpful to use a bedside masker to play soothing sounds, such as ocean waves, falling rain and white noise, as they prepare to sleep. These masking sounds help with relaxation and obscure tinnitus during sleep. You can find maskers as stand-alone devices for your bedside or even as apps for your cellphone or tablet.

Drug therapy

Although many medications have been studied, the Food and Drug Administration (FDA) has not approved a drug specifically for tinnitus. However, there are some antidepressant and anti-anxiety medications that can reduce the stress associated with tinnitus, improve your outlook and help you cope with the condition.

Music therapy

Researchers are studying many music therapy devices and methods for their long-term effects on tinnitus. These devices can often be fitted to your specific needs, combining relaxing music with customized sounds to help you reduce stress and potentially diminish the perception of tinnitus.

Cognitive behavioral therapy

Cognitive behavioral therapy tries to change your understanding and perception of tinnitus rather than change the physical effects that tinnitus may have on you. This approach is based on the idea that negative thought patterns lead to negative and adverse behaviors.

For example, you may come to believe that tinnitus will make it impossible to enjoy pleasurable activities and you begin to avoid social events and pastimes. A psychologist can use cognitive behavioral therapy to train you to overcome these negative thoughts and eliminate avoidance behaviors.

Learning to view the condition differently can give you a sense of control and allow you to have a positive outlook.

Self-help tips for tinnitus

You may consider using these measures to reduce the severity of tinnitus and better cope with its symptoms:

Protect your hearing. Avoid loud noises, which may decrease your hearing and worsen tinnitus. If you work in a noisy environment, wear hearing protective devices regularly.

Fill your environment with sound. If you're in a quiet setting where tinnitus may seem more obvious, use a masker, fan, soft music, low-volume radio or commercially available sound generator to produce soft background noise that masks the tinnitus. Listening to pleasant and relaxing sounds can be helpful.

Distract yourself. Many people say they don't hear tinnitus if they're not paying attention to it. Do things that you enjoy and that absorb your attention. This will help take your mind off the tinnitus and provide needed relief.

Manage your stress. Stress can make tinnitus seem worse. The basic principles of a healthy lifestyle go a long way toward reducing stress — get plenty of sleep and exercise, and eat a healthy diet. For example, reducing tobacco, alcohol, caffeine and salt intake may help you better cope with the aggravation of your tinnitus.

Practice good sleep habits. People who sleep well tend to better manage their tinnitus. Although you might not be able to control all the factors that interfere with sleep, you can adopt habits that encourage better sleep. For example, try to go to bed and wake up at roughly the same time every day, and keep your bedroom comfortable and dark.

Educate yourself. Learning about tinnitus can give you a sense of control over it. Resources such as the American Tinnitus Association are listed at the back of this book.

Tinnitus retraining therapy

Tinnitus retraining therapy (TRT) is based on the idea that a person can gradually lose the awareness of a sound if that sound poses no threat or demands little attention. People can become oblivious to the sound of a ticking clock or whirring fan, even a passing train. But if the sound carries some sort of meaning with it — for example, you associate a ticking clock with being late or behind schedule — it's likely to heighten your awareness and may make it stressful.

This concept is applied to coping with tinnitus. If you have tinnitus, you may have a constant urge to examine the sounds and find a cause for what you're hearing. Being unable to identify a source may leave you feeling frustrated and insecure, which further focuses your attention on the tinnitus. When this happens, it may seem as though you'll never lose your awareness of the sounds.

The goal of TRT is to get you accustomed to the tinnitus so that its steady, persistent sound becomes just like other nonthreatening sounds and blends into the background. If the effort is successful, you'll perceive tinnitus less often on a conscious level.

To start treatment you use noise generators, usually worn in both ears, for approximately eight hours a day. The devices are set such that the generated soft noise is audible but doesn't mask your tinnitus. In other words, the generated noise and the tinnitus are blended together.

You'll also receive counseling that helps you perceive the tinnitus in a rational, intelligent way so that it no longer causes fear or obsession. The audiologist will explain what's known about tinnitus and how you can become habituated to the sound.

This therapy takes time. Most people participate in the program for one to two years before stopping the use of the noise generators. Although it's not for everyone, a majority of people undergoing TRT report at least some success in reducing their perception of tinnitus.

Complementary, alternative and new treatments

Although Western science has yet to document all of the benefits and risks of many forms of alternative medicine, treatments that deal with the overall well-being of your body may be helpful. These may include meditation, journaling, deep breathing, tai chi and yoga. These usually aim to reduce the general stress of life and may help reduce anxiety.

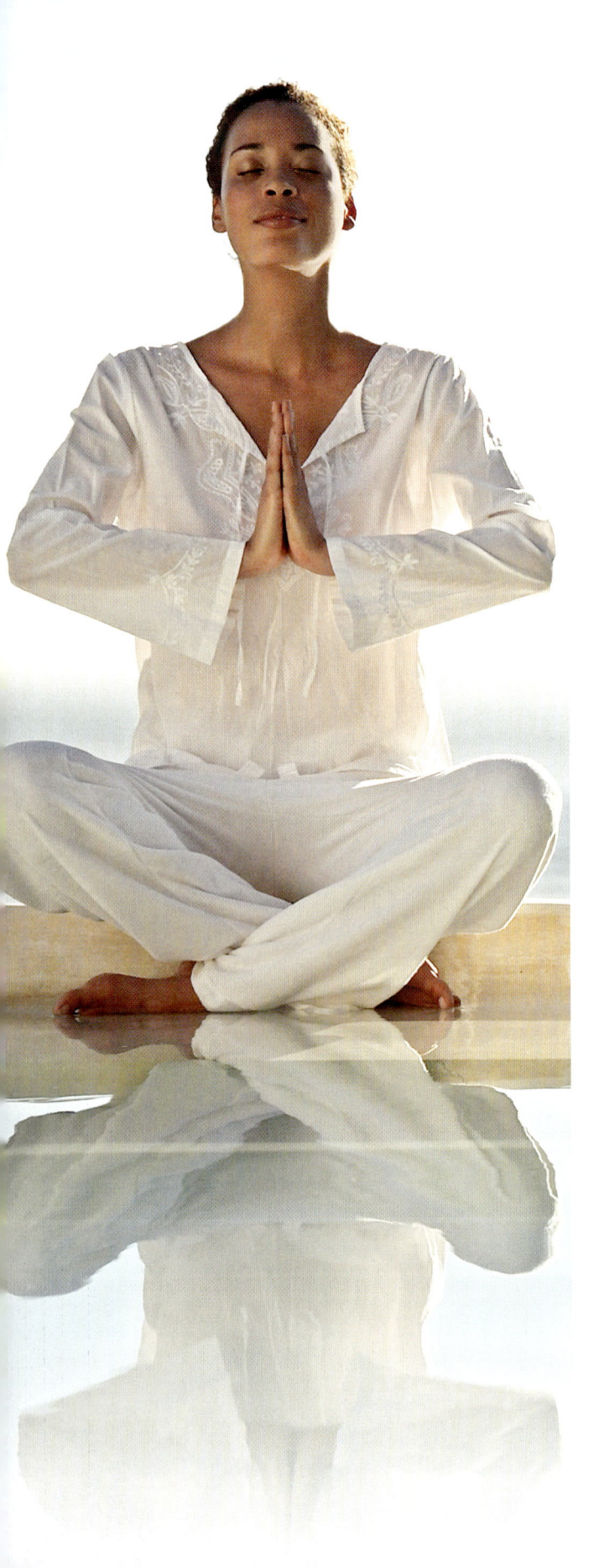

Scientists are working on new treatment approaches to reduce tinnitus. One promising therapy is repetitive transcranial magnetic stimulation (rTMS). In rTMS, pulses from a magnetic coil placed on the head suppress activity in regions of the brain that are thought to be involved in the perception of tinnitus. Treatment with rTMS is currently available at some medical facilities, but it is still considered to be experimental for tinnitus.

While you may have tinnitus, it does not define you. Many times it's not the tinnitus itself that is the problem, but rather your reaction to it. Educate yourself, practice healthy habits, seek help from experts, and choose a management strategy that fits your needs. There are ways to cope.

Part 2

The management of hearing loss

Chapter 6

Living with hearing impairment

Hearing loss isn't a condition that you can simply ignore. It's difficult to go about the responsibilities of your daily life pretending it's not there. Hearing loss can impact your quality of life, affecting family relationships, job performance and social interactions. It can diminish self-confidence and sense of identity. For many people hearing loss is an ongoing challenge, one that may result in feeling isolated from family and friends.

But hearing loss doesn't necessarily mean your life takes a turn for the worse. You can change that trend, starting with your attitude. Acknowledging that you have a hearing impairment — instead of denying it — is vital to overcoming its consequences. By doing so, you can start opening yourself up to help and solutions.

Dealing with the challenges of hearing loss may also require changing your behaviors. Many people are uncomfortable with change and find it difficult to adjust to new routines. But learning to live with hearing loss enables you to stay engaged with family and friends and to participate in and enjoy a wide range of activities. You may find that it opens up avenues or relationships in your life that you have neglected or let go because of hearing challenges.

This chapter presents strategies you may follow to improve your ability to communicate and find emotional and financial support. Assertive communication, speech reading and sign language also may help you. In addition, the chapter directs you to support groups and community resources. You're not alone.

Quality of life

Sound helps anchor you to the world around you. Sound gives you pleasure and a sense of belonging. Sound also alerts you to danger or opportunity.

Hearing impairment may deprive you of listening to the laughter and conversation between friends at a social gathering or the inspiring sounds of nature on a forest trail. Activities such as eating at a restaurant, traveling, attending religious services, classes or concerts, and watching movies become more difficult. Even something as routine as talking on the telephone, shopping for groceries and running errands can pose special challenges.

Frequently, hearing loss is gradual over several years. For that reason it may take time to recognize that you're having more difficulty hearing. In fact, family and friends may notice your hearing loss before you do.

Initially you may deny or try to minimize the hearing impairment, perhaps because you can still hear certain sounds well. You may convince yourself that other people only need to speak more clearly or slowly. But denying your hearing difficulties or blaming them on external factors doesn't make the problem go away and may just create additional problems.

Access

Have you ever strained to understand what's being said over a public address system? Have you found yourself unable to enjoy the theater because you can't hear the actors unless they speak in your direction? Have you struggled with schoolwork because the classroom either mutes or echoes the teacher's voice? Situations like these can be stressful for anyone in an active life. They present unique challenges for people with hearing impairment.

All too often, people with hearing impairment aren't provided with the communication tools they need for travel, entertainment, education and medical care. Few movie theaters provide captioning services or assistive listening systems. Many medical clinics and hospitals don't have interpreters on staff for the hearing impaired.

Organizations such as the Hearing Loss Association of America (HLAA) are working to improve access in a variety of situations for people who are hearing-impaired. Improvements in assistive technology are allowing more

In denial

Why do so many people deny having hearing loss? And why do so many put off getting help — sometimes for years? Denial happens for many reasons:

- Hearing loss usually develops over time, so you may not recognize the problem at first. Often, you find ways to compensate for hearing loss without even being aware that you're doing so. For example, you may become very adept at speech reading without realizing it.
- Many people underestimate the severity of their hearing loss. When people lose their hearing, they tend to lose their ability to hear high-pitched tones first, such as the consonant sounds. Consonants are the sounds of speech that provide clarity and crispness to what you hear. Voices may still sound loud, but they also seem unclear.
- People often associate hearing loss with old age. You may fear that there is a stigma associated with wearing hearing aids.
- You may fear being considered incompetent. A common concern expressed by people coming to terms with hearing loss is that others will assume they're also losing their ability to think and act independently.

When you're in denial about hearing loss, you're not able to admit to yourself that there's a problem. You may convince yourself that you heard what was said or that you just weren't paying attention. You may deflect attention from your hearing loss with expressions such as "You're mumbling again" or "I don't need to hear what they're saying" or "I'm too young for hearing aids."

Whatever the cause, denial won't help you for the long term. If you can't admit to hearing loss, you'll have trouble taking the steps to communicate better and make life easier. You'll only prolong the time it takes for making adjustments and finding solutions.

hearing-impaired people to participate in a greater range of activities. The advent of online learning has improved access to education. For more information about assistive listening devices, captioning and other communication aids, see Chapter 9.

Employment

Hearing impairment may cause problems at work. You may misunderstand a conversation with your manager or supervisor because of background noise in the office or shop. You may have difficulty hearing someone speaking to you through a glass partition, such as at a bank teller's window, or from another room. You may have trouble participating in meetings or conferences with several people talking rapidly at once.

Practical solutions to many common workplace problems such as these are available. It's also useful to know your legal rights. Almost every state has a statute making it illegal to discriminate in employment on the basis of disability, race, religion, sex, age or other minority status.

Under the Americans With Disabilities Act (ADA), it's against the law to discriminate against qualified people with physical and mental disabilities in job application procedures, hiring, firing, advancement, compensation and training. You can find more information about these important regulations at the Department of Justice website (*www.ada.gov*).

The ADA requires employers to make what's called reasonable accommodation for employees with disabilities. A reasonable accommodation can be any modification or adjustment to a work environment that enables the employee with a disability such as hearing loss to perform essential functions of the job.

For deaf or severely hearing-impaired employees, reasonable accommodations may include providing a text telephone (TTY or TDD), captioned telephone, videophone or even something as simple as a flashing ringer on the regular telephone.

Sound barriers or muffling can be added to office walls and floors to control background noise in the work environment. Assistive listening systems can be installed in auditoriums and meeting rooms. The services of a transcriber or sign language interpreter can be sought out. In addition, employers should change or add lighting to enhance visibility.

Dealing with hearing loss in the workplace

You'll benefit from the adjustments your employer can make to create a more accessible environment, but you too can take steps to reduce potential problems in the workplace:

- Use the communication aids that are provided. These may include assistive listening devices such as telephone amplifiers, FM systems, captioning and alerting devices. These resources are discussed in Chapter 9.
- Move away from the source of background noise. If possible, locate your desk away from busy hallways and noisy office machines, such as air conditioners and photocopiers.
- Ask co-workers to address you by name as they speak. This allows you to focus your attention, understand what's being said and participate in discussions.
- Sit up front at meetings and presentations. Arrive early or ask to be seated close to the speaker.
- Give yourself a break in between situations that require a lot of listening and communication. Otherwise fatigue may set in.
- Alert co-workers to situations that may cause problems. Let them know how they can help you communicate.

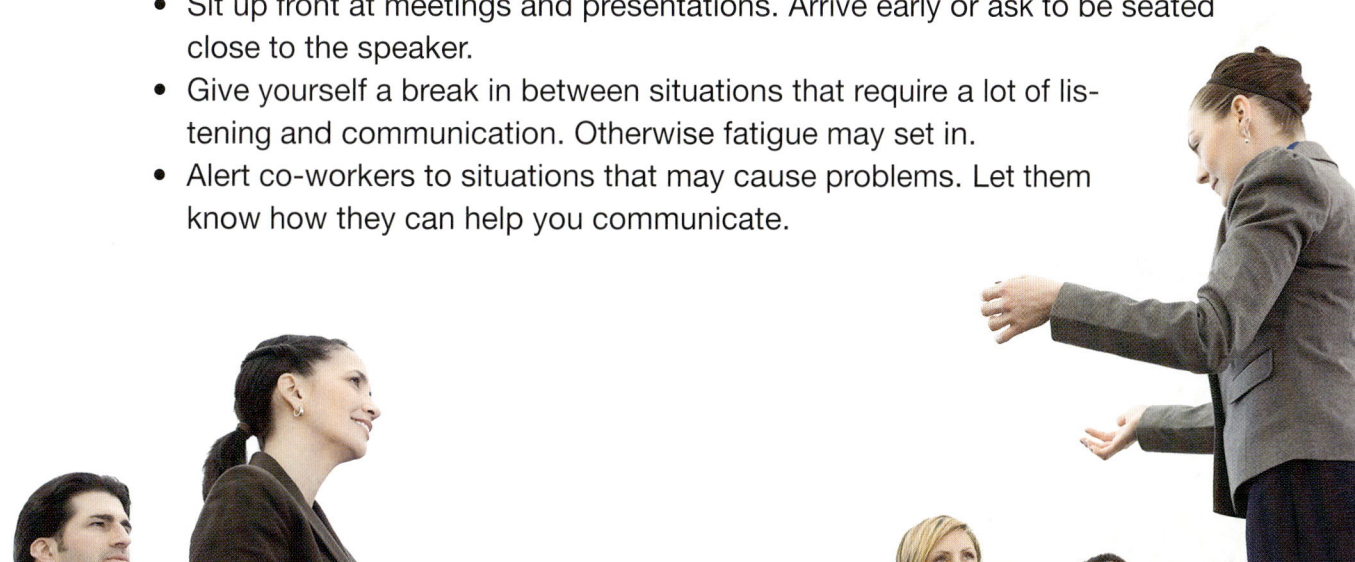

State governments operate vocational rehabilitation agencies to help people with disabilities retain their present jobs or, if that's not possible, retrain for other jobs. Rehabilitation means getting ready for useful employment and successful integration into society. Certified rehabilitation counselors and rehabilitation psychologists can help address your work-related concerns.

Relationships

Humans are social creatures — most people seek out connections with others and thrive on them. Living in an intensely social world can be difficult when your ability to communicate is hampered. Hearing loss can strain your relationships with family, friends, co-workers and anyone with whom you interact regularly.

For example, when you're unable to hear much of what's being said at a dinner party, you may tire quickly from the effort and feel left out. This may cause you to skip these events and stay home. At the store you may have trouble hearing your charge total from a soft-spoken clerk. If your spouse calls to you while you're working in front of a running faucet or dishwasher, you may not understand the words.

Other factors associated with hearing loss, such as social isolation, low self-esteem and depression, may further strain relationships.

Isolation

When you're struggling to hear, conversations can quickly become frustrating and tiresome. Although you want to spend time with your family and friends, interacting gets too stressful. It's natural to try to avoid situations that you know will be difficult. In so doing, you may cut yourself off from the world around you and the people who love you.

Social isolation is a serious problem for older adults with hearing impairment. Research by the National Council on Aging found that hearing-impaired older adults who don't use hearing aids are more likely to withdraw socially, become depressed, and feel that other people get upset and angry at them for no reason.

By contrast, hearing-impaired older adults who use hearing aids tend to have a higher quality of life, better relationships with their families and better feelings about themselves. They are more socially active, experience more interpersonal warmth and have greater emotional stability.

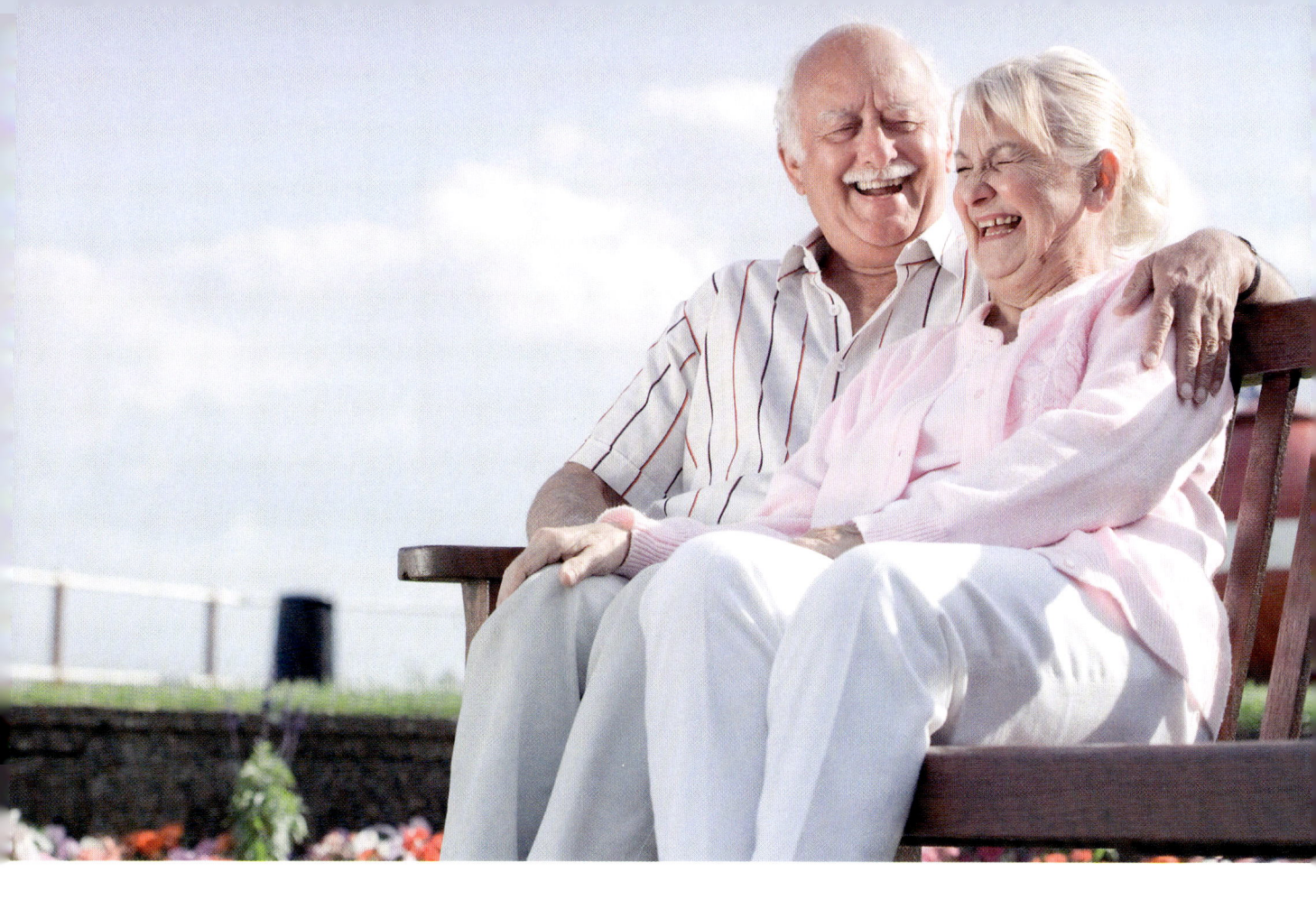

To minimize the negative effects of hearing loss, it's important to remain socially involved. Chats with friends, attendance at family gatherings, dinner parties and card games, and evenings at the movies or theater — these pleasurable activities keep us involved in the mainstream of life. Strategies to improve communication and social interaction — both for yourself and for people involved in your day-to-day life — are discussed starting on page 119.

Identity

Hearing loss affects how you perceive your place in the world. Many adults whose hearing loss occurred early in life have, over time, incorporated the impairment into their self-image — it's a part of who they are. As a result they're more accustomed to managing hearing loss in their daily lives and routinely cope with it.

But for adults who lose hearing later in life, the impairment can be more disruptive. Commonly, feelings of inadequacy accompany hearing loss and inhibit daily activities. These adults may worry about the potential social stigma with hearing loss and fear that others will treat them as incompetent.

To build your new identity as an adult with hearing loss, you may need to let go of some preconceived notions about aging and focus on the positive aspects of your life.

Emotional effects

Everyone's experience with hearing loss will be slightly different. But most people who endure any kind of serious loss — whether it's physical or emotional — go through the stages of denial, anger, bargaining, depression and acceptance. Other feelings associated with loss include frustration, embarrassment and sadness.

Two especially common emotional effects of hearing loss are depression and anxiety.

Depression
Depression isn't a weakness, nor is it something that you simply "snap out of." Depression is a medical condition that affects how you think and behave and can cause many emotional and physical problems.

Individuals who are depressed often deny or minimize the problem — which only delays treatment and can make the problem worse. Signs and symptoms don't always follow a particular pattern. But they can include persistent sadness and feelings of hopelessness, loss of appetite, sleep disturbance, extreme mood changes, irritability, and poor concentration.

Many studies have demonstrated a link between hearing loss and depression. Compared with peers who have normal hearing, older adults with hearing loss report significantly more signs and symptoms of depression. Most individuals experiencing depression will improve following treatment involving both medication and counseling.

It should be noted that depression is often considered a natural stage in the grieving process. In other words, it may represent a part of coming to terms with your hearing loss. Regardless, you should not delay seeking medical treatment for the condition.

Anxiety
Anxiety involves extreme worry and fear about a future event, whether or not it's likely to happen. The feeling often stems from misinformation and mistrust of the unknown. Anxiety can be influenced by other factors, including family history, personality and general outlook on life. Anxiety and depression often go hand in hand.

Signs and symptoms of generalized anxiety include restlessness, irritability, impatience, muscle tension, sleep problems, headache, shortness of breath and difficulties with concentration.

Hearing loss sets the stage for many anxiety-producing situations: On the way to a store, you may be anxious about understanding the cashier. When going to meet a friend, you may fear that you'll misunderstand the conversation. On your own, you may be concerned about hearing warning sounds of danger, such as traffic noise or the footsteps of someone approaching around a blind corner.

Research shows that as hearing loss progresses from a mild to moderate level, anxiety increases as well. People with hearing loss may develop deep anxieties toward social situations in which they believe it will be difficult to hear clearly. As a result, they tend to avoid these situations at all costs.

If you're concerned that you or someone you care about may have an anxiety disorder, talk to your doctor or a mental health professional. Treatments are available to help you get anxiety under control. Learning coping skills and using relaxation techniques also can help.

Improving social interaction

Although hearing loss may change your relationships with others, many strategies and tools can allow you to still communicate effectively and stay involved in a range of activities.

As you're learning new communication skills, you may work with health care professionals, other people with hearing loss, family and friends. Most people are eager to help you communicate better. But you must be more than a passive recipient of their services — learning requires your commitment and effort.

Effective communication can occur even if you don't hear each and every sound. Your remaining hearing along with visual information, context clues and life experience help you understand speech. With the assistance of technology, the impact of hearing loss can be considerably reduced.

Assertive communication

Good communication may require you to become more assertive. But being assertive doesn't mean being loud and intrusive. Assertiveness simply means letting others know your needs without ignoring their needs in the process. Often, without some assertiveness, you may not be able to hear and understand anything in a conversation.

Assertive communication means being forthright about what it will take for you to participate and interact. With assertive communication, you:

- Let others know that you have hearing loss. Then they won't misconstrue your behavior or think you're aloof or forgetful.
- Are aware that your hearing loss affects other people and are prepared to deal with their reactions.
- Are willing to use hearing aids and assistive listening devices.
- Ask for, but not demand, help when you need it.
- Tell people exactly what you need. You might ask individuals to slow their speech, look at you when they speak, move a hand away from their face or repeat a phrase.
- Take a break from conversation when you're tired.
- Show your appreciation when others make an effort to communicate better with you.
- Are willing to admit if you're taking out your emotions on others.
- Modify your environment to fit your hearing needs.

With assertive communication, you'll probably find it easier to cope with many social situations. Most people will be receptive if you tell them you're having trouble hearing and will ask what they can do to help.

Creating an environment for better listening

One of the most-effective strategies for better hearing and social interaction is to modify situations that make listening difficult. Often, by altering or stage-managing your environment, you can avoid communication breakdowns. Following are suggestions that might help you:

Move closer to the source of a sound you want to hear

This may include a television or stereo system, a public speaker or lecturer, or a visitor to your home. Arrange your home or office furniture so that guests or family members are seated nearby and facing directly toward you. In locations where you can't organize the arrangements, choose your own seating for minimum distance and maximum visibility.

Move away from distracting or overpowering noise

When you're in public places, try to avoid sitting in locations close to machinery, appliances or busy hallways. In a restaurant, request a table away from the kitchen, lobby, bar or other noisy spot, and sit with your back to the wall. Avoid sitting close to music speakers or ventilation ducts.

At home, turn off or mute the television or radio when you're conversing with someone. Seat yourself away from open windows that let in traffic noise and outdoor sounds.

Position yourself so that the speaker's face is visible and well-lit

Visual cues, such as facial expressions or the position of the speaker's head, provide clear indications of what's being said. Good lighting helps your speech reading.

Plan in advance for social activities

Before attending an event in a busy or crowded setting, such as a theater or place of worship, call ahead to see if the facility is equipped with assistive listening devices. Arrive early to pick up the devices and so that you have a choice of seats.

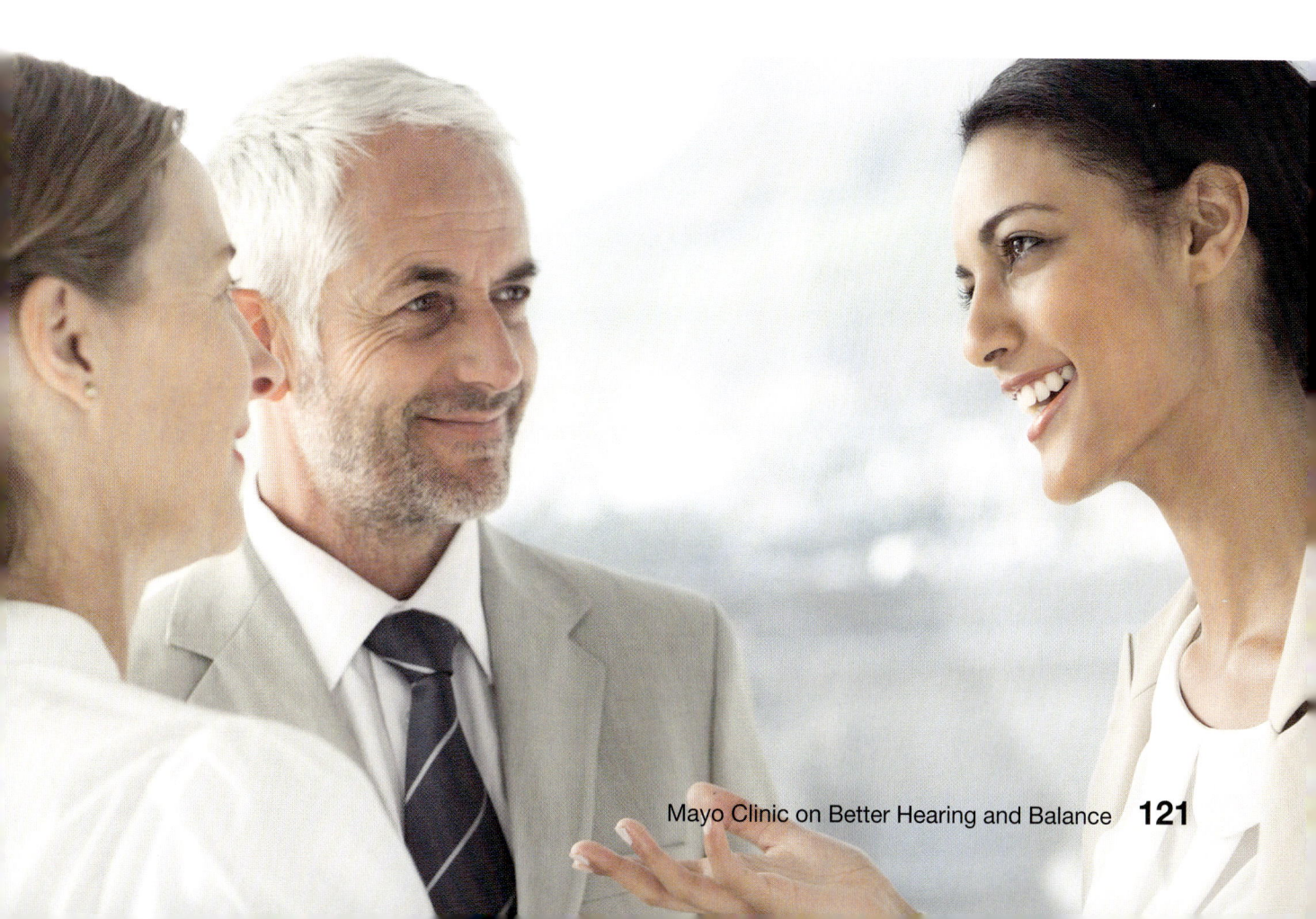

Communicating with a hearing-impaired person

Communication is the lifeblood of any relationship. When you're conversing with someone who's hearing-impaired, keep in mind that what to you is simple communication may be a tiring effort for your companion. He or she has to make an active effort to understand. Hearing aids may help, but turning up the volume won't make distorted sounds any clearer.

You can enhance communication with a hearing-impaired person by following a few practical suggestions:

- Before starting to talk, reduce the level of background noise. Turn off the television, radio, air conditioner or other noisy appliances. Don't leave a faucet running. If you can't reduce background noise, try to move to a quieter area.
- Make sure you have the person's attention before speaking. You can do this by saying his or her name or touching his or her shoulder.
- Talk face to face. Speak at eye level, and no more than a few feet away. Don't chew gum, smoke, talk behind a newspaper or cover your mouth while you're having the conversation.
- Speak at a normal conversational level, especially if the person is wearing hearing aids or has a cochlear implant. Don't shout. If necessary, modestly increase your volume.
- Speak clearly but naturally. Slow your speech a little, using a few more pauses than usual.
- Use facial expressions, gestures and other body language cues to make your points.
- Watch your listener's face for signs that comprehension is a problem. Rephrase your statements if the listener is unsure of what's been said.
- Alert your listener to changes in topics of conversation.
- Show extra consideration in a group situation. What's known as cross talk is one of the most difficult situations for someone with hearing loss. Try to structure the event so that only one person is speaking at a time. At meetings it's helpful to display an agenda on a board or overhead transparency and, as the meeting progresses, to indicate which item is under discussion.

Speech reading

Speech reading, also called lip reading, is a tool that individuals with hearing loss can use to navigate many social situations. With this technique, you learn to recognize spoken words by watching the movements of the speaker's lips, tongue, lower jaw, eyes and eyebrows, as well as facial expressions, body stances and gestures. These visual cues are critical for understanding the words being said.

Most people, whether they hear normally or not, rely on speech reading to some degree. In fact, many individuals are unaware that they can speech read. For example, when background noise is extremely loud, people with normal hearing may try instinctively to match the motion of the speaker's lips to the sounds they hear.

Speech reading works best if you still have some hearing ability left and use hearing aids or other assistive devices. It's accomplished primarily by following lip patterns — the shapes made by people's mouths when they speak. For example, the vowel *o* is formed with rounded lips, the consonant *m* is made by pressing the lips firmly together, and the consonant *l* requires placing the tongue behind your teeth.

But even the most skilled speech reader can't pick up every word. Not all sounds are visible on the lips, and some sounds look exactly alike. For example, the consonants *b*, *m* and *p* look similar on the lips. So the words *ban*, *man* and *pan* are almost impossible to distinguish.

Other factors — rapid speech, poor pronunciation, bad lighting, averted face, covered mouth, facial hair — can make speech reading more difficult. You often need to rely on the context of the sentence and other nonverbal cues to understand what's being said.

As with any new skill, learning the basic techniques for speech reading takes time and patience. For people with hearing loss, including those with hearing aids, speech sounds may be muted or distorted. And you must learn to focus on the lip movements.

But your skill usually improves with practice, and the more you practice, the more confident you'll become. Many proficient speech readers find that the technique allows them to follow conversations more easily. In fact, some people who are profoundly deaf choose to communicate using speech reading and speech rather than sign language.

Tips for speech reading

Rather than trying to catch every word that's spoken, focus on the overall intent and context. Here are other suggestions for making speech reading easier:

- Position yourself so that a light source is behind you and the speaker's face is clearly visible. Any factor that reduces the visibility of the speaker's face will interfere with your ability to speech read.
- Identify the topic being discussed as quickly as possible. If you're familiar with the topic and can identify key words, you won't need to analyze every phrase.
- Watch for clues in the speaker's facial expressions, body language and gestures.
- Before you enter a conversation, inform the person who's speaking that you have hearing loss. Encourage him or her to speak normally, but maybe a little slower.
- Try to relax as much as possible. Don't try to understand everything, or you may become tense, which can only make speech reading that much more difficult.
- Use your remaining hearing in combination with speech reading. Diminish background noise by turning off the television or radio, closing the door or window, or sitting in a quieter section of a restaurant, away from the bustle.
- Focus on the message rather than specific lip movements. You'll find that subsequent sentences may clarify the words you've missed.
- If you can't fill in a missing word, ask the speaker to rephrase the sentence in a different way.
- Take frequent breaks, especially when you're first learning to speech read. The technique requires deep concentration, and you may tire quickly from the effort. When you get the chance, close your eyes and relax for a few minutes.

Cued speech

Another useful technique that can help people with hearing loss to listen and communicate is known as cued speech. This system supplements the basic principles of speech reading (lip movements) with the use of "cues" — specific hand shapes and hand placements around the mouth.

The eight hand shapes represent different consonant sounds. The placement of the hands represents vowel sounds. So, by combining a hand shape and hand placement, you create a visual cue for an individual syllable. Using this technique in combination with lip reading can greatly improve your understanding and communication.

Cued speech was developed as a way to improve literacy in children with severe hearing impairment. Its success is due to making the sounds of spoken language look different.

Sign language

Sign language uses hand signs — made with hand shape, position and movement — as well as body movements, gestures, facial expressions and other visual cues to form words. It's often the first language of many individuals who are deaf or have severe hearing impairment.

Sign language is a complete language with distinct grammar, semantics and syntax. This is unlike cued speech, which is based on the sounds and structure of a spoken language.

Different sign languages are used in different countries and regions of the world. American Sign Language (ASL) is commonly used in the United States and Canada. And like the English language, ASL allows for regional differences and jargon.

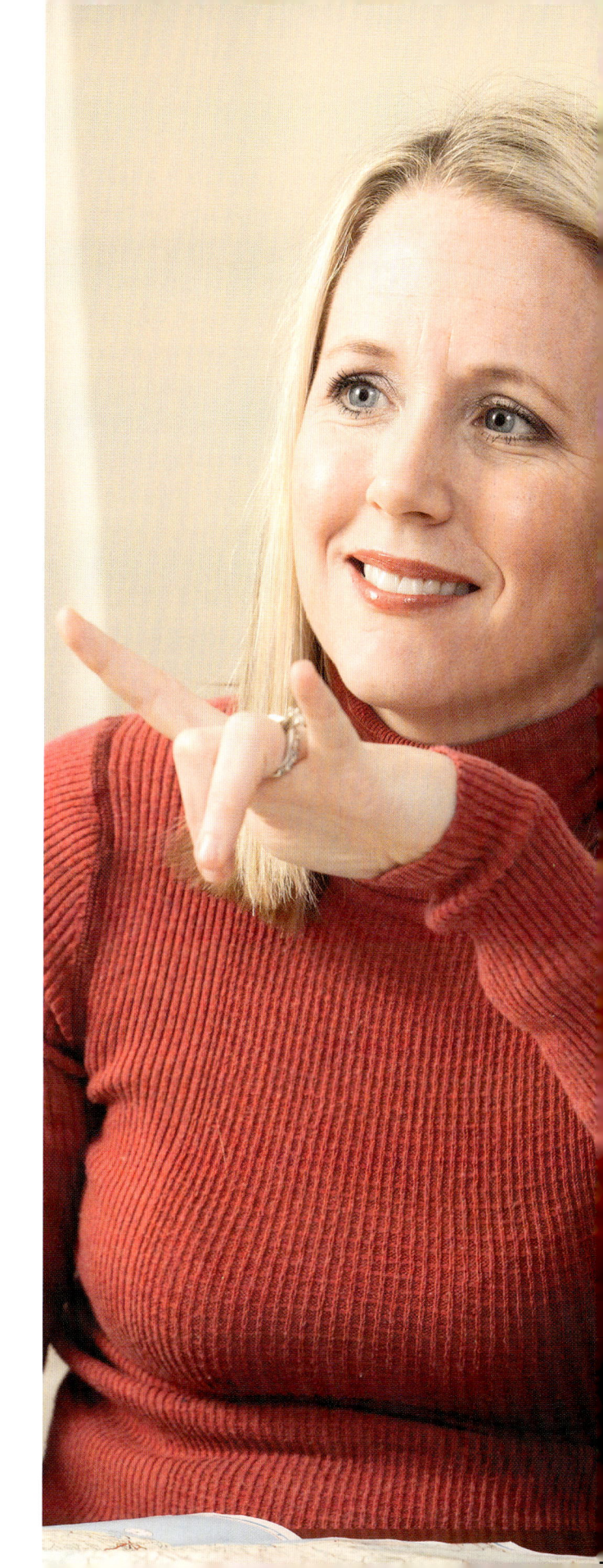

Sight is considered the most valuable tool for using sign language. Each sign in this language may be broken down into parts — in the same way that spoken words can be broken down into individual sounds and intonations. Each ASL sign is, in fact, a distinct combination of hand shape, hand movement and hand location. Changing any one of these parts changes the meaning of the sign.

Facial expressions and body movements also are very important in sign language. For example, English speakers usually signal that they are asking a question with a raised tone of voice. ASL users ask a question by raising their eyebrows and widening their eyes. Stating a command may require them to sign more emphatically.

Learning sign language

Using sign language takes time and practice, and learning from a book is difficult. It's generally recommended that you enroll in classes and meet with other people who use sign language. Picking up enough signs for basic communication can take a year or more of training.

Community colleges, universities, libraries, continuing education programs and vocational rehabilitation centers are some of the institutions that may offer sign language classes. The American Sign Language Teachers Association (ASLTA) certifies qualified teachers. The ASLTA website (*www.aslta.org*) has information about state and local chapters.

Hearing dogs

You're probably familiar with guide dogs for people who are blind. Did you know that service dogs are also available to help people with severe or profound hearing loss? Hearing dogs can alert you to everyday sounds such as a doorbell, ringing telephone, oven timer, alarm clock, and smoke and fire alarms. A dog can even respond when someone calls your name.

Hearing dogs don't bark to get your attention. Rather, they're trained to use their noses or paws to nudge you, then lead you to the source of the sound. Hearing dogs can also carry messages or notes between you and another household member.

Paying attention to your hearing dog's reactions in public spaces can help you be more aware of car traffic and pedestrians, especially when they approach you from behind or around a corner.

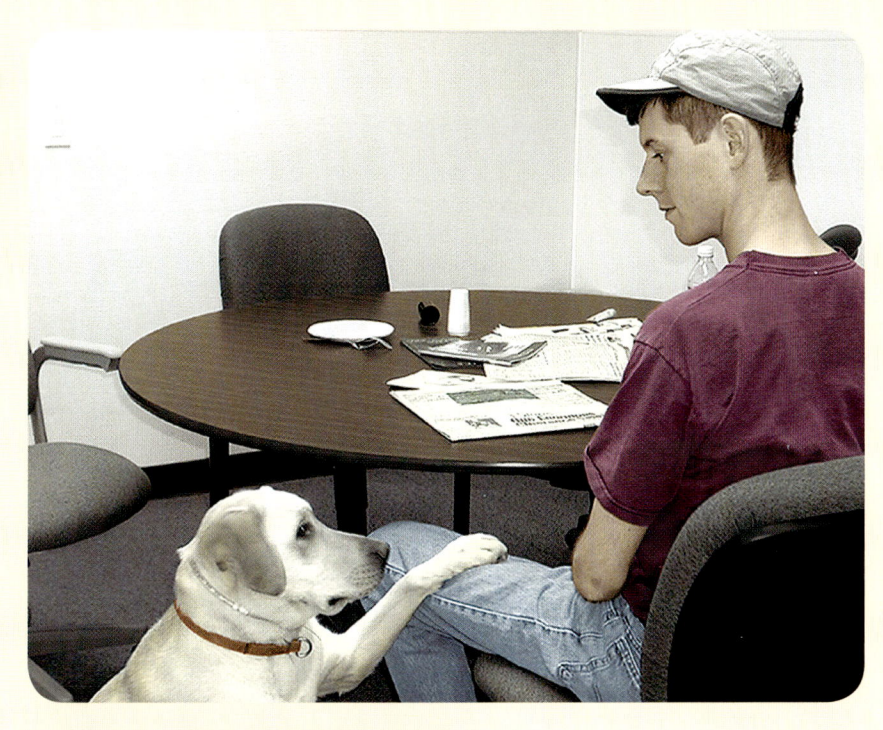

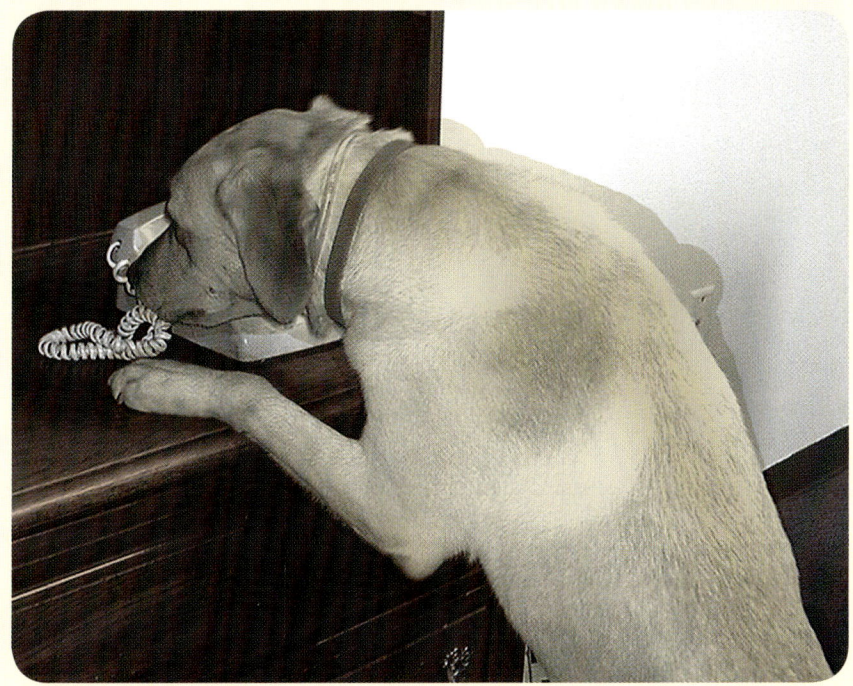

To alert you to a sound, a hearing dog will first nudge you to get your attention (top), then lead you to the source of the sound, such as a ringing telephone (bottom).

Mayo Clinic on Better Hearing and Balance **127**

According to the Americans With Disabilities Act, hearing dogs must be allowed to accompany their owners into businesses and other places that serve the public. Often a bright orange or yellow leash identifies a hearing dog. But the dog doesn't have to have special identification to accompany you into a business or public space.

Getting a hearing dog

Hearing dogs come in all shapes and sizes. Many are taken from animal shelters and given three to six months of training — obedience training as well as special service training. There's no national training standard, and the dogs aren't required to be certified.

Some people with hearing loss choose to participate in the training, working directly with a private trainer and the dog. Others prefer to get a dog that's already trained. Regardless, you may have to wait two or more years before getting a canine companion.

In the United States, the two largest hearing dog organizations are Paws With A Cause and Canine Companions for Independence. Most service-dog organizations are nonprofits that provide the dogs at no charge to the people who need them.

Finding support

Even under the best circumstances, living with a hearing impairment will have its frustrating moments. There will be times when you feel overwhelmed by the effort of staying connected to the hearing world. You'll also sometimes feel isolated by your inability to hear certain sounds.

You don't have to cope with all of the challenges alone. Various options are available that provide support to people with hearing loss, such as aural rehabilitation or a support group. Many national, state and local organizations provide information on preventing hearing loss and resources for living with hearing impairment.

Aural rehabilitation

If you don't feel comfortable with your hearing impairment, consider aural rehabilitation, also called hearing rehabilitation or auditory training. Aural rehabilitation helps you adjust to hearing loss and tries to reduce the difficulties. Advocates say that by making the best use of hearing aids and assistive listening devices, you can take charge of your communication needs.

An audiologist, a speech-language pathologist or both typically provide aural rehabilitation services. For rehabilitation, you may work one-on-one with a therapist or as part of a group or in both settings. Group therapy can be especially helpful because you'll meet others facing the same issues as you are.

The overall goal of aural rehabilitation is to maximize your self-confidence and your ability to communicate with others in everyday situations. This can be achieved by a number of helpful steps, including:

- Understanding your hearing loss
- Learning how to listen
- Learning skills in speech reading
- Building confidence in communication situations
- Dealing with emotional problems related to hearing loss
- Learning about all the options among different hearing aids and assistive listening devices
- Understanding your legal rights and being your own advocate
- Promoting your family's understanding of your needs
- Making it easier for your family to communicate with you

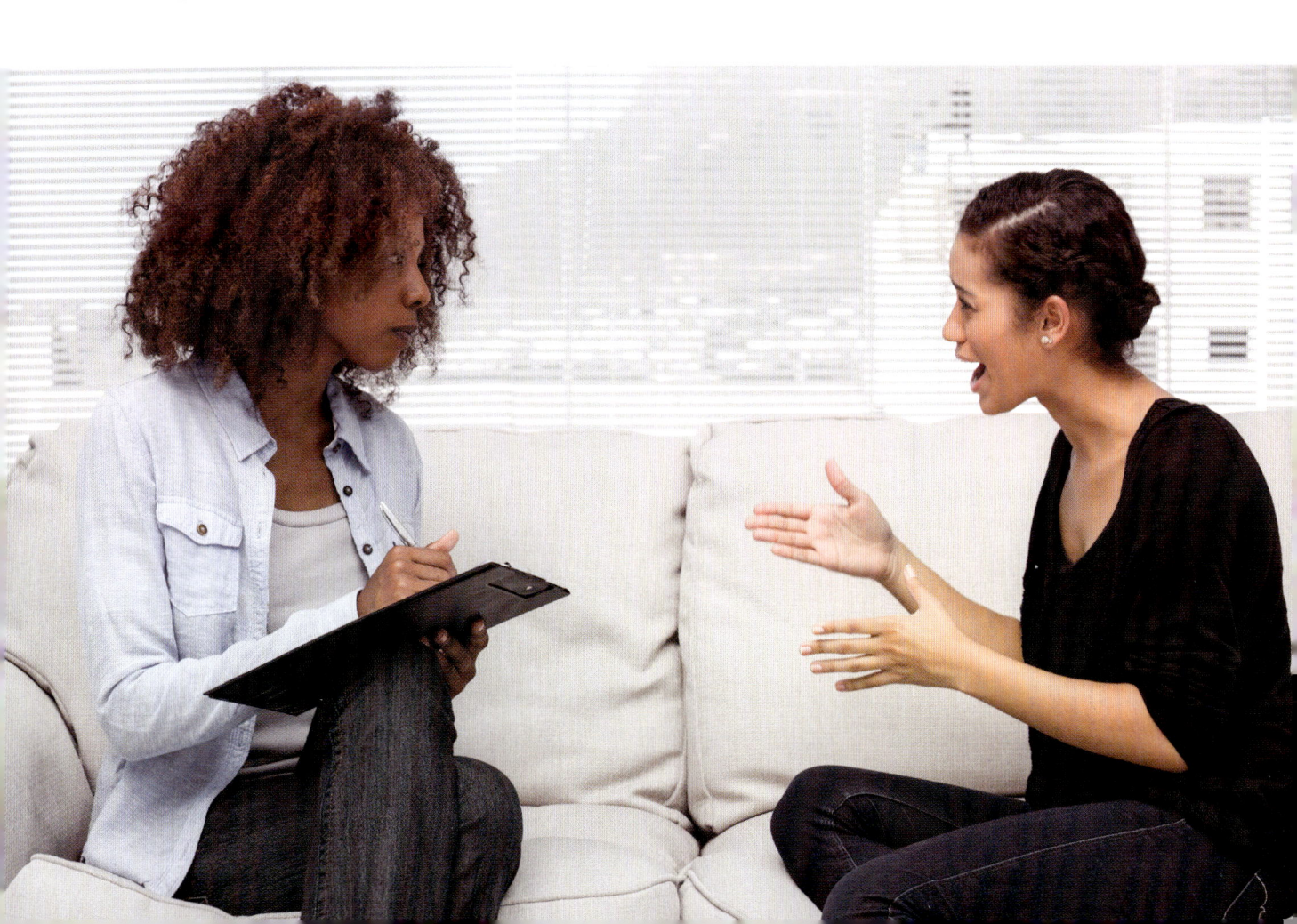

Evaluating information

You can find hundreds of products, publications, services and websites devoted to hearing impairment. But be careful. The information ranges from solid research to outright quackery.

When evaluating information you find on the Internet, consider these guidelines:

- Look for websites created by national organizations, universities, government agencies or major medical centers.
- Search for the most recent information you can find.
- Check for the information source. Notice whether articles refer to published research. Look for a board of qualified professionals who review the content before it's published. Be wary of commercial sites or personal testimonials that push a single point of view.
- Double-check the information. Visit several sites and compare the information offered.

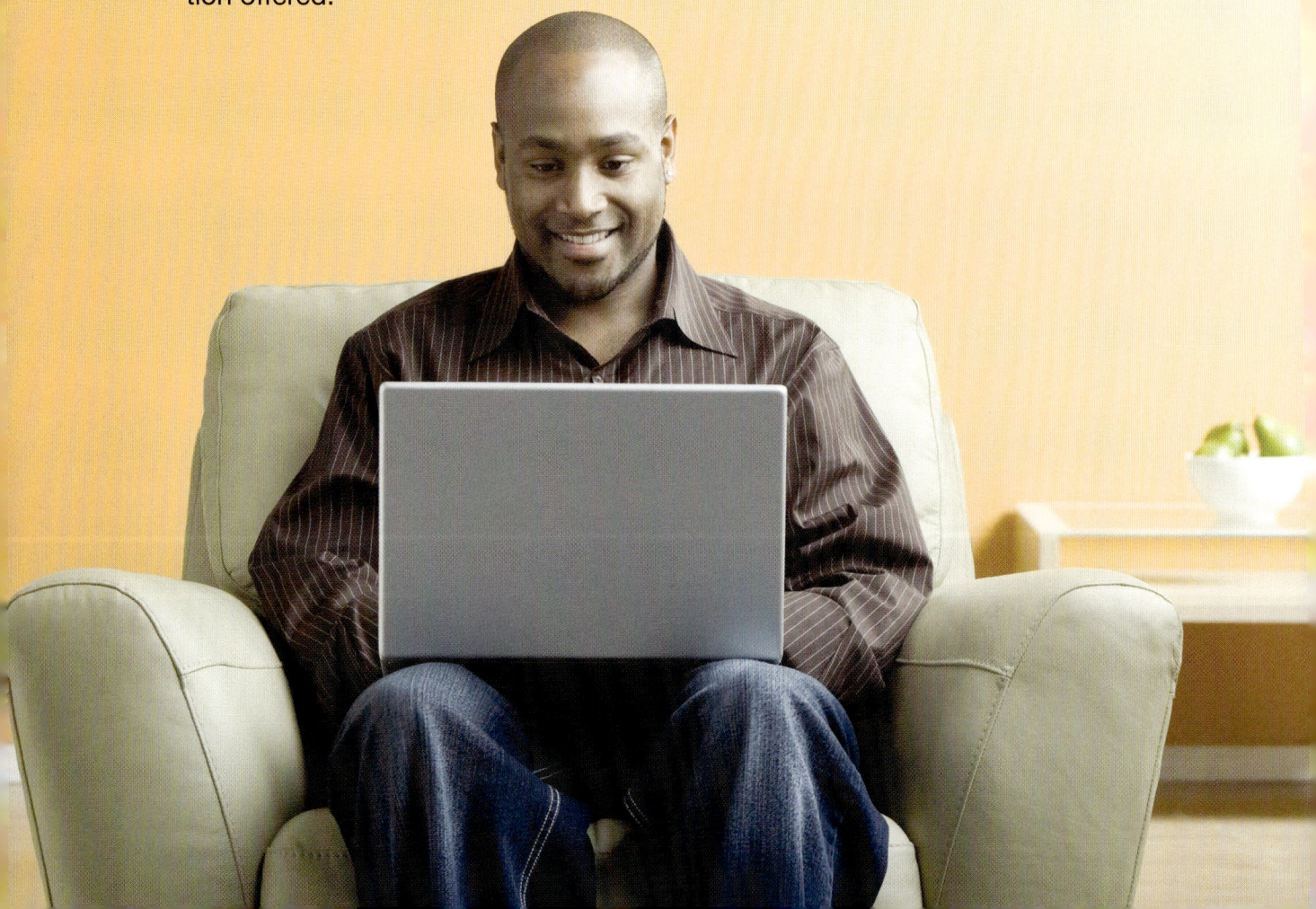

A typical rehabilitation session lasts from one to two hours a week. The session may be held at a medical clinic, rehabilitation center, community college or private office. Aural rehabilitation sessions generally last over a period of four to 10 weeks.

There are now commercially available aural rehabilitative software programs that can be used at home and at your own pace of learning. Your hearing health care provider can discuss these programs with you.

Support groups

Sharing experiences with other people with hearing impairments is a great way to find support. Belonging to a group can remind you that you're not alone in dealing with this problem.

Support groups aren't the same as group aural rehabilitation. An audiologist leads an aural rehabilitation group. Peers frequently lead support groups.

Support groups are an excellent resource for problem-solving and mutual support. They're also a way to meet potential new friends. How have others handled traveling, meetings, telephone conversations, communicating in public places or dealing with difficult work colleagues? What problems have they had with hearing aids? Have they used assistive listening systems?

Many national organizations with local chapters provide support groups for people with hearing loss. These include the Alexander Graham Bell Association for the Deaf and Hard of Hearing, the Association of Late-Deafened Adults, the National Association of the Deaf, the Center for Hearing and Communication, and the Hearing Loss Association of America (HLAA). See "Additional resources" at the back of this book for contact information for these organizations.

National, state and local resources

Dozens of national, state and local organizations provide services for people who are deaf or hearing-impaired. These resources include advocacy, education, financial aid, referral, advice on medical issues, and counseling on professional and work issues.

There are also opportunities for self-help and support groups, recreational and social activities, and spiritual needs. Most organizations have websites and publications about hearing loss that offer easy-to-understand information for the public.

The federal government provides information on affirmative action programs, reasonable accommodation and improving accessibility for disabled people. For example, if you feel your legal rights have been violated, you may contact the Equal Employment Opportunity Commission for advice, either by phone (800-669-4000) or on the Web (*www.eeoc.gov*).

States provide services for individuals who are deaf and hearing-impaired. The state office might be a commission or vocational rehabilitation program for people with disabilities. Offices that provide rehabilitation services often provide counseling and job retraining and may help pay for hearing aids.

Some states have programs to provide amplified telephones to people with hearing impairment. A state human rights or human relations commission or a governor's committee on employment of people with disabilities can provide information on related laws.

Chapter 7

Hearing aids

Hearing loss doesn't mean you're cut off from the world of sound. But you may need a little help to make the sounds you hear audible and understandable. If you feel like you're missing out because of hearing loss, you'll likely benefit from a hearing aid.

Hearing aids are sophisticated electronic devices that make sounds louder. They don't restore your hearing to what it was, but they can improve your ability to hear and communicate in daily activities. Hearing aids are the single most effective treatment for a majority of people with hearing loss.

Hearing aids can greatly enhance personal interactions. They assist with many problems associated with hearing loss, such as difficulty understanding conversations — face to face or on the telephone — and being aware of signals, timers and beepers. Hearing aids can help reduce feelings of social isolation and problems with self-image.

Hearing aid technology has improved tremendously in recent decades. Many years ago hearing aids were large and cumbersome. They had a harsh, distorted sound quality, like that of a cheap transistor radio. Newer hearing aids are compact and provide far better sound quality. Many options are available to match your lifestyle and your communication needs.

As you adjust to a new hearing aid, you'll start to enjoy your improved ability to hear and communicate in a variety of social situations. You may feel a little safer when you can hear environmental sounds around you.

You'll likely notice improvements in your quality of life by regularly wearing the aid and taking good care of it.

Setting priorities

Motivation is the key to success with hearing aids. People with a positive attitude and commitment to hearing better are often the best hearing aid users. They're also more likely to continue wearing the devices.

There are a variety of hearing aid styles. Selecting which type to use is often a personal choice based on your specific needs — each person and each type of hearing loss is different. In making the selection, it helps to be informed, patient and open to the suggestions of your audiologist or hearing aid dispenser.

There are several things you can do to increase your satisfaction with hearing aids. You've probably already taken the first steps — acknowledging your hearing loss, having your hearing tested, and seeking out the best solutions to the challenges this loss presents.

It's also important to know what you can realistically expect from a hearing aid. Identify the situations in your life when communication is most difficult. When are the times when it's important for you to hear especially well? Are there occasions when you have to concentrate so hard on hearing that you become fatigued? Perhaps you want to make sure you can hear your children or grandchildren when they visit, or to understand conversations during a weekly card game.

When considering which type of hearing aid to buy, you'll typically face trade-offs among many factors, such as performance, style, size, technology and cost. For example, you may simply want the smallest device available. Or maybe you prefer a hearing aid that's easy to operate, regardless of size.

If you're retired and spend most of your time at home, the most expensive model with all the latest technology may not be required. Prepare a list of priorities, ranking the various considerations by their order of importance.

Everyone experiences varying degrees of success with hearing aids. How well they function for you personally will depend on many variables, including the type and severity of your hearing loss. But if you expect a hearing aid to restore perfect hearing, you're bound to be disappointed.

Resistance to hearing aids

Despite the benefits of hearing aids, many people with hearing loss haven't ever bothered to try one. Some estimates say that only 1 in 5 people who could benefit from hearing aids actually uses them. Others put the rate much lower, especially for working-age adults — less than 1 in 20 of hearing-impaired adults in their 50s.

People reject the notion of wearing an aid for many reasons, including an unwillingness to accept hearing loss, the cost of the device, the lack of insurance coverage, and reports of bad experiences with hearing aids from friends or relatives. Often the biggest deterrent is fear of the social stigma — concern that a hearing aid is a sign of old age, incompetence or unattractiveness. But such concerns have little basis in fact.

In addition, the advances in technology and design are making hearing aids stylistically more appealing and functionally more effective. Each improvement, big or small, seems to have only increased user satisfaction with the devices.

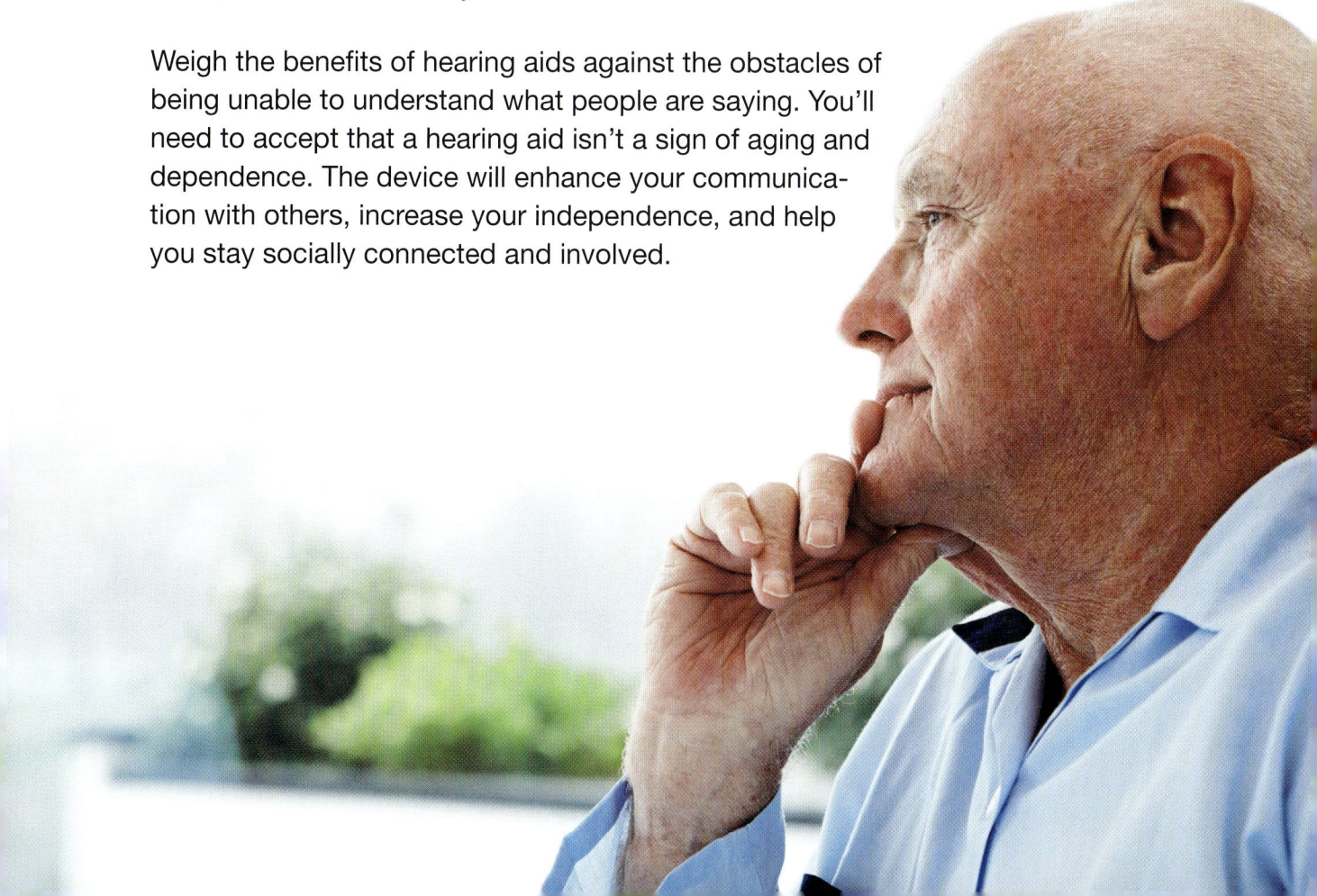

Weigh the benefits of hearing aids against the obstacles of being unable to understand what people are saying. You'll need to accept that a hearing aid isn't a sign of aging and dependence. The device will enhance your communication with others, increase your independence, and help you stay socially connected and involved.

One way to develop realistic expectations is by educating yourself about your type of hearing loss. Another is by talking to other people who have coped with hearing loss and used hearing aids. It's also important to work closely with your audiologist or hearing aid dispenser.

How hearing aids work

There are many types of hearing aids available, and the technology is continually improving. But the fundamental purpose of all hearing aids is the same: to make sounds stronger and thus more audible. They allow more sounds to be heard.

Hearing aids collect sounds from the environment via a small microphone. The sounds are then amplified and directed into the user's ear via a speaker. The amplified signal stimulates the inner ear, activating nerve fibers that carry the sound impulses to your brain.

The illustration on the adjoining page labels the parts of what's known as an in-the-ear style of hearing aid.

With hearing aids, you should be able to understand a conversation without needing to strain as much. They should make it easier for you to hear people talking in a soft voice. You'll probably be able to turn down the volume of your television to a level that's more comfortable for others in the room who don't have hearing loss. Hearing aids can also help you hear environmental sounds, which gives you a better sense of what's taking place around you.

Hearing aids may help you in situations where you've had difficulty hearing, such as a theater performance or worship service when the speaker is far away or the sound is weak. They can help you feel more at ease when you're on your own — for example, while shopping — or at times where speakers may not be talking directly to you.

Hearing aids may improve your hearing, but they don't provide a completely natural sound. They're electronic devices, after all, which can slightly change the quality of what you hear — just as a radio might slightly change the quality of music being played.

When you first listen through a hearing aid, you may notice that many things sound a little different. But you'll likely adapt to this change quickly.

Microphone
Microphones pick up sounds, convert them into electrical energy (signals) and deliver them to the amplifier. This aid utilizes a directional microphone, allowing you to pick up the sounds directly in front more than sounds coming from the other directions.

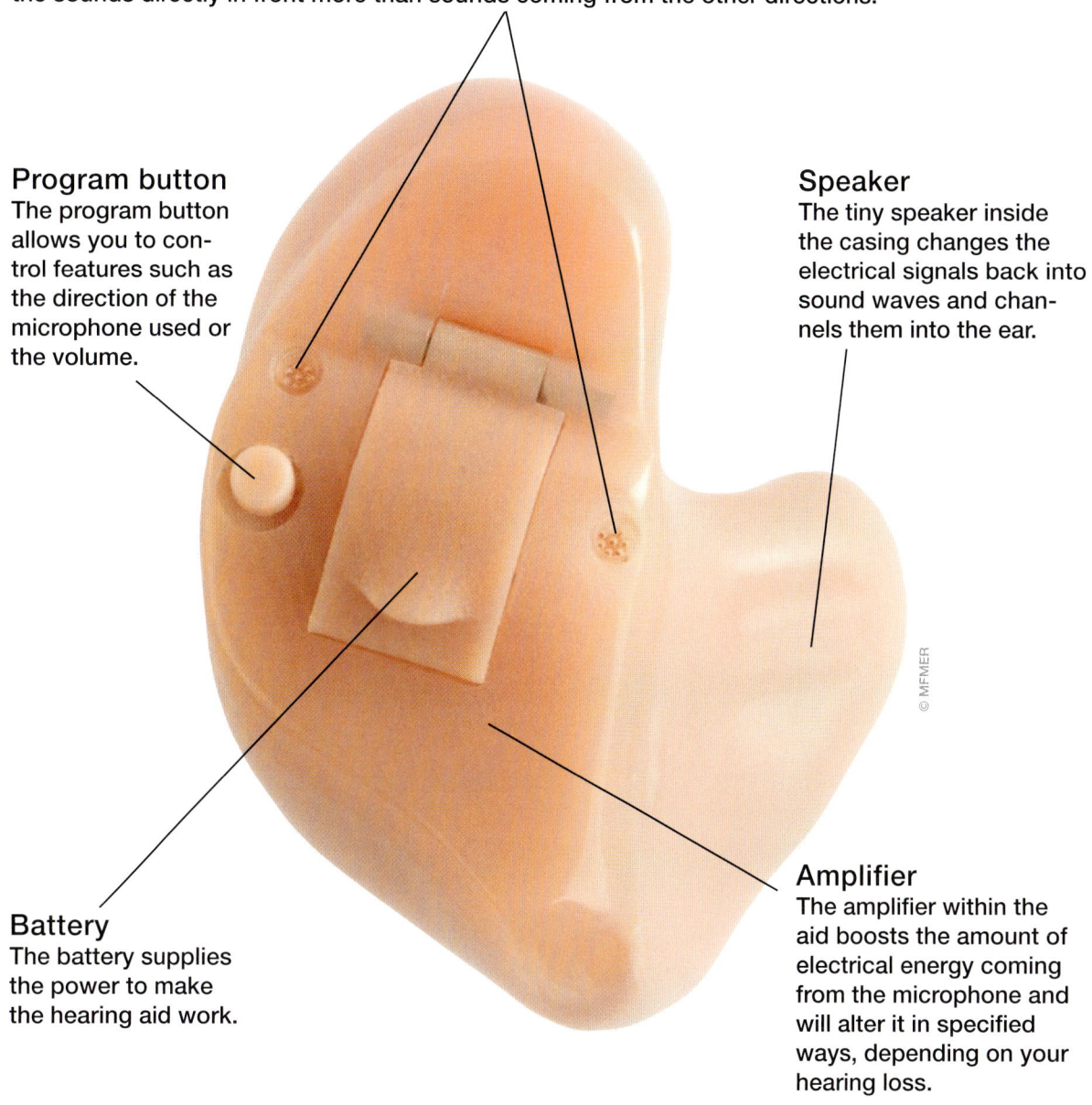

Program button
The program button allows you to control features such as the direction of the microphone used or the volume.

Speaker
The tiny speaker inside the casing changes the electrical signals back into sound waves and channels them into the ear.

Battery
The battery supplies the power to make the hearing aid work.

Amplifier
The amplifier within the aid boosts the amount of electrical energy coming from the microphone and will alter it in specified ways, depending on your hearing loss.

All the components of this in-the-ear style of hearing aid are held in a small plastic container called the casing. In a behind-the-ear style of hearing aid (see page 140), the casing rests behind the ear and is connected to an ear mold by a plastic tube. The ear mold is custom fit to direct sound into your ear canal.

Are two hearing aids better than one?

Can you hear better with a hearing aid in each ear? The answer, in most cases, is yes. Wearing two (binaural) hearing aids has many advantages over wearing one (monaural) aid. More auditory information is sent to your brain, and the signals reaching each ear will be slightly different. This makes it easier to hear speech in situations where there's background noise.

Two aids also provide more balanced hearing. You won't have a bad side, where sound is muted. Having two ears to listen with helps you locate the origin of sounds more easily, so you won't have to turn your head around to figure out who's talking. Another advantage of wearing two aids is that neither device needs to be turned up as loudly as when you're wearing only one. This helps reduce feedback and increases comfort.

Financial constraints and inability to wear an aid in one ear keep some people from wearing two aids. Talk to your audiologist about your options.

Furthermore, hearing loss typically causes the ear to distort some of the sounds you hear. Hearing aids can't eliminate that distortion, so some sounds may not be crystal clear.

You may continue to have problems understanding speech in certain situations. For example, when there's background noise or many people talking at once, hearing aids can't isolate the voice that you want to hear from other sounds. Remember that even with normal hearing, background noise often affects your understanding.

Some newer hearing aids have additional features that may help you in challenging listening situations. These attachments are discussed on pages 147-149.

Hearing aid styles

The type and severity of your hearing loss will help determine what style of hearing aid may be best for you. Most people will be a candidate for either conventional (air conduction) hearing aids or hearing devices that work through bone conduction.

Conventional hearing aids

Conventional hearing aids work by air conduction — they amplify sounds and then channel them into your ear canal for better processing inside the ear.

These aids come in various styles, which differ in size and the way in which they fit in the ear. Some conventional aids are small enough to fit deeply in the ear canal, making them almost invisible. The most widely sold aids are those that fit behind the ear — accounting for approximately half of all the hearing aids that are dispensed.

With different styles to choose from, keep in mind that the choice of a hearing aid concerns more than just looks. The style that may best suit you will depend largely on your hearing test results. In general, the smaller a hearing aid is, the less powerful it is and the shorter its battery life.

Also, some styles of hearing aids tend to not work as well when your hearing remains good at the low frequencies but decreases substantially at the higher frequencies.

The size and shape of your outer ear, especially the ear canal, may eliminate certain style options. For example, in-the-canal styles can be difficult to fit in smaller ears. In addition, your ability to handle a small hearing aid may be a factor if you have limited finger dexterity. Medical conditions also may dictate which style is appropriate.

Completely in the canal

The smallest hearing aid commonly available is called a completely-in-the-canal (CIC) aid. All parts, including the battery, are contained in the tiny casing that fits deep inside the ear canal. A thin, plastic pull cord on the aid sticks out into the bowl-shaped part of your ear to help in removal. The CIC aid is appropriate for mild to moderate hearing loss. It's not used for children or infants.

Hearing aid manufacturers are developing progressively smaller versions of CIC aids. This style may be referred to as a mini CIC, micro CIC or an invisible-in-the-ear (IIC) hearing aid.

Advantages. The CIC aid is the least visible hearing aid. It may help reduce problems with wind noise.

Disadvantages. The CIC style can have power limitations and some may not be suited for severe hearing loss. CIC aids have less space for options such as volume control or directional microphones. In addition, the batteries are small, so battery life will be shorter. They're susceptible to problems with earwax clogging the speaker and microphone openings.

In the canal

An in-the-canal (ITC) hearing aid fits partly in the ear canal but not as deeply as a CIC aid. The outer edge of the ITC aid extends into the bowl of your ear. ITC aids can accommodate mild to moderately severe hearing loss, but they're not appropriate for use with infants and children.

Advantages. Like CIC aids, ITC aids are hardly visible. An ITC aid is likely to be more powerful than a CIC aid, with more opportunity for add-on features.

Disadvantages. Like CIC aids, ITC aids can be difficult to handle and insert into the ear. Some users may also find them difficult when replacing batteries.

In the ear

An in-the-ear (ITE) hearing aid fills most of the bowl-shaped area of your outer ear. It's also known as the full-shell style. ITE aids are suitable for mild to severe hearing loss.

Advantages. ITE aids can be more powerful than smaller aids, and they can accommodate more options, such as a telecoil and directional microphones (for more on options, see pages 147-149).

They're appropriate for a wider range of hearing loss. The battery may be larger and easier to insert than are batteries for the in-the-canal styles.

Disadvantages. ITE aids may pick up more wind noise than the smaller in-the-canal styles do.

Behind the ear

Behind-the-ear (BTE) aids have two parts. A small plastic casing that rests behind the ear contains the hearing aid circuitry: the microphone, amplifier and speaker.

The casing is often connected by plastic tubing to a custom-made ear mold (earpiece) that directs the amplified sound into your ear canal. BTE aids are suitable for almost all types of hearing loss and for people of all ages.

BTE aids are often perceived — erroneously — as old-fashioned and not technologically advanced. In fact, BTE aids contain the latest digital technology of the other styles and may offer the greatest improvement in hearing.

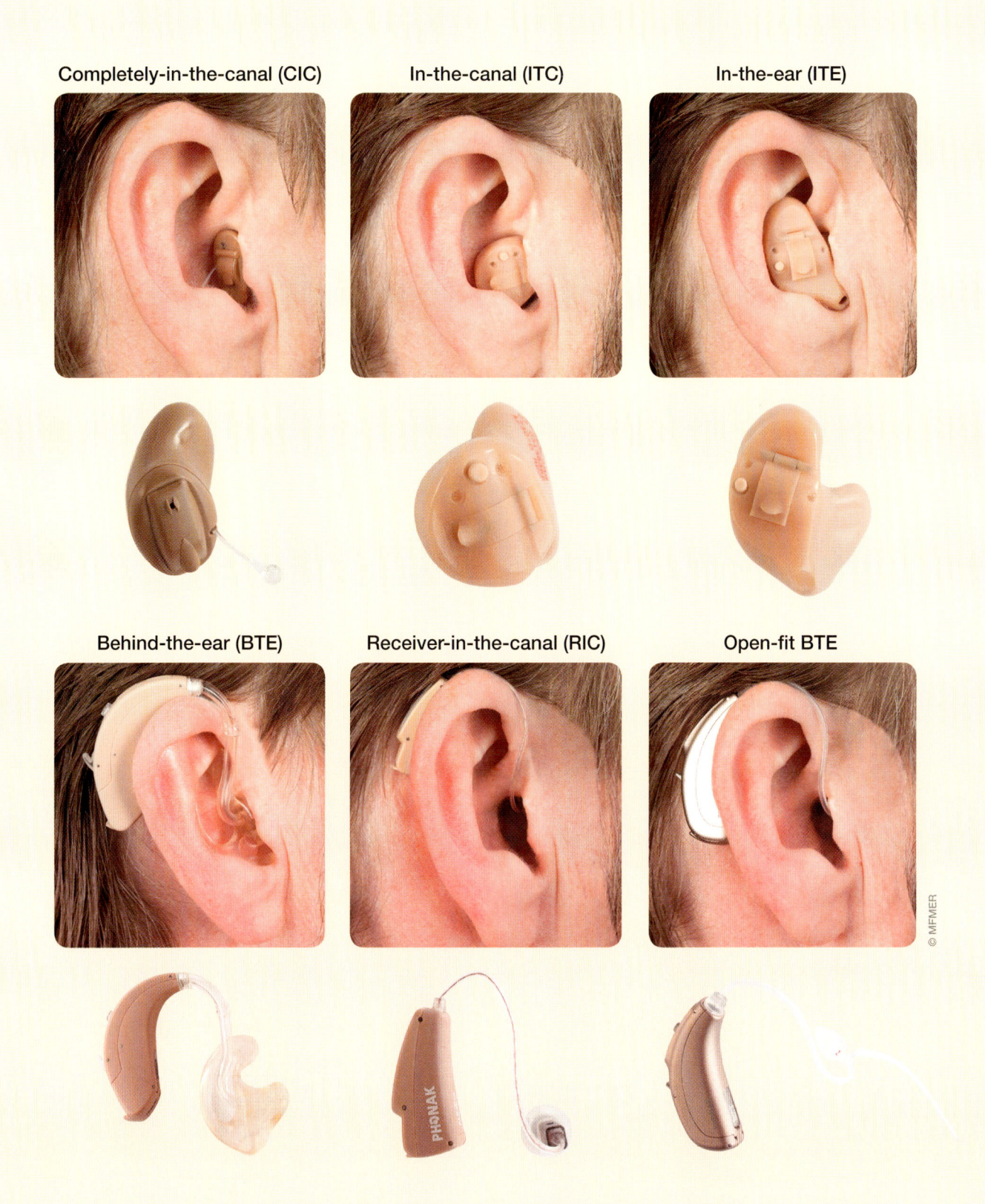

Completely-in-the-canal (CIC)	In-the-canal (ITC)	In-the-ear (ITE)

Behind-the-ear (BTE)	Receiver-in-the-canal (RIC)	Open-fit BTE

Mayo Clinic on Better Hearing and Balance **141**

Advantages. These are the most powerful hearing aids available, and they can be programmed for any level of hearing loss. There's also plenty of space for options. BTE aids are the best style for infants, children and people with severe hearing loss. BTE aids are the easiest to maintain, partly because battery replacement is easier. These aids usually require fewer repairs than other styles.

Disadvantages. Some individuals simply don't have enough space between their ear and the side of their head to accommodate a BTE aid. This style may pick up more wind noise than the smaller aids do.

Receiver in the canal or receiver in the ear

Receiver-in-the-canal (RIC) or receiver-in-the-ear (RITE) hearing aids typically have a very small casing that fits behind the ear and houses the microphone and amplifier. The casing is connected by a tiny wire to the speaker that sits in the ear canal. The speaker can be fitted into the ear canal with a custom ear mold or a soft, flexible dome-shaped tip.

Advantages. This type of hearing aid is small and less obvious, making it more cosmetically appealing for some people. Because the receiver is close to the eardrum, feedback is less problematic than it is with open fit BTE aids. And the speaker can be replaced in the office, avoiding a factory repair.

Disadvantages. The receivers of RIC and RITE hearing aids can be susceptible to wax. Smaller aids use a small battery, which means shorter battery life.

Open fit

Both BTE and RIC (or RITE) aids can be fit with a dome-shaped tip in the ear canal, leaving the ear canal largely open. This style has recently become popular for mild hearing loss and mild to moderate high-frequency hearing loss where hearing in the low frequencies is normal. However, people with more severe hearing loss can't use the open-fit style because of inadequate volume.

Because most of the ear canal is left open, individuals can use their remaining hearing for lower pitched sounds — which are able to pass directly to the eardrum — and the hearing aid selectively amplifies higher pitched sounds.

Advantages. The ability of the casing to fit behind your ear, and the use of very thin tubing, makes the open-fit style very attractive to individuals who have cosmetic concerns. Leaving the ear canal open often makes the individual's own voice sound more acceptable.

Disadvantages. Due to the open ear canal, this style is limited in how much volume it can produce before whistling or squealing (feedback) problems occur.

Bone conduction devices

There are several devices that can be used to overcome conductive hearing loss when a conventional hearing aid is not an option. A convention aid may not work due to ear malformation or medical problems of the ear — for example, when there's a physical abnormality or chronic drainage from the ear that makes the use of ear molds a problem.

These devices can also be used for profound inner ear hearing loss in one ear with normal or near-normal hearing in the better ear (single-sided deafness). These devices bypass the outer and middle ear and stimulate the inner ear directly through bone conduction.

Bone-anchored hearing aid (BAHA)

The BAHA stimulates the inner ear with an external device that has a microphone and amplifier and changes

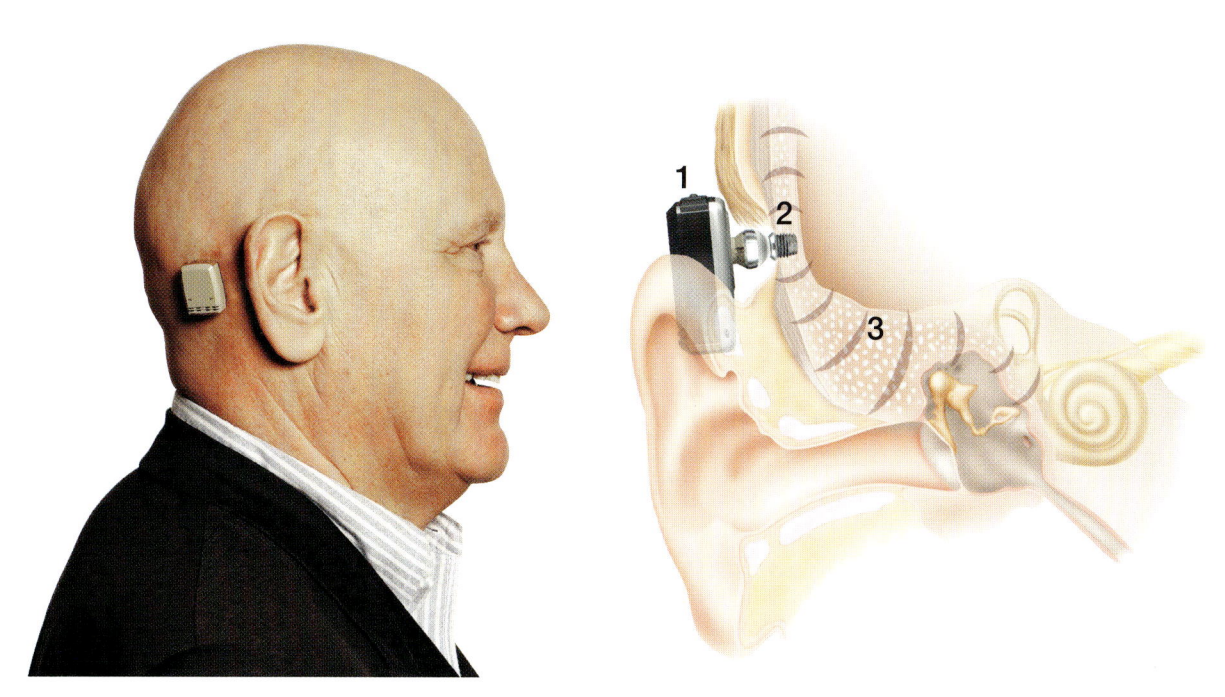

How BAHA works: 1. Sound waves are received by the BAHA sound processor and changed into vibrations. 2. Vibrations from the sound processor are transferred from the abutment to the titanium implant. 3. The implant uses direct bone conduction to transfer the sound vibrations to the functioning cochlea.

sound to a vibration that is then picked up by the inner ear. The external device is attached to either a titanium post that is surgically placed behind the ear or to an elastic or metal headband.

Advantages. BAHA aids can be used when more-conventional hearing aids that use air conduction cannot function. A BAHA aid is more comfortable than bone conduction hearing aids that are mounted on a headband.

Disadvantages. Typically, there is a three-month wait time after surgery for the surgically placed post to grow into the bone before the device can be attached to the post. Feedback can be more problematic when using a headband. Repairs to the external device can be costly.

Magnetic bone conduction

This type of aid consists of a surgically implanted magnet near the ear, which is paired with an external device consisting of a microphone and amplifier and a transducer. Like a BAHA, the external device changes sound to a vibration that is picked up by the inner ear.

Advantages. Unlike a BAHA, there's no wait time needed after surgery.

Disadvantages. Because this is a newer technology, there isn't much information available on longevity or overall effectiveness of the device.

In-the-mouth bone conduction

For this type of aid, you wear a device that looks like a BTE hearing aid that has a microphone and transmitter. However, the transmitter sends the signal to a receiver that is built into a customized retainer-like device. This device fits in the mouth around the upper back teeth. The receiver converts sound to a vibration that is sent through the teeth via bone conduction to the inner ear.

Advantages. This is the only nonsurgical option for bone conduction devices other than those that use a headband. Both the external device and in-the-mouth receivers are rechargeable.

Disadvantages. Feedback may be problematic, both through air conduction (from the open mouth to the microphone) and bone conduction.

Implantable aids

Implantable hearing aids may be an option for people with moderate to severe sensorineural hearing loss, that is, loss associated with damage to the inner ear.

These devices use a tiny electromagnet that's attached to the bones of the middle ear and an external unit that stimulates the magnet. This type of aid is less commonly used, and ongoing research is still needed to determine its overall effectiveness.

Other selection considerations

When selecting a hearing aid, your decisions primarily involve different styles, sizes and circuitry features. You may also be faced with choosing whether one or two devices are necessary to improve your hearing. This process can become confusing because the decisions regarding style, size and circuitry can be made somewhat independently of each another.

For example, you may have heard that digital hearing aids provide the best sound. What may not be clear is that digital refers to the electrical components and not to a particular style of hearing aid.

Style and circuitry — along with size — are separate issues. Any circuitry can be placed in any style or size of hearing aid.

Hearing aid electronics

The circuitry of hearing aids refers to the electronic components inside the casing. Hearing aid electronics are specially programmed to amplify certain frequencies more than others. And the frequencies that are programmed correspond to the locations where hearing is impaired.

Nearly all of today's hearing aids contain a small computer chip — so they're referred to as digital hearing aids. This type of aid converts incoming sound into a digital code, which is analyzed and adjusted based on your hearing loss and listening needs. Then the code is converted back into sound waves and delivered to your ear canal. Computer chips provide many new options in sound processing and make the devices more comfortable for use in various sound environments.

The computer chip allows the audiologist to program your hearing aid to fit both the objective characteristics of your condition as well as some of your own subjective preferences. For example, the chip allows the audiologist to adjust how much amplification is required for you to hear at different ranges of frequency or pitch. This will depend on the type and severity of your hearing loss.

In addition, the computer chip can allow for several different settings for amplification. The audiologist can program one setting for use in quiet situations and another setting for use in loud, noisy situations such as restaurants or parties. You can select which setting you want by pushing a small button on the outside edge of the hearing aid or, in some cases, with the use of a remote control.

Often, special features in the circuitry can be activated for use in certain settings. For example, in noisy situations, you can activate directional microphones in the hearing aid that reduce the amount of noise that's picked up behind you — typically, background noise. Special noise-reduction circuitry also may be included.

With most aids, the computer chip itself can automatically adjust the settings based on the amount of noise and on how loud the sounds are.

Some new circuitry is available to help those who have severe or profound high-frequency hearing loss for which conventional amplification may not be beneficial. These hearing aid circuits shift or move high-frequency sounds to mid or low frequencies where the listener has better hearing and can "hear" the high-frequency sounds.

Some hearing aid circuitry allows devices worn in the right ear and the left ear to communicate with each other to make joint setting adjustments. Furthermore, hearing aids are available that incorporate wireless technology. This permits better communication between the hearing aids and cellphones or other electronic devices.

Digital hearing aids are available across a wide price range, from relatively inexpensive to very expensive. The cost is determined primarily by how many special features and adjustments are included on the computer chip.

Typically, more-expensive hearing aids have more frequency bands or channels. The number of channels determines how well a hearing aid can be adjusted for the hearing loss and how the noise reduction, feedback and other parameters are controlled.

Feedback refers to a high-pitched whistle, squeal or crackle that occurs when amplified sound is inadvertently picked up by the microphone and then reamplified. This is similar to the loud noise you may hear over a public-address system when the volume is set too high. New technology is helping to reduce feedback problems in hearing aids.

For many users, the less expensive aids may contain enough features to suit their hearing loss and their lifestyles. Other users may prefer to include all possible features and are willing to pay for them accordingly.

Special options

Other considerations when choosing a hearing aid are options that can help you in difficult listening situations.

Directional microphones

A hearing aid may have a microphone with dual sound inlets or be equipped with multiple microphones. Either arrangement allows the hearing aid to switch between directional and omni-directional modes. In fact, most recent hearing aid circuits are equipped to make this switch automatically as the acoustic environment changes. All but the CIC aid can accommodate directional microphones.

In noise, most directional microphones function to pick up the sounds directly in front of you more than the sounds coming from other directions. This can diminish the background noise processed by your hearing aid and improve your understanding of face-to-face conversations. Some new hearing aid circuits can be programmed to focus on sounds coming from other directions. For example, the aid can be right focused for driving a car, left focused when riding in the passenger seat, or rear focused when driving with others in the back seat.

Telecoils

Many BTE hearing aids, as well as some ITE and ITC aids, contain a built-in telecoil circuit. A telecoil is a tiny metal rod encircled with a coil of copper wire. The coil generates an electric current when it receives naturally produced electromagnetic signals from the telephone receiver. The hearing aid converts the current into sound, allowing you to hear clearly when someone talks to you on the telephone.

The telecoil can be manually activated with a switch, but many hearing aids now have an internal switch that picks up the electromagnetic signal automatically when a hearing aid-compatible phone is held up to the hearing aid. When the telecoil is switched on, the microphone in your hearing aid is usually turned off and only the telecoil signal is amplified. This avoids the feedback or squeal that often happens when a telephone is held close to a hearing aid with the microphone switched on.

Telecoil

A telecoil picks up electromagnetic signals directly from the telephone receiver, allowing you to hear the caller's voice.

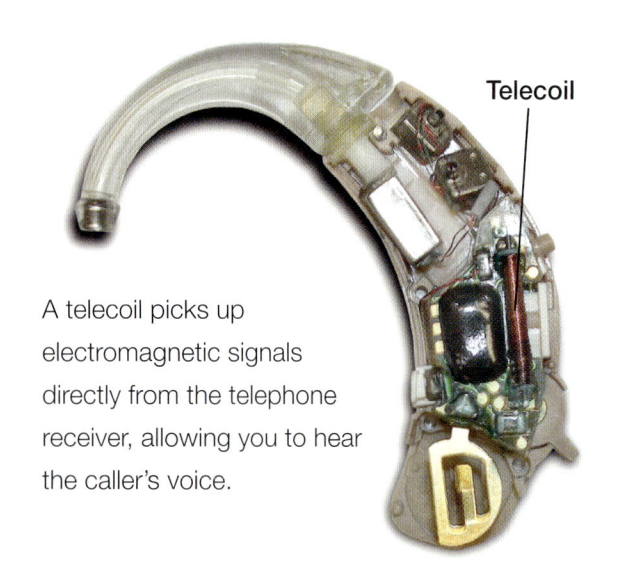

Besides telephones, telecoils can be used with assistive listening systems (see Chapter 9). Telecoils may not work with cellphones that are not hearing aid compatible. However, current cellphones generally come with compatibility ratings for telecoils. The higher the number, the more compatible the cellphone is for hearing aids with a telecoil.

Remote microphone

Some hearing aid companies offer a remote microphone that can be used in conjunction with some hearing aid circuits. The microphone is typically small and portable and can be passed to someone you're talking to. By putting the microphone closer to the speaker's mouth, there is an emphasis on the speaker's voice with significant reduction of environmental noise.

Remote control

Some hearing aids can be operated with a remote control device. This feature allows the user to turn the hearing aid on or off, and to adjust settings without touching the hearing aid or trying to find a small button or knob on the casing.

Bluetooth interface

Some hearing aids have a type of streamer that is used as a wireless interface between Bluetooth devices, such as cellphones or other electronic devices, and the hearing aid. The streamer picks up the signal from the wireless device and sends it directly to the hearing aid. Streamers need to be kept close to the hearing aid and may come with a clip or cord to allow them to be worn around the neck.

Some streamers can serve as a remote control. Most of these devices also have options for connecting to televisions, computers and other nonwireless devices.

Audio input

An input jack on the aid allows you to connect a wire directly to a television, stereo, separate microphone or assistive listening device. This is an option on some BTE hearing aids, but not styles worn inside the ear.

Ear-level FM systems

FM listening systems are particularly helpful for overcoming the impact of background noise, reverberation and distance on your hearing (see Chapter 9). Some BTE hearing aids combine regular circuitry with an FM receiver in the same casing. The receiver responds to a direct signal from the FM transmitter.

Buying a hearing aid

If you're planning to use hearing aids, you'll want to consult first with an audiologist or a hearing aid dispenser, also known as a hearing instrument specialist.

Audiologists must earn a doctoral degree in audiology (Au.D. or Ph.D.) to enter the practice. Licensing is required in all states in which they practice, and they may be certified by professional organizations such as the American Speech-Language-Hearing Association or the American Academy of Audiology. The practices of many ear, nose and throat (ENT) specialists include audiologists on staff to provide testing and rehabilitation services and to dispense hearing aids.

Although nonaudiologist hearing aid dispensers aren't required to have a college degree in order to practice, many have completed course work in the field. They're registered in the state they work in. Most states require hearing aid dispensers to be licensed, which means that they've passed state-administered written and practical examinations in the field. Dispensers should be certified by the National Board for Certification in Hearing Instrument Sciences.

To find a reputable and qualified audiologist or hearing aid dispenser, ask your doctor for recommendations. In addition, you can get lists of qualified hearing professionals in your area by contacting hearing organizations such as the American Academy of Audiology or the American Speech-Language-Hearing Association (see "Additional Resources" at the back of the book for contact information). Several Internet sites that sell hearing aids will refer you to dispensers within their network — but this practice is illegal in several states.

Don't buy hearing aids by mail or over the Internet from makers who claim you don't need to see an audiologist or dispenser in person. Proper testing and individualized fitting and adjustments are essential.

Hearing aids for children

It's particularly important to identify hearing loss in a child as soon as possible — before the loss has significant impact on speech and language development, social development, and education.

After the hearing loss has been diagnosed and the child has been seen by an ENT specialist to rule out medically treatable problems, hearing aids will likely be recommended. Just as for adults, the goal of hearing aids for children is to make speech and environmental sounds loud enough to hear.

Some factors that need to be taken into account include:

- The type of hearing loss
- The degree of hearing loss
- The child's age
- The child's ear size and shape

Behind-the-ear (BTE) aids with soft custom earm olds are most often recommended for children. With this style, the ear mold can be easily remade to fit the growing ear. BTE aids are generally more durable, are not exposed to earwax, and have less feedback and better battery life. Parents and caregivers can easily check the aid's function and make needed adjustments. And the soft ear mold is less likely to cause injury to the ear in the case of an accidental blow to the ear with play or during sports.

In school and at home, children frequently connect their hearing aids to FM systems or other assistive listening devices, which are described in Chapter 9. The hearing aid chosen should have features to allow for this connection.

In general, hearing aids need to be adjusted more often in children because of changing physical characteristics as the ear grows. Because of their smaller ear size, children may have some difficulty keeping hearing aids in place. There are many types of cords, clips and skin-safe tapes that can help make the aid more secure, which an audiologist can recommend.

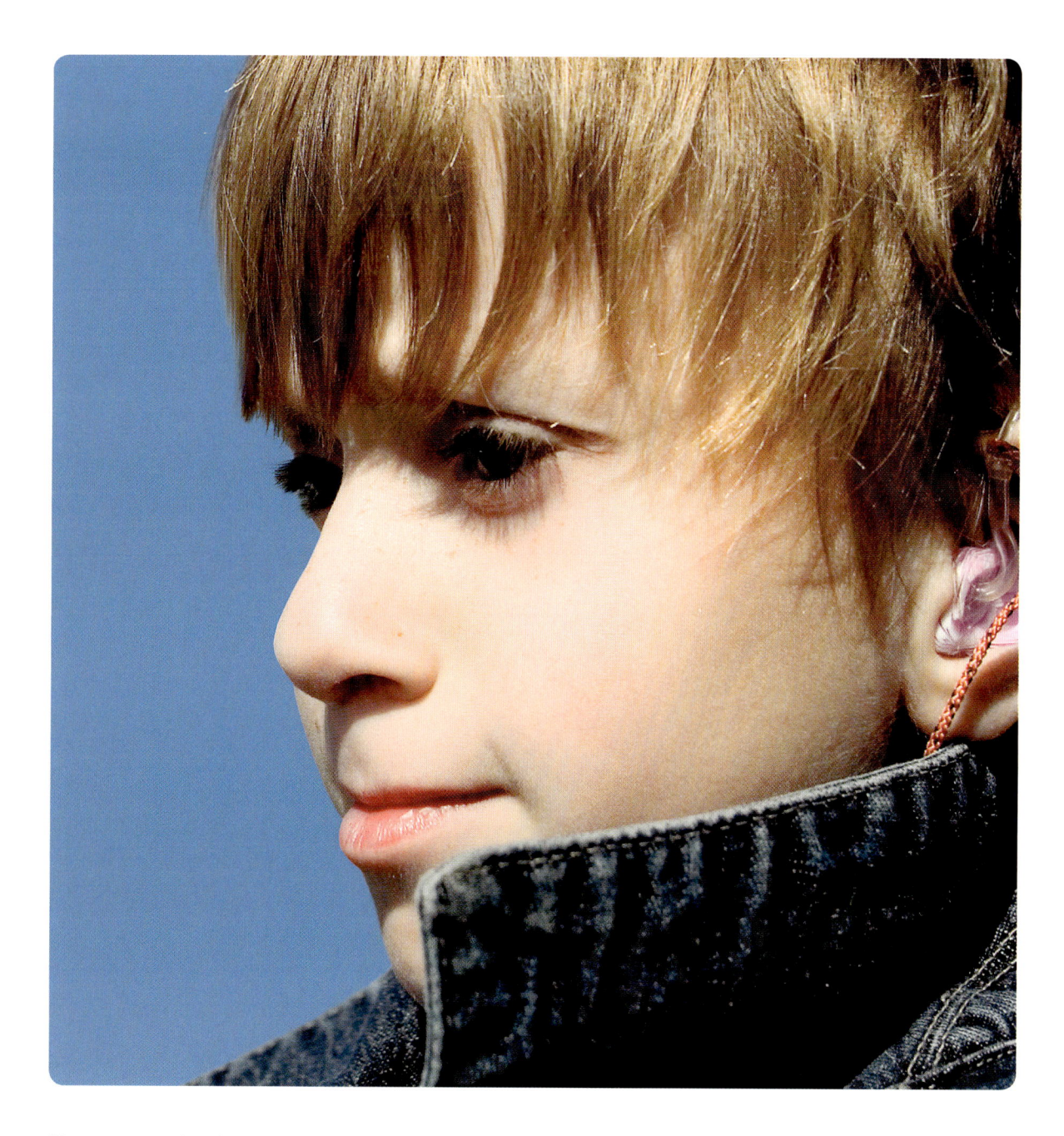

Parents and other caregivers play a critical role in helping children get the best experience out of their hearing aids, especially for younger children. Fortunately, with fun colors to choose from and easy links to the latest technology, today's hearing aids are much more appealing for children and adults alike.

Purchasing tips for hearing aids

Keep the following suggestions in mind when selecting a hearing aid:

- Consider all the options available, since more than one type of hearing aid might work for you. If your first selection is unsatisfactory, try a different type.
- Don't assume that the newest, most expensive model is also the best — a less expensive aid might improve your hearing just as much.
- Be cautious of "free" consultations and dispensers who sell only one brand of hearing aid. Look for a dispenser who offers plenty of options.
- Be alert to misleading claims. Be wary of advertisements that claim hearing aids can eliminate background noise or restore normal hearing. Most aids can help you, but no hearing aid can completely filter out one voice from other voices or restore your hearing to normal.
- Ask what the cost of a hearing aid includes. Most dispensers offer a single fee that bundles the cost of the aid with the costs of follow-up visits, the warranty and one pack of batteries.
- Get the terms of the trial period and the warranty in writing. This should include the return policy, the amount that can be refunded, how long the warranty lasts (preferably one or two years), and specifically what is or isn't covered — the warranty should cover both parts and labor.
- During the trial period, keep a detailed list of what you like or dislike about your hearing aid. Take the list with you when you return to the dispenser or audiologist.

The buying process

In the discussion that follows, the terms *hearing aid* and *aid* are used in the singular form. But keep in mind that frequently the most improvement results from a hearing aid in each ear.

To start the process, plan on being examined by a physician, preferably an ENT specialist. Children under age 18 are required by federal law to have a medical examination and an audiological examination prior to obtaining hearing aids. Audiologists and hearing aid dispensers are required to obtain a medical clearance — indicating that you've had a hearing examination within the past six months — before they can sell an adult a hearing aid. Otherwise, you'll have to sign a waiver.

Schedule a complete hearing evaluation by an audiologist. The hearing examination helps decide whether any medical treatment can improve your hearing or if a condition prevents you from using a hearing aid. Although few health insurance plans pay for hearing aids, many that offer coverage require a medical clearance prior to purchasing the device.

Get a copy of your audiogram if you're not buying a hearing aid at the same place where you've been tested. The audiogram provides an accurate guide for selecting the hearing aid. If you waived a medical examination, your audiologist can also identify if a medical condition is affecting your hearing and recommend a specialist.

Discuss all of your needs and expectations with the audiologist or chosen hearing aid dispenser. Indicate which situations cause you the greatest amount of difficulty with hearing. The primary goal is to match your lifestyle and your communication needs as closely as possible.

After studying the evaluation of your hearing loss and your lifestyle needs, the audiologist or dispenser will discuss various options with you and offer some recommendations. Makre sure you understand why a specific type of hearing aid has been recommended. Before you make a final decision, make sure you're aware of all the features included, as well as the cost of your selection and the terms of the trial period and return policy.

Regardless of which type of hearing aid you buy, always purchase it with a return privilege. The aid should come with a 30- to 60-day trial period and a return policy. You may use that time to adjust to using the device and decide whether it helps your hearing.

After you've made a selection, the audiologist or dispenser will need to fit the hearing aid. For most types of aids, an impression will be made of your ear, using a putty-like material to create an accurate mold of its shape. This mold helps the manufacturer make a custom ear mold or hearing aid that's comfortable and fits properly in your ear.

After one or two weeks, you'll return to the audiologist or dispenser's office to resume the fitting with your actual hearing aid. This visit will also involve programming the aid to provide maximum assistance for your particular hearing loss.

Once the aid is fitted, the audiologist or dispenser should instruct you on how to operate and maintain the hearing aid — how to insert and remove the device, check the battery, adjust the controls, and keep it clean and operational.

The trial period mentioned earlier allows you to adjust to the hearing aid. You'll probably schedule a return visit to the office within a few weeks. Until that time, write down questions or concerns and take them with you to the appointment.

If during the trial period you can't adjust to the aid or you decide that your hearing doesn't benefit enough from its use, notify your audiologist or dispenser. Under the agreement, you're entitled to a refund for the cost of the device.

Costs

The cost of a hearing aid varies considerably. Most digital aids range from $1,000 to $3,000 apiece. Your costs will be about double if you get two aids. Although this may seem expensive, if hearing aids can help you hear better and improve your quality of life, they're worth the investment.

Medicare and most private insurance policies don't cover the cost of a hearing aid. But some employer- or union-sponsored policies will provide limited reimbursement.

Qualified veterans may be eligible for free hearing aids and services, as well as batteries and other accessories, through the Veterans Affairs. Some fraternal and charitable organizations provide financial assistance for hearing aids for people who meet financial eligibility requirements.

Wearing your hearing aid

You should notice immediate improvement in the first days of wearing a hearing aid, but more benefits for your hearing come after you've become more accustomed to using the device.

Getting used to a hearing aid takes patience and practice. Your brain requires time to readjust to sounds that you may not have heard for a while.

Some sounds will seem different when they're amplified by the device.

To get the maximum benefit from your hearing aid, it's important to understand how it works, learn to insert it properly and use it regularly. A positive attitude also helps.

Schedule return appointments. After you've had your hearing aid for a week or two, you may wish to have it adjusted for more or less loudness or for better fit and control. The audiologist or hearing aid dispenser will help you achieve the best possible fit and greatest benefit for your hearing.

The audiologist or hearing aid dispenser will continue to counsel you on operating and maintaining the aid. Practice using the device in his or her presence. If you use two aids, insert and remove both to learn how to distinguish between the device for your right ear and the one for your left ear. Practice adjusting the controls, cleaning the aid and changing the batteries.

Readjustment

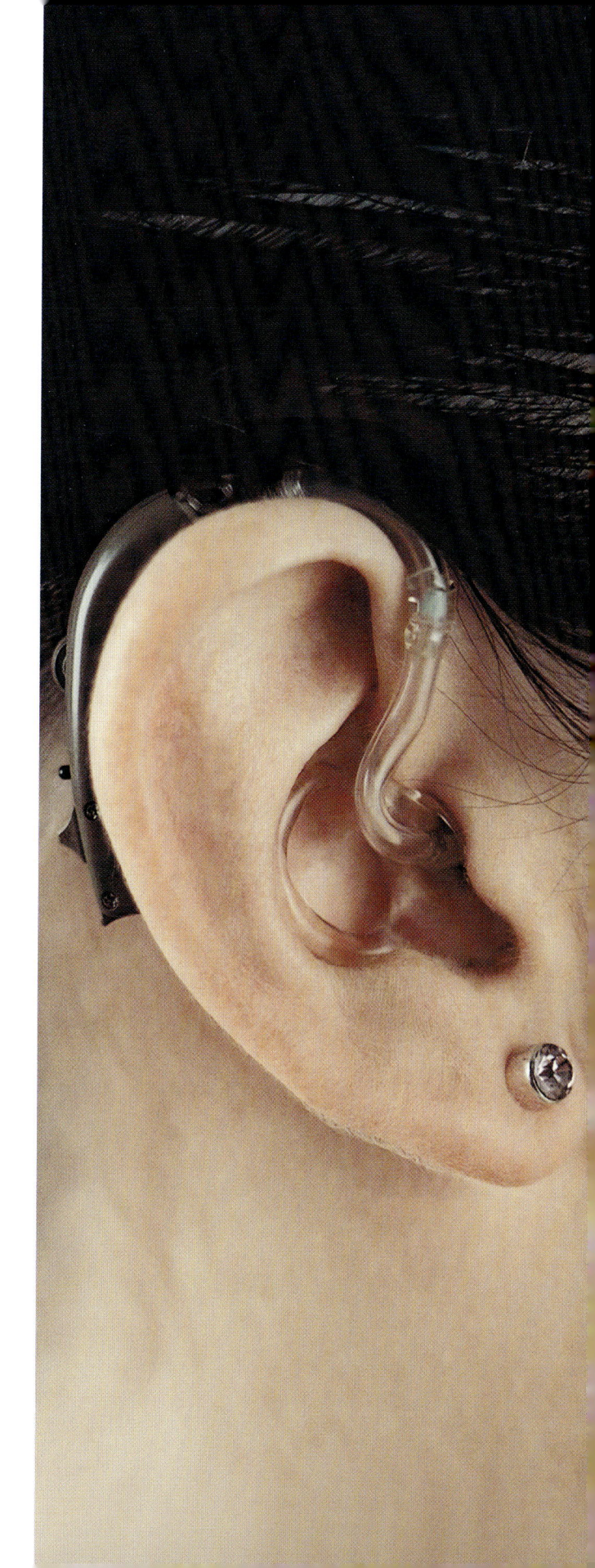

When you first use a hearing aid, some sounds may not seem natural. You may have come to think of what you hear with hearing loss as normal. Now, with the use of an aid, you're exposed to more sounds and louder sounds, as well as different patterns of sound.

Many first-time users of hearing aids say that people's voices, including their own voices, sound strange. In fact, the voices you hear are being picked up by a microphone and amplified. Hearing aids are often programmed to amplify certain pitches more than others depending on your type of hearing loss — so you may be hearing pitches that you haven't heard for some time. However, the more you wear the aid, the quicker the sounds will seem normal to you.

As your hearing has decreased over the years, you've probably become more accustomed to a quieter life. Many common environmental sounds, such as appliance motors, clocks, dripping faucets, a car's running motor, footsteps, even your own chewing or breathing, were soft or inaudible when you weren't using a hearing aid.

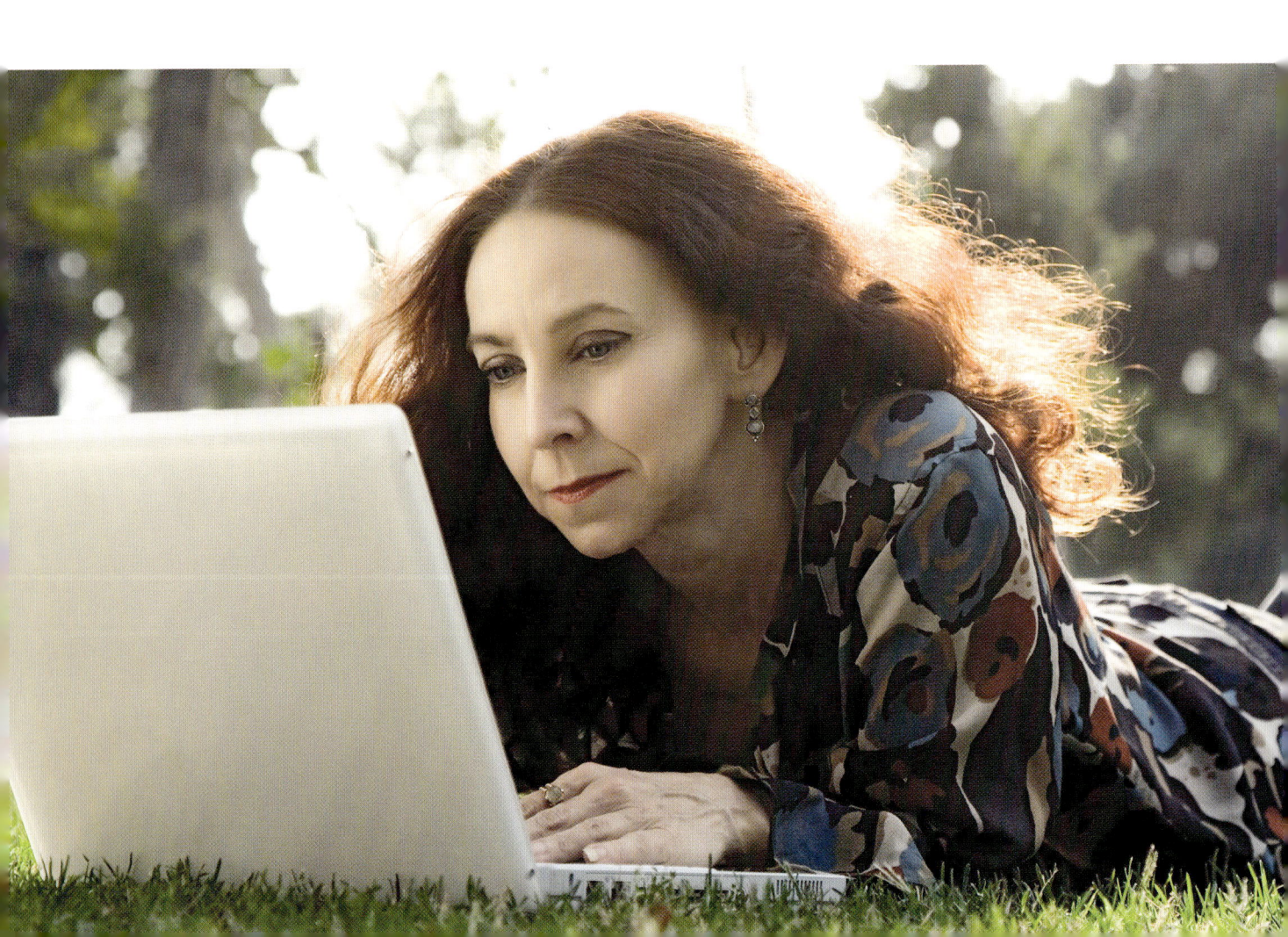

During the first days of wearing a hearing aid, you'll start noticing these sounds again. Because you haven't heard them for a while, your brain is more aware of them. The change may annoy you. But after several months, your brain will shift these sounds to the background where they belong and you'll notice them less.

Some hearing specialists recommend that new hearing aid users build up their listening experiences gradually, wearing their aids for only a short time in quiet situations. New users often make the mistake of immediately wearing hearing aids in the most difficult listening conditions, such as loud restaurants. Starting off in this way can be frustrating and discouraging.

If you're having a problem adjusting to the aid, consider using it only for a few hours a day in your home, where you can control the noise level. Practice conversing with one or two people in a quiet place. Gradually increase the amount of time you use your hearing aid each day.

As your comfort level builds, expose yourself to different listening situations until you're able to use your aid all day in any environment. It will take some time, perhaps months, to get used to new sounds and achieve the maximum benefit from your hearing aid.

Discuss any problems you experience with your audiologist or hearing aid dispenser. You may be directed to a group orientation session for new hearing aid users. This session provides information about hearing loss and hearing aid use. You may also contact an organization such as the Hearing Loss Association of America.

Remember that hearing aids are meant to improve your communication, not to give you new ears or the normal hearing of a healthy 20-year-old. You'll inevitably encounter circumstances in which hearing aids don't give you all of the benefits you'd like. In these situations you may need to rely on other methods for improving communication.

Tips for better communication

Difficult listening situations may require you to use other, simple techniques in addition to your hearing aid. Consider these strategies to improve your hearing in these circumstances:

Talk face to face
Supplement what you hear with what you see. When you're talking to someone, make sure you can see his or her

face and lips. Converse on a one-to-one basis or in small groups rather than large groups.

Don't talk to people from a different room
Distance and physical barriers such as walls reduce the amount of sound that reaches you.

Control background noise
Talk in locations with the least background noise. Steer clear of noisy restaurants, or go during off-peak times to avoid a crowd. You may also ask for a booth in a quiet corner with good lighting. In meeting rooms and lecture halls, sit in the front row. At home, turn off the television or stereo while conversing on the telephone or in person.

Ask others to help
People are usually glad to accommodate you if they understand your needs. Let others know how to help you and what listening strategies work for you. Start by telling people that the circumstances are making it difficult for you to hear. Ask them to talk directly to you face to face and to speak clearly and slowly, but it's not necessary to shout.

Educate yourself about other assistive tools, including devices and listening systems

Resources such as a telephone amplifier, FM transmitter, Bluetooth technology, induction loop or closed captioning service may prove helpful in difficult listening environments. These resources are discussed in Chapter 9.

Common problems

As with any complex piece of equipment, things can go wrong with a hearing aid. Most hearing aid problems are minor and easily corrected.

It's always important to inform your audiologist or hearing aid dispenser of any problem. Before calling, however, check to make sure the problem isn't something that you can easily fix:

- Is the hearing aid turned on?
- Are all switches or controls in the correct position?
- Is the battery fresh and inserted properly?
- Is the sound outlet plugged with wax or debris?
- Is the microphone opening plugged?
- If you have a remote control for the aid, is it functioning?

Here are tips for some of the most common problems with hearing aids.

Feedback

Discordant sounds such as whistling and squealing are usually the result of a poorly fit hearing aid, an improperly inserted device or an ear that's plugged with wax. The more powerful a hearing aid is, the more critical the fit is for receiving and amplifying sound. When you experience feedback, always check for the following:

- Make sure the aid is inserted properly in your ear.
- Make sure the volume control isn't set too high.
- Have your audiologist or doctor check your ear for wax buildup.

Dead or defective batteries

Weak and faulty batteries are one of the most common causes of hearing aid failure. Signs of a failing battery include weak output, distortion, increased feedback, and other strange or unusual sounds, such as crackling static or fluttering.

Hearing aid batteries

Use only the size and type of battery recommended by your hearing aid dispenser. Most hearing aid batteries are zinc-air. They're activated when an adhesive tab is removed and air gets into the battery. Never remove the tab until you're ready to insert the battery into your hearing aid. Zinc-air batteries have an excellent shelf life, so you can keep several packages on hand. Store them at room temperature, not in a refrigerator.

Battery life depends on the style and circuitry of the hearing aid, the size of battery and how many hours a day the aid is used. Most hearing aid batteries last from one to two weeks, although small batteries last only about three to seven days. Discuss a battery replacement schedule at your initial fitting.

You can buy batteries from your audiologist or hearing aid dispenser, or in drugstores, grocery stores and electronics supply stores. Make sure to keep them out of reach of children and pets, and dispose of them properly.

If any of these signs become evident, try inserting a new battery. Make sure that the battery is placed correctly with the plus and minus signs facing in the right direction. Many new hearing aids will give you a warning tone that your battery soon needs replacing.

Wax blockage

Placing a hearing aid or ear mold in your ear seems to stimulate wax production. People who don't wear hearing aids also can get wax buildup, but it gradually loosens, moves to the edge of the ear canal and falls out. The hearing aid or ear mold can compress the wax and cause it to stay in the canal. The wax can block the speaker and shut it down.

The best way to prevent wax buildup is to visit a doctor or audiologist regularly to have the wax removed. It's a simple procedure. Don't try to remove the wax by yourself using cotton swabs. This may only pack the wax deeper into the ear canal and damage your eardrum.

Ask your audiologist or hearing aid dispenser about a means to keep wax from getting inside your hearing aids, such as a wax guard. He or she can show you the best way to clean wax from the aid. Every day, inspect the end of the hearing aid where the sound comes out and look for wax blockage.

Ear discomfort

The ear mold of a BTE aid or the shell of custom hearing aids (ITE, ITC or CIC) should fit snugly but not uncomfortably in the ear. Initially, the ear mold or hearing aid may feel slightly uncomfortable, but it shouldn't cause soreness, redness or irritation. Discomfort may also result from a poorly fitting aid or from an aid that's positioned incorrectly in the ear canal. Difficulties with correct placement are fairly common among many new hearing aid users.

If you experience constant discomfort from wearing a hearing aid, consult your audiologist or dispenser about the problem. The ear mold or hearing aid may need to be modified or remade.

Moisture

Moisture often collects in the tubing between the ear mold and the BTE casing — as warm air from the inside of your ear travels into the cooler tubing, water vapor condenses and collects in the tubing. Condensation usually isn't a problem unless the tubing becomes plugged. Moisture can also affect the BTE itself due to perspeiration of skin behind the ear — it can affect ITE hearing aids, as well. Storing the aids in a dehumidifier pack may help. Electronic drying devices also are available.

Maintenance

Proper care is a key to keeping your hearing aid in good working order and ensuring that it'll last as long as possible. Here are a frew suggestions:

Keep your hearing aid clean and dry

Wipe your hearing aid with a tissue or soft cloth every time you take it out of your ear. Gently scrub it with a soft brush every morning before inserting, when wax is dry and more easily crumbles and falls out. A dry, soft-bristle toothbrush works well.

Don't wear your aid while bathing, showering or swimming

Keep it away from steamy kitchens or bathrooms where someone has just taken a shower, and don't spray it with hair spray.

Keep the hearing aid in safe, dry, dust-free storage

You may want to buy a dehumidifying container to store it in at night. Ask your dispenser to recommend a container that would work for you.

Check the small holes at the tip of the hearing aid or custom ear mold

Carefully clean out any wax with a small brush, a wire looped around the end of a piece of plastic (a wax loop) or a pick. Most custom hearing aids that fit in the ear have a built-in wax guard, as does the RIC or RITE hearing aid receiver that fits in the ear canal.

Don't expose the hearing aid to intense heat

Don't leave the aid on the top of a radiator, and don't leave it in the car in the sun.

Open the battery door when the hearing aid isn't in use

This ensures that the hearing aid is turned off. It also lets dry air in and moisture out.

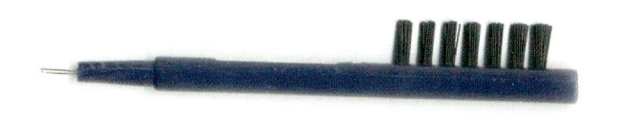

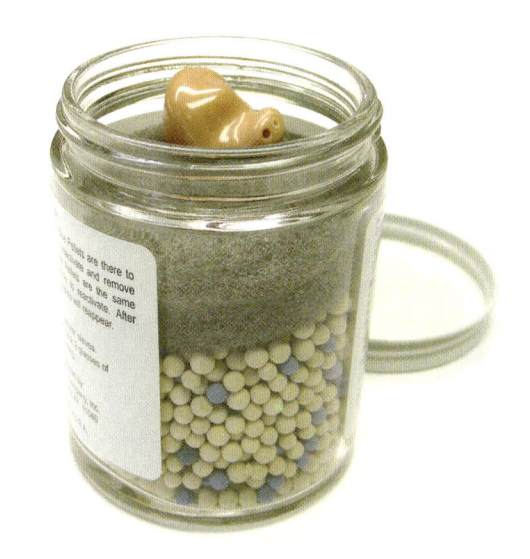

Don't drop the hearing aid. Develop the habit of inserting and removing your aid over a soft surface, such as a bed or sofa, or over a hand towel on a table. Never leave the aid where it could be knocked to the floor.

Have the hearing aid cleaned and serviced regularly. Never attempt to repair a hearing aid yourself. This can damage the aid and void the warranty. If the hearing aid breaks or malfunctions, contact your audiologist or hearing aid dispenser.

Always keep the hearing aid and the batteries away from small children and pets. They can choke on an aid or swallow a battery.

Chapter 8

Cochlear implants

Sensorineural hearing loss results from damage to the inner ear and to the auditory nerve that carries signals to the brain. The damage is usually permanent, and the hearing loss is irreversible.

At present, the most effective treatments for adults and children with moderate to profound sensorineural hearing loss is a cochlear implant. A cochlear implant is an electronic device that generates a sense of sound by stimulating the hearing nerve. This can help people who would gain little to no benefit from the amplified sound of hearing aids.

A cochlear implant is something like an artificial inner ear, taking over the job of the cochlea. A healthy cochlea converts sound waves into electrical signals and sends those signals along the auditory nerve. If the cochlea is damaged, an implant can be surgically placed in the inner ear that directly stimulates the auditory nerve. An external device then picks up the sound and transmits it to the internal device.

Research on cochlear implants began in the 1950s as scientists looked to help people with sensorineural hearing loss. They began experimenting with ways to compensate for the damaged hair cells in the inner ear. The first devices were approved for adults in 1985, and for children in 1990.

Cochlear implant technology has improved tremendously since its introduction 30 years ago, and new developments are on the horizon. Hundreds of thousands of adults and children around the world have benefitted from the procedure and are using the implant in their daily lives.

Although a cochlear implant doesn't restore normal hearing, it can dramatically improve your ability to hear and to understand speech. Benefits vary from person to person, but some users find that it allows them to perform many tasks that previously were difficult, such as talking on the phone or listening to classroom lectures.

Hearing with a cochlear implant is different from normal hearing, and it takes the brain time to make sense of the information it's receiving. With consistent use, understanding will improve. After a month or so of using the implant, the recipient usually finds that the sound of other voices begins to seem natural. For children with hearing loss since birth or a very young age, cochlear implants provide enough input to develop hearing that allows for speech and language development.

Many recipients of cochlear implants feel that their quality of life improves following the procedure. The new sense of sound helps reduce feelings of isolation and increases their ability to participate in social situations. They're able to enjoy pleasurable sounds such as the laughter of babies and — sometimes with time — the harmonies of song. They feel safer because they can hear fire alarms, warning sirens and traffic noise. They can better perform their jobs by being able to hear the ring of a telephone or the beep of a timer and to participate more at one-on-one or group meetings.

Cochlear implants and hearing aids

A cochlear implant is very different from a hearing aid. Hearing aids amplify sound waves, making them stronger when they're delivered to the ear. This amplification helps make more sounds detectable, louder and understandable.

A cochlear implant doesn't make sounds louder. Rather, it bypasses the damaged or nonworking parts of your inner ear and directly stimulates the auditory nerve. The implant gathers acoustic information from your environment and converts it into a form that your brain can understand.

Normally, the sensory hair cells in your inner ear convert sound vibrations arriving from the middle ear into nerve impulses. These impulses are relayed to the brain, which interprets the impulses and gives them meaning as sounds.

In order for a person to hear sounds correctly, thousands of tiny hair cells must be functioning in the inner ear in order to fully detect the vibrations. A person with normal hearing will typically have 20,000 to 30,000 healthy, delicate hair cells in each ear.

In most people with sensorineural hearing loss, some hair cells are damaged and don't function properly. They're unable to stimulate the auditory nerve effectively. Although many nerve fibers are intact and able to transmit electrical impulses, these fibers are unresponsive because of the hair cell damage.

People with mild or moderate hearing loss still have a sufficient number of healthy hair cells. Sounds that are amplified by a hearing aid can be converted into electrical impulses by the undamaged hair cells, in the same way that sounds are transmitted in a normal-hearing ear.

But if you have moderate to profound sensorineural hearing loss, extensive hair cell damage prevents your auditory system from processing the information, no matter how much hearing aids amplify the sound.

Cochlear implants help resolve this sensorineural problem because they're able to stimulate the intact nerve fibers directly. This allows you to still communicate auditory information to your brain and perceive sounds.

How cochlear implants work

Different cochlear implant systems are available. The Food and Drug Administration (FDA) has approved several systems and is doing clinical investigations to test others.

All systems work by converting sounds into electronic impulses that are transmitted to your brain. The implants aren't single units — they have both internal and external components. The external components are a microphone, speech processor, transmitter and connecting cords. The internal components are a receiver-stimulator and electrodes. These parts work together as follows:

- The microphone picks up sounds from the environment. It's located in a headpiece or casing that's typically hooked over the ear, similar to a behind-the-ear hearing aid.

Transmitter

Receiver-stimulator

Cochlea

Electrodes

Transmitter

Microphone and speech processor

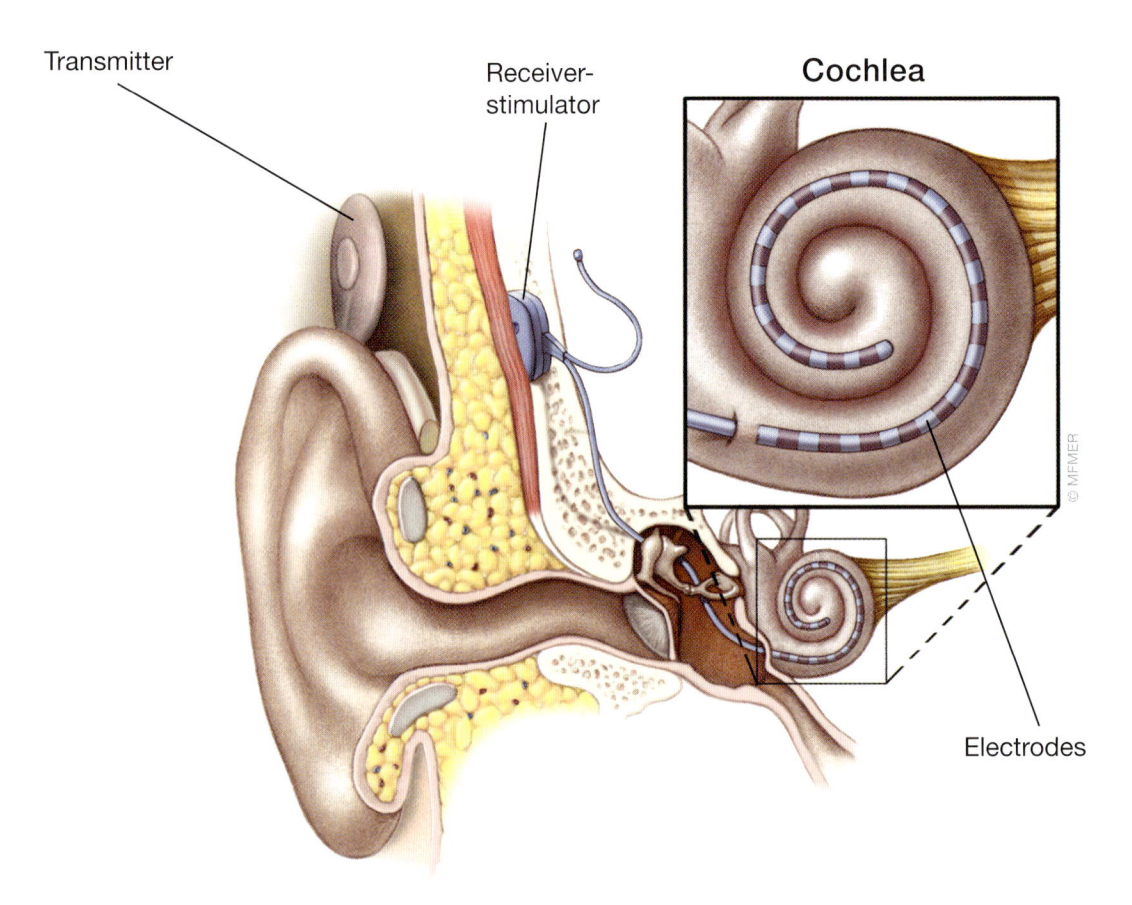

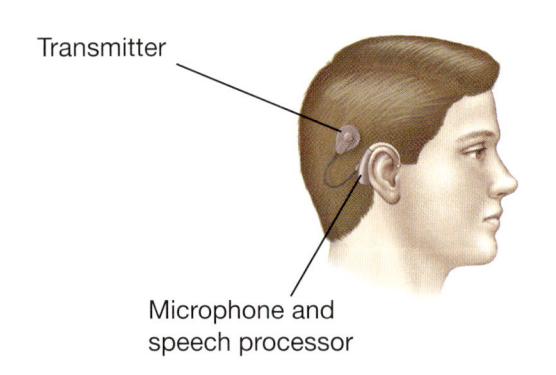

Cochlear implants use an external microphone and speech processor that you generally wear behind or near your ear. A transmitter sends radiofrequency signals to a surgically implanted electronic chip, the receiver-stimulator, that stimulates the auditory nerve with electrodes that have been threaded into the cochlea.

- The speech processor includes a small, powerful computer chip that digitally converts the sounds from the microphone into electronic impulses. The impulses will be directed to specific locations in the cochlea based on pitch and loudness. Processors most often are worn behind the ear, similar to a large hearing aid. Another style of processors is waterproof and is worn using a clip pinned to a shirt, armband or hat. A newer style incorporates the microphone, processor and transmitter into a single casing that is worn on the head over the internal receiver-stimulator.
- Impulses from the speech processor are sent to a transmitter — sometimes called a transmitting coil. A magnet holds the transmitter in place behind the ear, directly over a receiver-stimulator that's implanted beneath the scalp.
- The receiver-stimulator receives the impulses as radiofrequency waves from the transmitter. It relays the impulses as electronic signals through electrodes to the inner ear. The electrodes have been threaded directly into the cochlea on a bundle of tiny insulated wires.
- The electrodes stimulate the intact nerve fibers in the cochlea. This triggers the creation of electrical impulses. The impulses travel along the auditory nerve to the brain for processing and interpretation.

Although this multistage process seems complicated, the time it takes is quite short. The length of time between when the microphone first picks up a sound and when the brain receives this information is just a few thousandths of a second. Any processing delay that occurs as a result of the cochlear implant isn't noticed by the user.

Current research efforts are devoted to increasing the amount of sound delivered to the implant user's ear. This includes research on using cochlear implants in both ears (bilateral implants), coordination of stimulation between the two ears, and using cochlear implants in conjunction with hearing aids when preservation of any low-frequency hearing function exists.

Implant candidates

Cochlear implants aren't alternatives to hearing aids. Rather, these devices best serve individuals for whom hearing aids will provide little or no benefit.

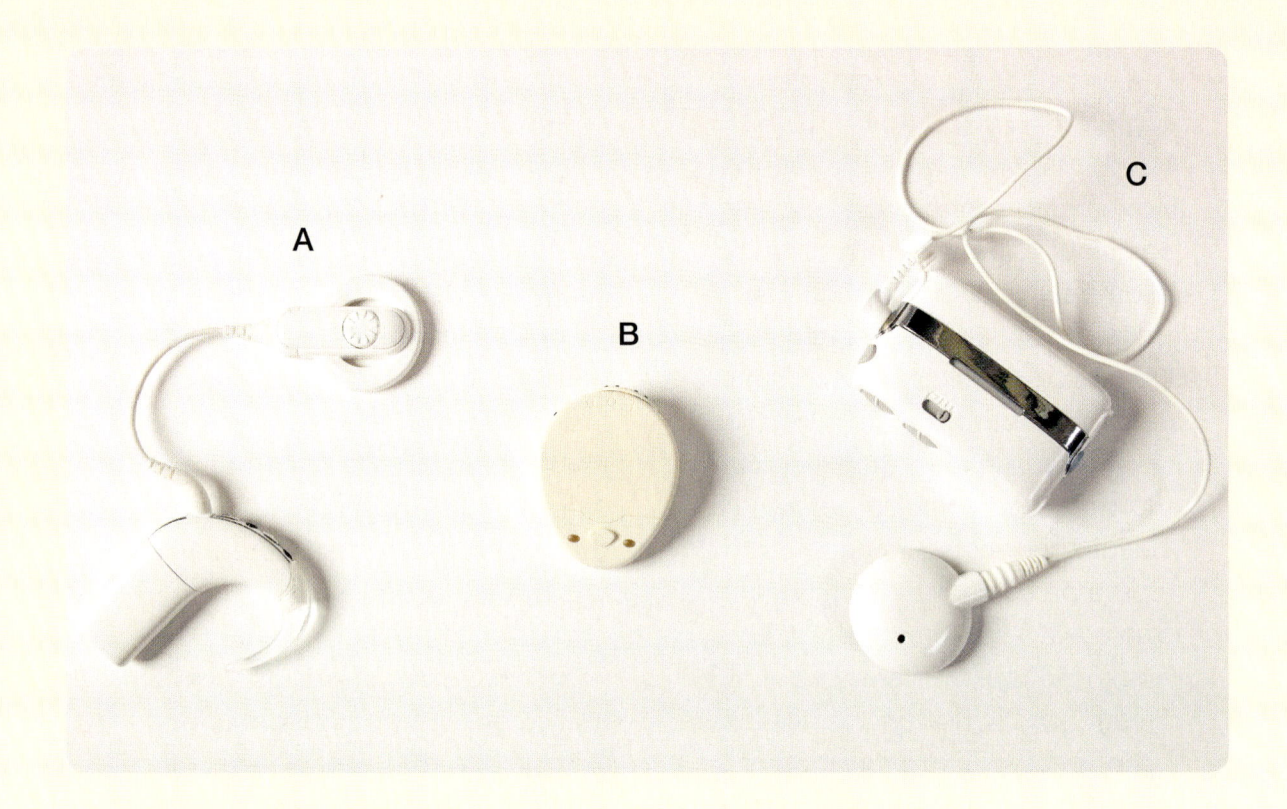

Above are three different external component styles for cochlear implants. Processors are most often worn behind the ear, similar to a large hearing aid (A). A newer style of processor incorporates the microphone, processor and transmitter into a single casing that is worn on the head over the internal receiver-stimulator (B). Yet another style of processor is worn using a clip pinned to a shirt, armband or hat (C).

At right is a typical receiver-stimulator used with the different types of cochlear implants. The receiver-stimulator receives impulses as radiofrequency waves from the transmitter. It relays the impulses as electronic signals through electrodes to the inner ear.

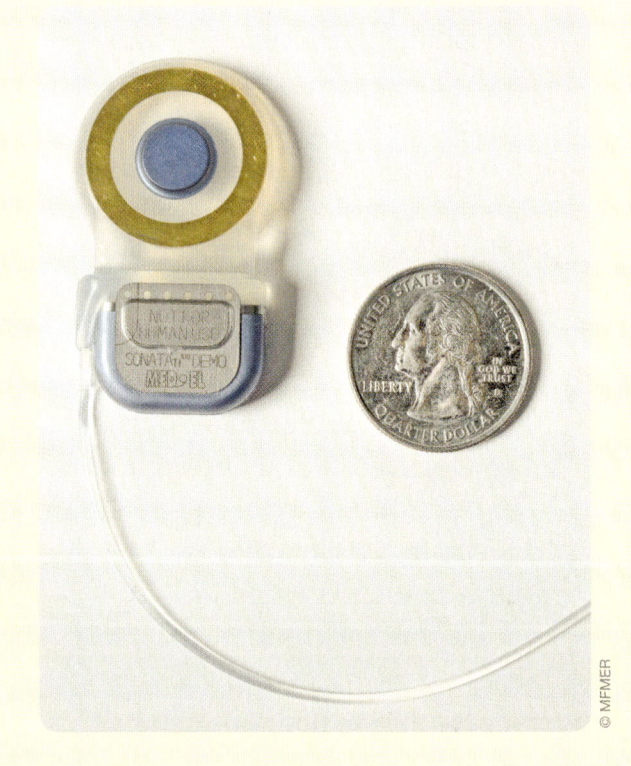

168 Chapter 8: Cochlear implants

Cochlear implants and the Deaf community

To the surprise of many people in the hearing world, many members of the Deaf community object to cochlear implants. For them, deafness isn't regarded as a disorder that needs to be treated or altered. They're often content within their unique culture, which includes a shared language (American Sign Language), social customs and lifestyle, and educational, economic, artistic and recreational institutions and organizations.

However, not all people who are deaf participate in Deaf culture. This has been a contentious issue for parents with children who are born deaf. Some parents have received negative reactions if they choose a cochlear implant for their children rather than resources of the Deaf community.

Headway has been made in reconciling the two perspectives because many people recognize the value of being fluent in both worlds. Deaf and hearing-impaired people can continue to remain part of Deaf culture, but a cochlear implant allows them to have greater participation in hearing culture. However, research also indicates that the more heavily you rely on sign language, the less benefit you'll likely receive from a cochlear implant.

If you have profound hearing loss, you may find it helpful to talk to people with different viewpoints, such as those who use cochlear implants, those who use both sign and spoken language, and those who oppose implants. Such discussions can help you better understand the different perspectives and choose the best option for yourself.

Candidates for a cochlear implant typically have moderate to profound sensorineural hearing loss in both ears or have great difficulty understanding speech. However, the criteria for implantation have changed significantly over the years. Recently, individuals with significant residual hearing remaining also are receiving implants. These implants, known as hybrid devices, combine the technology of a cochlear implant and a hearing aid in the same unit. Your audiologist can provide detailed information on this technology.

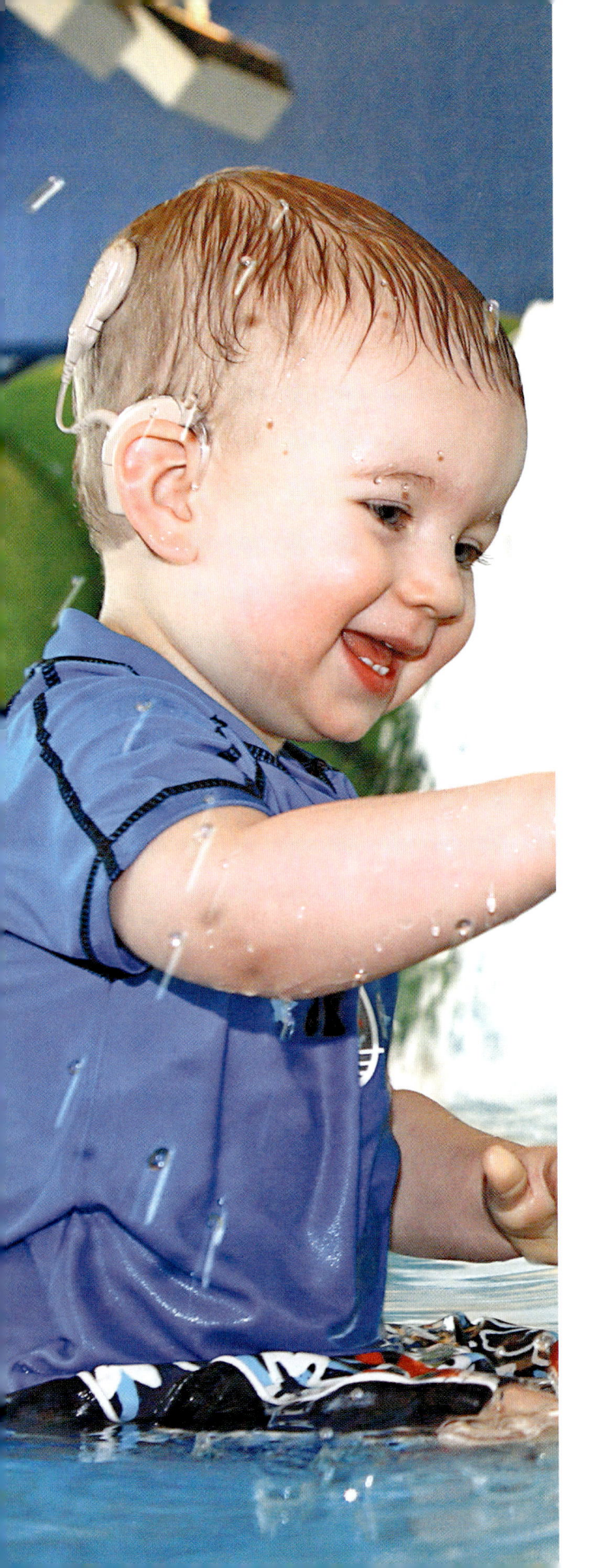

The earliest age for implantation in children can vary between centers. Although the FDA has offered guidelines for implantation in children as early as 12 months, some large centers have implanted children at 6 months.

In general, the younger a child is at the time of implantation, the less delay there will be in speech and language development — so long as appropriate therapy and education are provided after the procedure. Research indicates that getting a cochlear implant before age 2 typically provides the best outcomes.

Among adults, there's no upper age limit for implantation — even individuals in their 90s have received cochlear implants. Studies indicate that people older than age 65 can experience excellent outcomes, providing significant benefits for both communication and awareness of the environment.

In addition to having hearing loss, candidates for a cochlear implant must:

- Have realistic expectations — a clear understanding of the benefits and limitations of the implant

- Be willing to commit to the pre-implant evaluations and post-surgical follow-up services
- Be motivated for the change, with the support of family and friends
- Be committed to being a part of the hearing world

The decision to receive an implant should be made only after talking to a cochlear implant audiologist and an experienced cochlear implant surgeon.

Contributing factors

Although thousands of people have received cochlear implants, no one can predict how much a given individual will benefit from the procedure. The results depend on several factors:

Duration of hearing loss

Individuals who have experienced a relatively short period of moderate to profound hearing loss will typically adapt to an implant more readily.

In contrast, individuals who have had profound hearing loss since birth or at a young age typically have a harder time adjusting. In general, the shorter the duration of hearing loss, the better the outcome. Also, individuals with some residual hearing or progressive hearing loss tend to have better outcomes.

Auditory nerve fibers

People with a greater number of functioning nerve fibers in their cochlea may benefit more from a cochlear implant. No test can determine an exact number or location of functioning fibers, but imaging tests such as magnetic resonance imaging (MRI) and computerized tomography (CT) may provide valuable clues to the cochlear implant surgeon.

Sometimes, an electrical stimulation test can check if the auditory nerve will respond to small electrical signals.

Motivation

Much of the success of a cochlear implant depends on personal motivation and support. This commitment requires you to use the implant full time, maintain the equipment, keep follow-up appointments and take advantage of rehabilitation strategies.

Counseling is an important element of the implantation process. It can provide you with realistic expectations of the procedure. A cochlear implant is a tool, not a miracle cure. It will not restore normal hearing, but will give you the means to hear.

Benefits

According to reports from new users, hearing with a cochlear implant can range from "tinny" and "computer-like" to sounding almost normal. Generally, implant recipients notice the most improvement in their first year of using the device. But improvements can continue for many years after.

Generally, adult users are able to communicate more effectively and with less effort. Most recipients who are completely deaf are able to detect soft sounds, including low-level speech, and recognize many everyday noises.

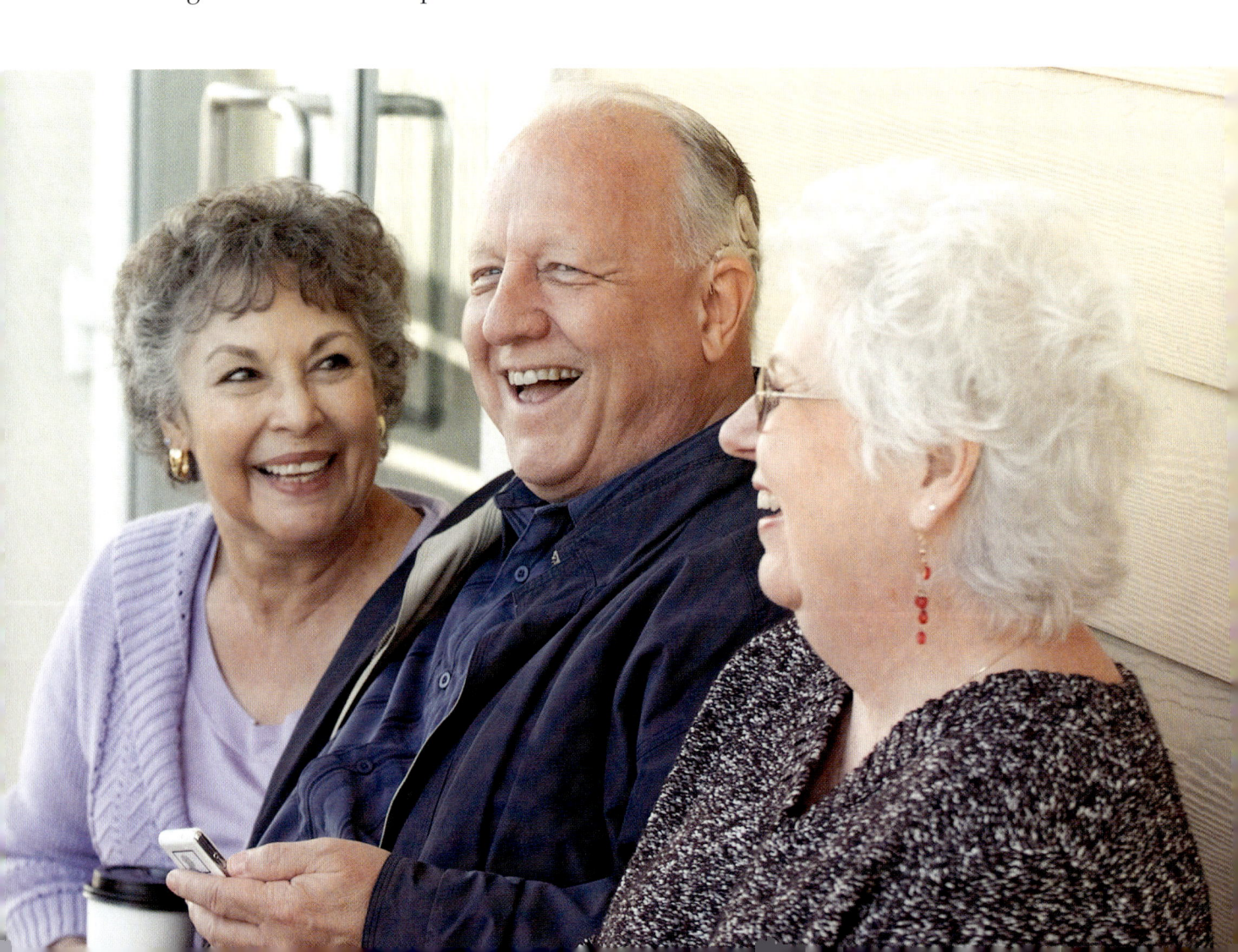

Some individuals can receive greater benefits from their implants. Detecting voices in an adjoining room, talking on the telephone and enjoying music is within the realm of possibility.

For many children, a cochlear implant has an impact on their potential to develop spoken language. Many can receive most of their education without the use of sign language or other methods of speech representation.

In general, adults with cochlear implants can understand about 70 percent or more of full sentences and about 55 to 60 percent or more of single words that are spoken. When the speech occurs in a personal conversation or within a familiar context, the level of understanding is even better — especially if the conversation is direct and face to face.

The implant procedure

A cochlear implant work-up starts with a thorough evaluation of your hearing, which will guide many decisions made by you and your doctor. After the device has been implanted and activated, a series of follow-up sessions are necessary for fine tuning of the device and speech perception testing.

Helping you through this process will be a team of specialists. Implant surgery is generally performed by an otolaryngologist, commonly known as an ear, nose and throat (ENT) doctor, or a neurotologist who has had specialty training in ear surgery. (However, not all otolaryngologists perform the procedure.) Other team members generally include an audiologist, speech-language pathologist, psychologist and educational consultant.

Your doctor can refer you to a cochlear implant center for evaluation. Cochlear implant centers are located throughout the United States and in other countries. There are many issues to consider as you proceed with implantation, and the initial testing these centers provide may help you.

Pre-implantation

A pre-implantation evaluation is undertaken by the implant team. The evaluation process can be stopped at any time that you or the implant team feel it's not appropriate to continue. The evaluation process includes the following tests:

Costly procedure

The cost of getting a cochlear implant — including pre-implant evaluation, surgery and hospital fees; medical personnel fees; implant hardware; and post-surgical fittings and training — is expensive, averaging around $60,000 for a single implant. Some estimates range from $40,000 to $100,000.

Unlike hearing aids, cochlear implants are covered by most private insurance plans, as well as Medicare and Medicaid programs. In some states, coverage is provided by children's special services, Tricare or state vocational rehabilitation agencies. Many patients receive the support of community or charitable organizations that hold special fundraisers, such as the Lions Club, Kiwanis, Sertoma and Jaycees.

Implant centers will likely have an insurance or reimbursement specialist who can help you determine the coverage provided by your health plan, and assist you with obtaining pre-authorization for coverage. It's important that you start the process early and allow your insurance company sufficient time to review your information before proceeding.

Medical evaluation
The ENT doctor will examine the health and function of your ear (otological examination) to ensure that no active infection or any type of abnormality precludes the use of an implant. An internist may be asked to do a general physical examination to make sure you can safely undergo general anesthesia.

Imagery
The physician reviews X-rays, computerized tomography (CT) scans and magnetic resonance imaging (MRI) to study the auditory nerve and to see if the cochlea is suitable for inserting implant electrodes.

Audiological evaluation
The audiologist performs an extensive series of hearing tests to determine how well you can hear with and without appropriately adjusted hearing aids. The audiologist will also help you understand the benefits and limitations for a cochlear implant.

Speech and language evaluation

A speech and language evaluation is done for children to assess their capacity to use cochlear implants to develop spoken language skills. A baseline of the child's development can be determined prior to surgery. The baseline results are essential for monitoring their development in follow-up sessions after surgery.

Psychological evaluation

Some people may benefit from a psychological evaluation that may help them cope with lifestyle changes following the procedure. Many issues could affect their satisfaction with the implant.

If the results from these evaluations indicate that you're a candidate for implantation, you can be scheduled for surgery. You and the surgeon will determine together which ear would be best for the implant.

The surgeon may recommend bilateral implants as your best option. It's becoming more common to implant devices in both ears of children and some adults. There's evidence that two implants help users identify the source of sounds and improve understanding of speech.

Before the surgery your implant team will discuss with you the benefits and limitations of a cochlear implant, care and use of the device, the surgery itself, and post-surgical follow-up. If you or a family member feels anxious during this process, feel free to ask questions and express your concerns.

Surgery

Cochlear implant surgery is performed under general anesthesia and lasts from one to four hours. Your doctor may do the procedure on an outpatient basis, or you may be asked to stay overnight.

After anesthesia is administered, the surgeon makes an incision behind the ear and exposes the mastoid bone. A small depression is created in the bone, and the receiver-stimulator is placed in this depression.

A portion of the mastoid bone is removed that allows access to the middle ear and the cochlea. A small opening is made in the cochlea, and tiny wires with the electrodes are inserted. Other times the surgeon inserts the electrodes through a natural opening called the round window.

Electronic tests are performed to make sure the stimulator is functioning properly with the intact nerve fibers. Then the incision is closed.

Cochlear implants and meningitis

Cochlear implant recipients are at a slightly greater risk of bacterial meningitis, an infection in the lining of the brain's surface. Although the risk is considered very small, the incidence is taken seriously and has been thoroughly studied.

The cause of meningitis in implant recipients hasn't been firmly established, but the design of earlier generations of implants is thought to be a factor. An implant, because it's a foreign body, may act as a breeding ground for infection — and the bacteria causing the infection may gain access to the brain via the pathway created by the implant electrodes. Some people may simply be more predisposed to meningitis due to abnormalities of the inner ear.

If you have a cochlear implant or are considering getting one, you should be vaccinated against the organisms that commonly cause bacterial meningitis. Pneumococcal vaccines are recommended for children and for adults older than age 65.

In the opinion of the Food and Drug Administration, the American Academy of Otolaryngology — Head and Neck Surgery, and the Center for Hearing and Communication, the cochlear implant remains a safe, effective device that provides many benefits. Thousands of recipients have had cochlear implantation with no adverse side effects.

When you wake up from anesthesia, you'll find a bulky bandage wrapped around your head. This will help reduce swelling around the incision.

You may experience some pain and nausea, but you can take medications for either form of discomfort. On the day of surgery, most people are able to get out of bed for short walks.

The day after surgery, the head bandage is removed. You may be given antibiotics to prevent infection, and will likely take prescription pain medication for the first three to four days.

Complications of cochlear implant surgery are uncommon. Some people report experiencing a bitter or metallic taste or other differences in their sense of taste immediately after surgery. But this sensation eventually goes away.

Because the surgery involves your inner ear, your system of balance may be disrupted. This can cause dizziness or vertigo, which will usually improve over the first three to four days, followed by a period of mild unsteadiness for a few weeks. By gently increasing activity, even though you may be slightly dizzy, your balance should gradually return to normal.

The nerve controlling facial expressions runs through the surgical area. Rarely, the nerve may be weakened after surgery due to temporary swelling. You may notice that your smile isn't quite straight or you have trouble closing an eyelid. These signs can be treated with cortisone-type medication.

It takes up to four weeks after surgery for the incision to heal. Most cochlear implant recipients are able to resume normal activity within a few days to two weeks after surgery. Once the incision heals, the implant is noticeable on the outside only as a slight bump to the touch.

Activation

A cochlear implant is inactive while it's being implanted. Deciding the time to activate the device signals the next step in the implantation process.

It's preferable to wait at least one to two weeks before activating a cochlear implant. This allows time for the incision to heal, and for you to recover from the anesthesia. You'll then meet several times with the audiologist to complete the process of fitting the external components and programming (mapping) the speech processor.

For some adults, activation soon after surgery may be an option. This recourse is taken to decrease anxiety about the procedure. But at the same time, early activation may be somewhat uncomfortable and programming the device less precise.

At your initial programming session with the audiologist, the headset or speech processor containing the microphone is placed on your head. The processor is connected to the audiologist's computer and programming equipment. The transmitter also is positioned, held in place by a magnet that couples with the magnet in the implanted receiver.

Care and handling

When you get a cochlear implant, members of your implant team will provide detailed instructions on how to take care of the external components of the system. The following tips may assist you:

- Try to avoid extreme heat and conditions that could cause breakage.
- Remove external components before participating in activities that generate high levels of static electricity, such as using trampolines or plastic slides. Like other electronic devices, the speech processor can be damaged by static electricity.
- You can wear the implant while participating in most sports. While it doesn't require extraordinary precautions, it's always a good idea to wear protective headgear for activities for which a helmet is recommended, such as bicycling, in-line skating, football and skiing.
- Turn off the speech processor before changing batteries, replacing cords or plugging something into it.
- Don't store batteries in the refrigerator. Putting a cold battery in a processor may cause condensation problems.
- Keep the microphone and processor in an anti-humidity kit when not in use. This is sometimes called a dryer or dry-aid kit.
- Most current controllers and processors are either water-resistant or waterproof. Depending on the processor, it may not be necessary to remove the external components before participating in water activities. Confirm with your implant team what to do when bathing or swimming.

The amount of electrical stimulation required for a hearing response will then be determined for some or all of the electrodes. You'll be asked to respond each time you hear a sound and to signal when the loudness of each sound is most comfortable.

The audiologist will feed the information you provide into special computer software that programs your speech processor. The speech processor is set to certain levels of stimulation for each electrode, based on your responses to the sounds.

After the programming is complete, the processor is disconnected from the audiologist's computer. Rechargeable or disposable batteries are inserted into the processor, and you're now able to take the system home.

Your audiologist will schedule more visits to fine-tune the speech processor. Repeated adjustments are necessary because it takes time for your auditory nerve to adapt to the signals from the electrodes and for your brain to interpret these signals. (See "An implant programming schedule" on page 180.)

Complete programming varies among different users and different implant systems. During the first year of use, the processor is reprogrammed often — you may have six or more appointments. Fewer visits are required after that. Experienced users usually visit just once a year.

Adjusting to an implant

Everyone who receives a cochlear implant seems to have a different experience. Some users quickly appreciate sounds they haven't heard for many years. Other users need a gradual period of adjustment.

Typically, the sounds you first hear with a cochlear implant will seem unnatural. Often, speech will be unclear and hard to understand. With time, however, these sounds become more familiar as your brain relearns how to hear with the implant.

The process of adjustment is slow and can take anywhere from weeks to years. Users who haven't had a long period of hearing loss can often understand speech rather quickly without speech reading. Users who have never had hearing before often need a longer time to adjust to the sounds.

Learning to listen and make sense of sound requires dedicated effort. It also requires consistent exposure to sound. Adjusting to a cochlear implant will be easier — and you'll gain greater benefit — if you wear the device full time.

Start out with easier listening situations, such as a conversation with one person in a quiet setting. With time, work up to more challenging situations, such as group conversations or listening in places where there's lots of background noise. Also practice listening to the radio and television.

Adult users can benefit from various support services. Working with an audiologist, speech-language pathologist or teacher of the hearing-impaired, you can practice identifying sounds, recognizing speech and using speech reading. Speech training can help you speak more clearly and with good voice quality.

Your training may include listening-only activities and practice with a telephone. You may be given instructions on how to continue auditory training at home. Many Web-based training programs are available over the Internet for free or at a marginal cost.

Rehabilitation training and education are essential for children who receive a cochlear implant. Without such training, a child will obtain only partial benefit from the device. Your child must learn to associate meanings to all of the new, unfamiliar sounds. Children must be taught to understand the sounds and integrate them into language.

Speech-language pathologists, educators and family members can help reinforce

An implant programming schedule

Below is the typical programming schedule for the first year of an adult receiving a cochlear implant.

- Initial stimulation (two sessions)
- Three weeks after activation
- Three months after activation
- Six months after activation
- Twelve months after activation

After the 12-month session, you may only need to have your implant programmed once every year or two.

The programming schedule recommended for children varies based on their developmental level.

the skills that your child is learning. The process takes time, dedication and a lot of hard work. But throughout childhood, training will usually continue to improve his or her performance.

Additionally, your audiologist or speech-language pathologist can provide you with other strategies to improve communication and handle difficult listening situations (see also Chapter 6).

Stay positive

Individual personality and many psychological factors can have strong impacts on your level of satisfaction with a cochlear implant. For example, whether you're a pessimist or an optimist, whether you carry moderate or high expectations of the procedure, and whether you have a weak or strong support network — all of these traits can influence your outcome with the implant.

You can boost your chances of success with a positive attitude. A person who's inflexible and pessimistic may look for — and find — all the wrong things about an implant, regardless of how well it functions.

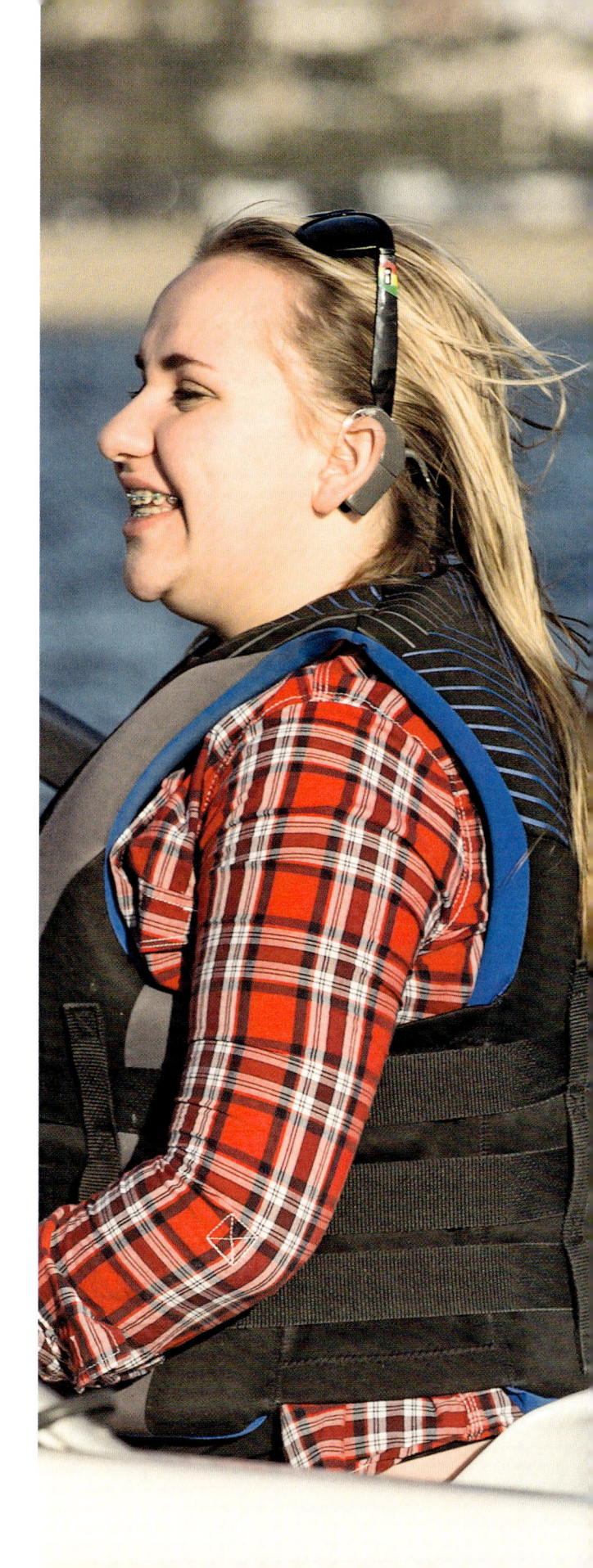

In contrast, an optimistic person will keep the adjustment period in perspective and focus on positive improvements that can be made. If you expect to hear speech clearly in the first days after your implant is programmed, you'll likely be disappointed.

A good support system is also very important. Let your family and friends know how they can help you succeed with an implant. You can also talk to your audiologist about any problems you're having as you adjust. At least once a year, return for a checkup at the cochlear implant center or clinic where you had your surgery.

Staying positive won't prevent you from experiencing a wide range of emotions about the implant, both positive and negative. Having the procedure triggers many emotions — and no one's reaction is the same. Whatever your experience, give yourself time to adjust and become used to hearing again. Most people adapt in their own way in their own time.

Chapter 9

Other options to communicate better

Hearing aids and cochlear implants are valuable tools if you have a hearing impairment. But other options, including special listening devices, wireless technology and even your cellphone, can help you in many challenging situations.

These technologies can resolve common problems you face every day and make your life easier and safer — by alerting you to a doorbell ring, by allowing you to listen to television at a reasonable volume and converse on the telephone, and by giving you the freedom to participate in different kinds of public events and activities.

The communication technologies aren't meant to replace hearing aids or cochlear implants. Rather they support these devices and enhance your hearing in difficult listening environments — such as noisy restaurants or lecture halls where sound reverberates. They allow you to lead a more independent and flexible lifestyle.

Special devices are especially useful for the times when you aren't wearing your hearing aids, such as when you're in bed or in the shower. They can alert you to sounds you need to be aware of, such as an alarm clock, smoke alarm or security alarm.

A variety of devices and services are available for you to use, both at home and in public places, including offices, restaurants, hospitals, places of worship, hotels, theaters, airports, trains, buses, libraries and courtrooms. Information desks and facility websites can help you find out what's available.

Under the Americans With Disabilities Act (ADA) and other legislation, public places are required to make reasonable accommodation for people who are deaf or hearing impaired. What is meant by "reasonable" may vary according to the type of establishment and the circumstances but may include different types of assistive listening devices, captioning services and alerting technology.

Assistive listening devices

Many situations in daily life can disrupt your ability to hear and to function effectively. Three factors are often involved, either alone or in combination, to cause the problem.

Noise. The hum of an air-ventilation system, traffic sounds or the scraping of chairs on the floor may prevent you from understanding what's being said. This can be even more challenging with the competing background noise of other people speaking, such as in a crowd or restaurant.

Reverberation. Confined areas that have many hard surfaces, concrete block walls or uncarpeted floors are likely to be reverberant — they easily echo sounds. The surfaces reflect sound waves multiple times, so the sound persists, even after the sound source is cut off.

Distance. The farther away you are from a speaker — or the farther off to the side you are — the harder it can be to hear. The best distance for hearing speech is between 3 and 6 feet.

Even with the help of hearing aids, these factors in certain environments will create severe acoustic difficulties. The environments include:

- Places with a lot of commotion and background noise, such as restaurants, cafeterias, lobbies, malls, subways and airports. An office can be a noisy place with the sound of foot traffic, conversation, manufacturing equipment, printers, copiers, telephones and radio.
- Situations where several people are talking at once, such as parties and social gatherings.
- Large rooms and facilities where a speaker may be far away, such as places of worship, classrooms, theaters and stadiums.
- Locations that are highly reverberant where sound waves echo, such as classrooms, hallways, basements,

open offices, worship halls, arenas and warehouses.
- Situations where a steady, constant background noise is created by a fan, air conditioner, traffic or wind. This type of noise includes travel noise from highways or rails when you're riding in a car or train.
- Outdoor activities where sound waves are dispersed, such as sporting events, festivals, parades, picnics and barbecues.
- Telephone conversations, especially when the connection isn't clear. These conversations are especially difficult because you can't use visual cues to improve your understanding.

Many of these environments are difficult, if not impossible, to avoid and hard to anticipate. Yet circumstances often require you to participate in them as you go about your daily life. Your ability to function effectively can benefit greatly from specialized technology developed specifically for these challenging environments.

Assistive listening devices (ALDs) are designed to improve your ability to hear in situations where conventional hearing aids aren't sufficient. ALDs are useful for many social, educational and entertainment activities, as well as for personal use at home.

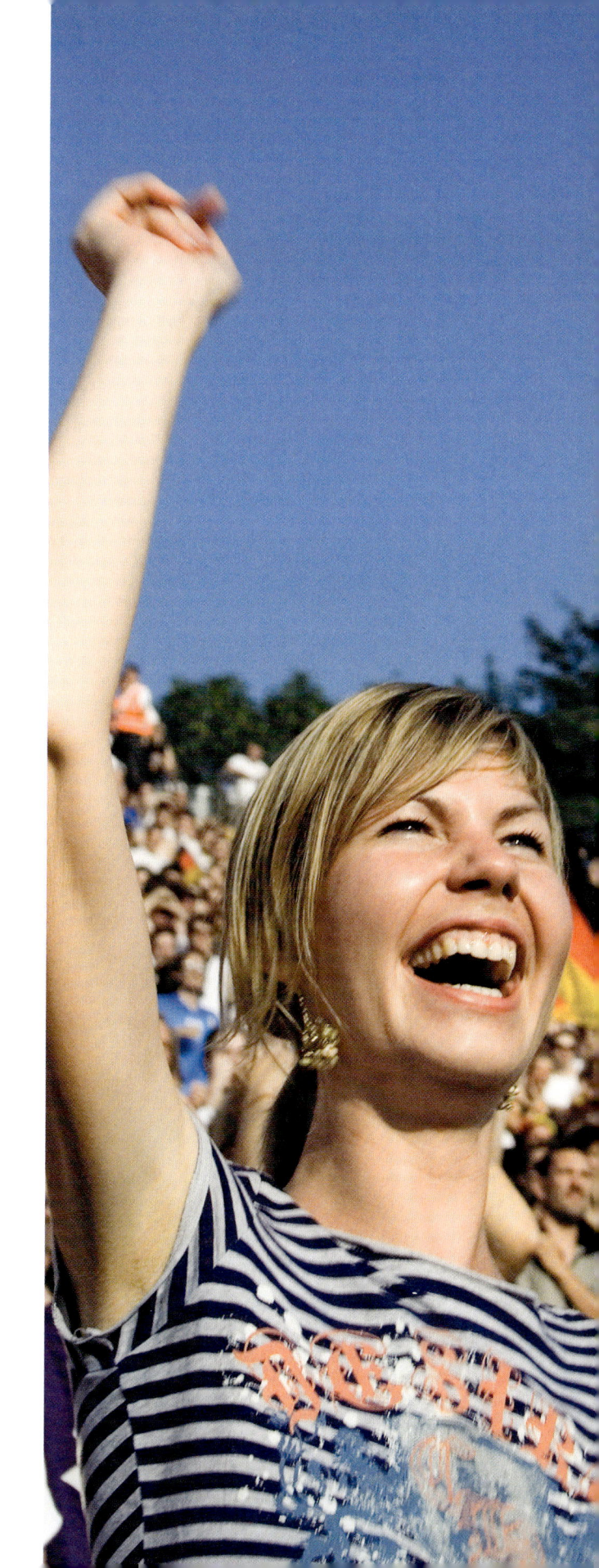

These devices can help you in noisy rooms and in group conversations. They make it easier to use a telephone. In addition, ALDs may be used in one-on-one conversations with a friend and for listening to television or radio while you're relaxing alone.

Several ALDs are designed for use in large rooms, where people with hearing loss may have trouble understanding a distant speaker at a podium or on a stage. Frequently, in these settings listeners face problems not only because of distance from the speaker but also because of reverberation and background noise.

In classrooms, teachers often move from side to side or turn away from the class, so the volume of their speech fluctuates. In these situations, asking the teacher to talk louder may not solve your problems. Turning up the volume

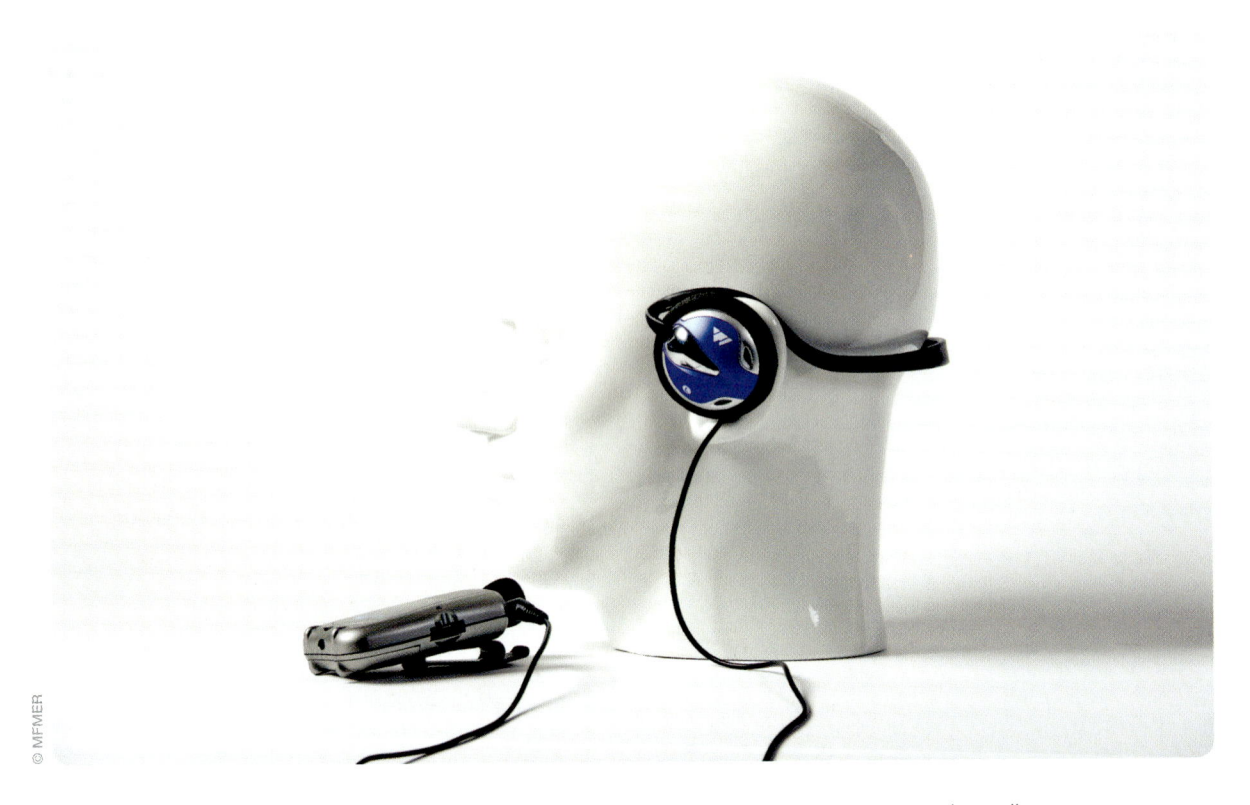

Personal amplifiers are a type of ALD used to increase volume in face-to-face and small group conversations. The small boxes have both a microphone and listening cord connected to them. Both talker and listener share the same device.

Buying ALDs and other communication aids

Many assistive listening devices (ALDs) are provided free of charge in public places. If you're planning to buy an ALD or another form of communication aid for personal use, discuss the different options with your audiologist. Various devices may be on display at a local audiological center or speech, language and hearing center, university, or community agency. Websites also offer a wide selection of products with in-depth information.

These devices vary in price, so it's wise to comparison shop and work with someone who's knowledgeable of the technology. Check the warranty before you buy — some products come with as much as a five-year warranty. The staff who dispense ALDs should provide you with training, including how to check and recharge batteries.

increases audibility, but it may not make speech more intelligible.

ALDs work by making the sound or signal you want to hear stand out from noises you don't want or need to hear. The signal might be a faraway voice coming over a static-filled telephone line, or a companion's voice that gets lost in the clatter of a noisy restaurant.

Although ALDs can usually amplify sounds, their primary purpose isn't to make sounds louder. Rather, they place a microphone close to the source of the sound you want to hear so that the sound is clearer and louder than other sounds in your environment.

ALD systems are equipped with different microphones, headphones and other features, but all systems are based on two components: a transmitter and a receiver.

The transmitter, located close to the person speaking, picks up the sounds and converts them to signals, then broadcasts the signals. Often, there's a direct hookup to a microphone.

The receiver, located close to a listener, picks up the signals and introduces them to the listener's ears. Receivers carried by different individuals in the same audience can pick up the same signal from a single transmitter.

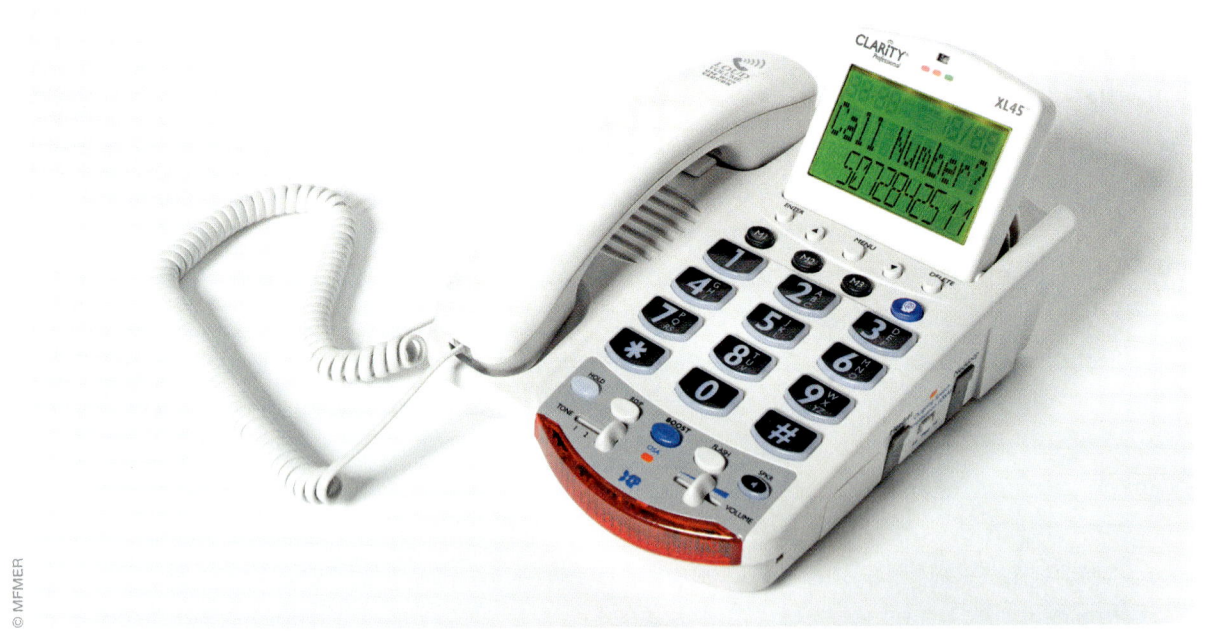

The controls at the bottom of an amplified telephone's body allow you to adjust the volume to your preference. A decal on the phone receiver indicates that this phone can amplify a speaker's voice.

Some ALDs are designed for use with hearing aids or cochlear implants. Many that are used with hearing aids require that the aid have a feature such as a telecoil (t-coil), telephone switch, hookup (port) for direct audio input or built-in Bluetooth compatibility.

Telephone devices

Using the telephone can be a special challenge. For one thing, a conventional telephone doesn't amplify sound loud enough for individuals with hearing loss. For another thing, the listeners can't see the speaker and therefore aren't able to use visual cues to help their understanding.

One of the most common and useful ALDs is a telephone amplifier, which may be used with a cellphone or with a wired, cordless or digital phone. The amplifier allows a user to adjust the volume of incoming calls so that even soft voices can be heard. It also allows a person with no hearing loss to easily use the device as well.

188   Chapter 9: Other options to communicate better

Many new telephones come directly from the manufacturer with a built-in amplifier. An amplifier may be installed in the telephone body or in the handset when the mouthpiece, receiver and buttons are included as one unit. An amplifier may also be added as an in-line unit between the telephone and wall jack.

Amplifier handsets may be installed in some public telephones, particularly at airports, train stations, museums and galleries, and hotel lobbies. A special telephone access sign on the receiver will identify whether amplification service is available.

Portable, snap-on amplifiers are small, battery-operated devices that can be carried with you in a purse or briefcase. When you're in situations where it's unlikely that you'll find a phone with an amplifier handset, you can slip the device over the receiver of most telephones. These portable amplifiers are especially helpful when you're traveling and on the run.

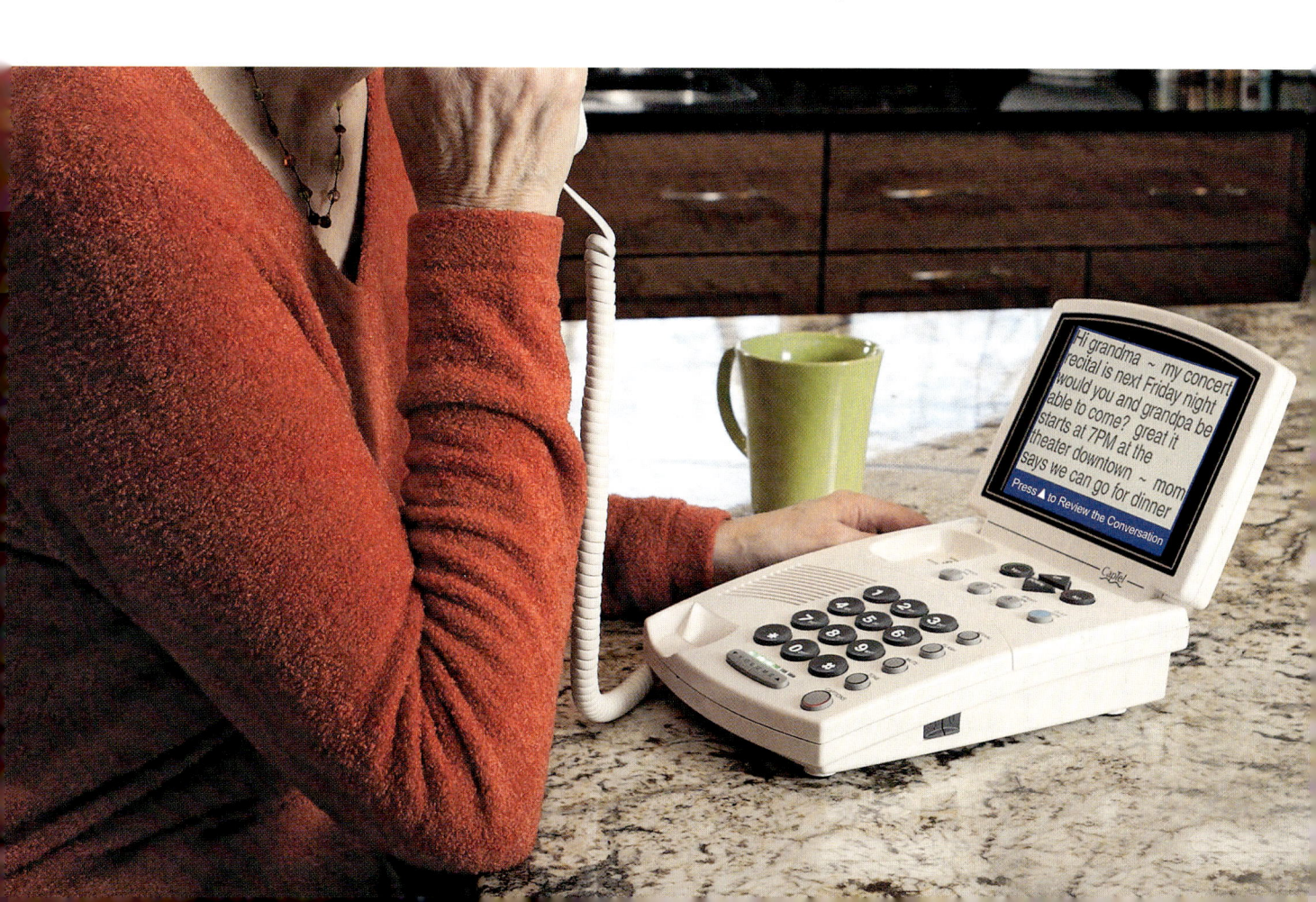

Telephone adapters are also portable devices that work with the telecoil in your hearing aids or cochlear implants. The adapter doesn't amplify sound but instead generates an electromagnetic field in response to sound waves. This allows the telecoil to pick up the sound directly. An adapter may work with some phones that aren't compatible with portable amplifiers.

When purchasing a new phone, be sure to verify with the supplier if the phone is compatible with a telecoil or portable amplifier.

Some telephones have special ringers that produce either an extra-loud ring or variable rings. Call indicators use a flashing light to inform you of incoming calls. Speakerphones can be useful in certain situations because they allow a person with hearing loss to listen with both ears.

Telecommunications Relay Service

People with severely limited hearing or no hearing at all can't use a standard telephone, even with an amplifier or adapter. They can still communicate over phone lines, however, by using a Telecommunication Relay Service (TRS).

TRS is a public service that comes at no cost to its users — the Americans With Disabilities Act requires U.S. telephone companies to provide the service free throughout the country. The phone companies are compensated with either state or federal funds.

Using TRS requires an individual with hearing loss to have a special phone that's equipped with a keyboard and text display monitor — a text telephone, or TDD — or a captioned telephone (see page 191). Certain types of relay services can also function with a personal computer.

TRS provides real-time communication by adding a third-party operator, called a communications assistant (CA), into your phone conversation. The CAs are on call 24 hours a day at TRS relay centers located throughout the country.

You provide the CA with the telephone number to be called, either by speaking it into the handset or by typing and sending it via the keyboard. The CA places the call and then relays the spoken and written messages back and forth between you and your correspondent.

The CA quickly converts spoken or written words into either text or voice. CAs are trained to be unobtrusive and to relay your conversations exactly as they're received. All calls through TRS are strictly confidential.

Telephones for hearing impairment

If you have severe or profound hearing loss, using text-to-voice or captioned forms of TRS with a communications assistant requires that you have a special telephone with a display screen for text.

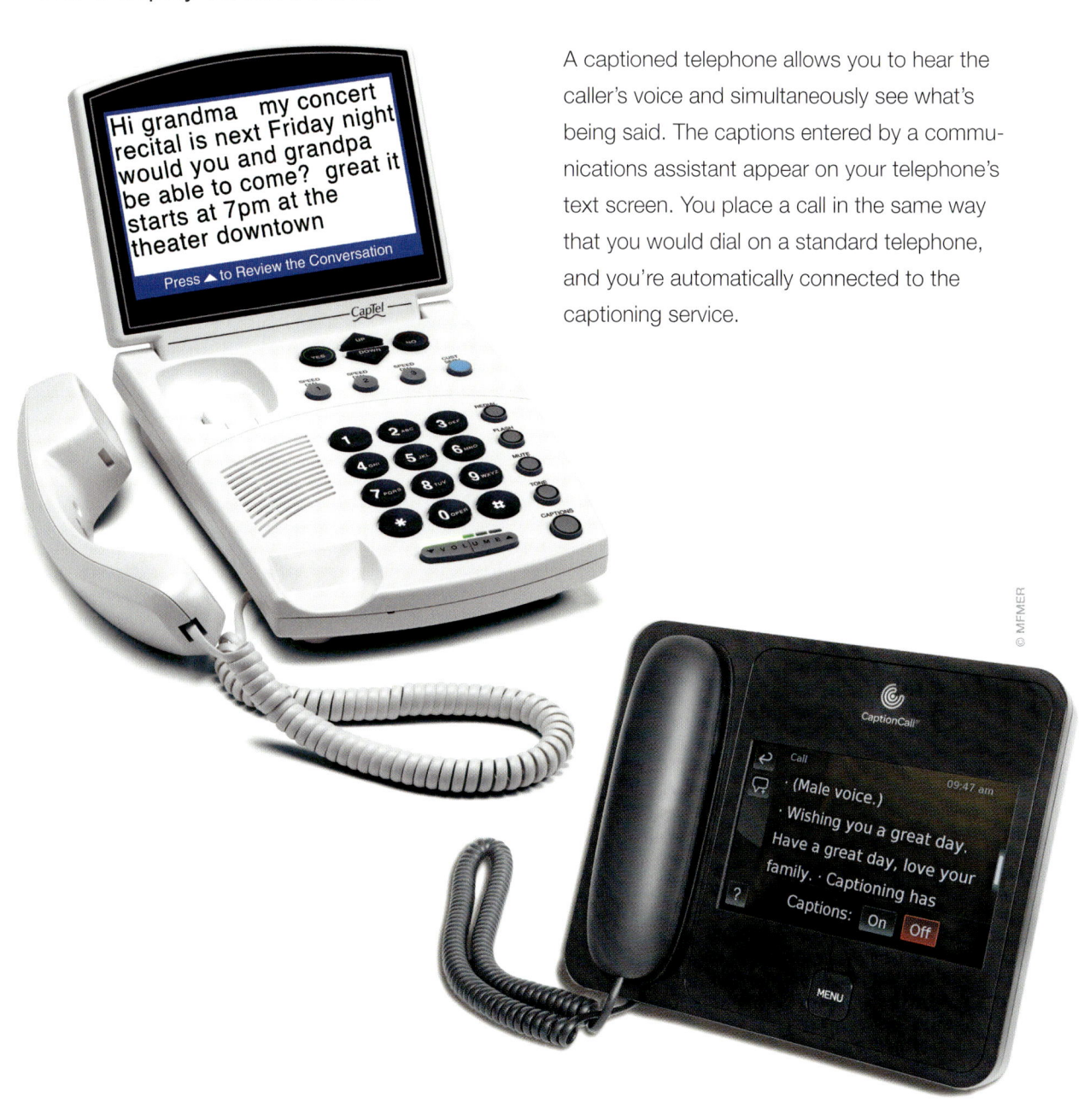

A captioned telephone allows you to hear the caller's voice and simultaneously see what's being said. The captions entered by a communications assistant appear on your telephone's text screen. You place a call in the same way that you would dial on a standard telephone, and you're automatically connected to the captioning service.

Mayo Clinic on Better Hearing and Balance

The Telecommunications Relay Service is easy to use. Anyone can initiate a call by dialing 711 — the number that the federal government has reserved for access to TRS. Callers pay only the normal cost of a phone call.

There are several forms of TRS to consider, depending on your hearing loss and your personal preference:

Text-to-voice
This is the standard method of TRS service, with a CA serving as an intermediary between the spoken and written portions of the phone conversation. The CA speaks what a text user types and types what a voice telephone user speaks.

A voice-carry-over (VCO) option allows a person with hearing loss to speak directly to the other person instead of corresponding through a CA. Similarly, with Hearing Carry Over (HCO) a person with speech impairment can still hear the other party's voice and then relay a typed response through the CA.

Captioned service
This form of TRS uses voice recognition technology to convert the CA's spoken voice into written text. The captions are transmitted directly to a text display screen on your telephone.

Internet protocol (IP) relay service
With this Internet-based form of TRS, a call goes from your computer to an IP relay center, which is usually accessed from a Web page. The CA relays your message via spoken voice over the regular telephone network.

You're not required to have a text or captioned telephone to use this service. A computer or any other web-enabled device such as a cellphone will do. The service connects directly to many forms of instant messaging and wireless text messaging programs.

IP-captioned telephone service combines the Internet-based system with a captioned telephone display. You speak directly to the called party and can listen to the response. At the same time, the CA repeats what's being said and speech recognition technology allows you to see the words almost instantaneously on your computer display.

Video relay service (VRS)
Another Internet-based form of TRS is a bridge between individuals using sign language and individuals using spoken English. A CA communicates with the sign language user via a computer monitor and video equipment. However, not all state TRS programs offer this service.

Multipurpose communication devices

Advances in computer hardware and electronics continue to create smaller and more-adaptable devices. This helps make many communication aids more portable, flexible and convenient.

Single devices have been developed that combine multiple functions. For example, a device that may look and function as a hearing aid — when needed — is also capable of other functions, serving as your wireless telephone with access to the Internet, voice mail and more.

Wireless technology takes these developments a step further. Wireless networks use low-power radio waves to link computers and other devices together — no wires or cable hookups are required for them to communicate. Generally, the different units must be located close together.

Bluetooth technology can connect as many as eight different devices together at the same time. That means

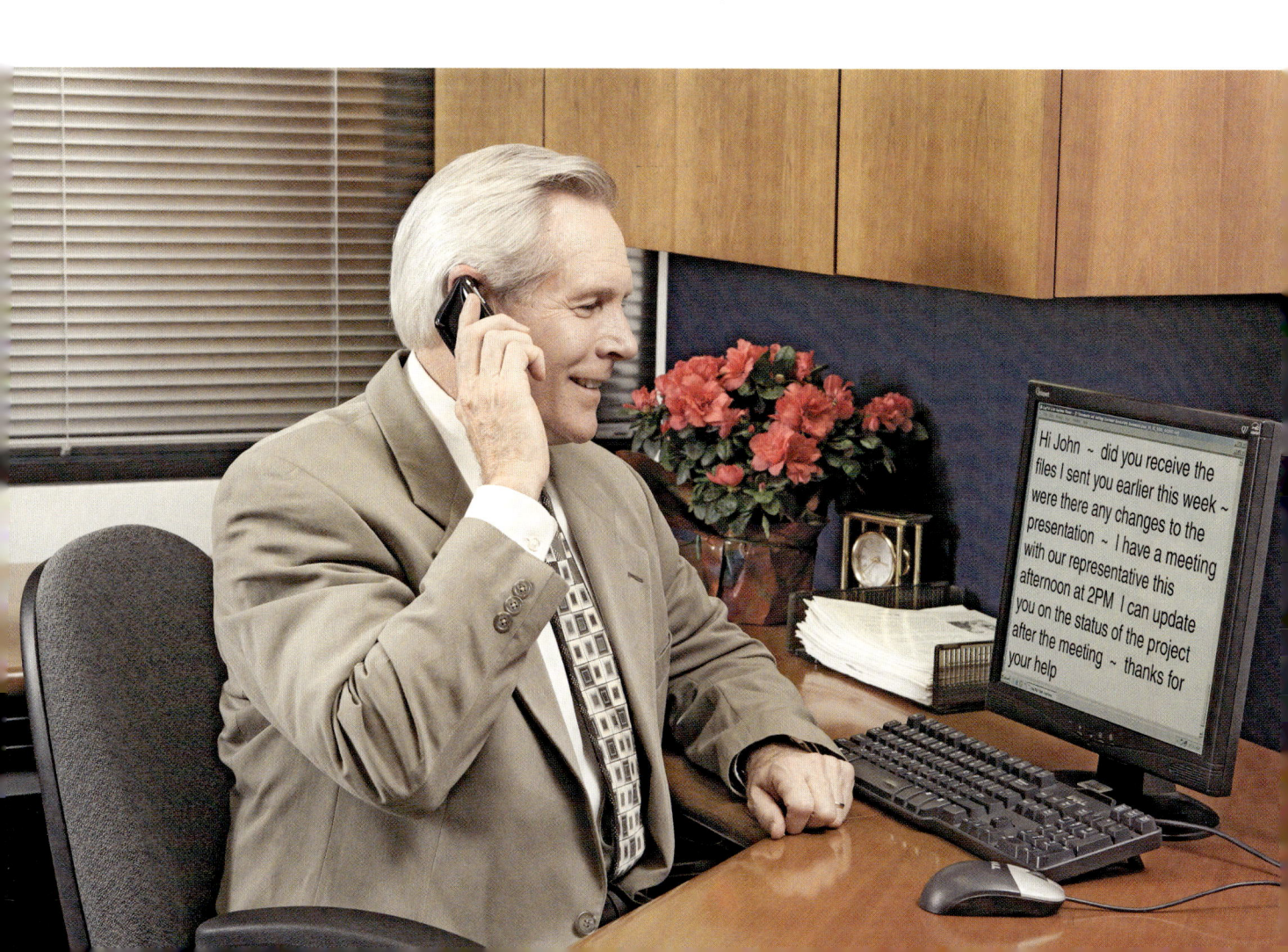

— so long as all the devices are Bluetooth-enabled — your hearing aid, computer, telephone and music player can be interacting simultaneously.

Text messaging

Cellphones have become exceedingly popular communication tools worldwide. People use these portable, easy-to-use devices not only for phone calls but also for checking email, taking pictures, accessing the Internet, and playing music and games.

Text messaging is another popular use of cellphones. Using the phone keypad as a keyboard, you can type text messages into your phone — generally up to 160 characters — and send them to one or more other phones. This means of communication is also known as Short Message Service (SMS).

SMS is a valuable tool for people with moderate to profound hearing loss, particularly because use is so quick and simple. You're able to communicate just about anywhere with many more people, and you're not tied to a TDD or computer. Furthermore, cellphones are so common that they call little attention to the fact that you have hearing loss.

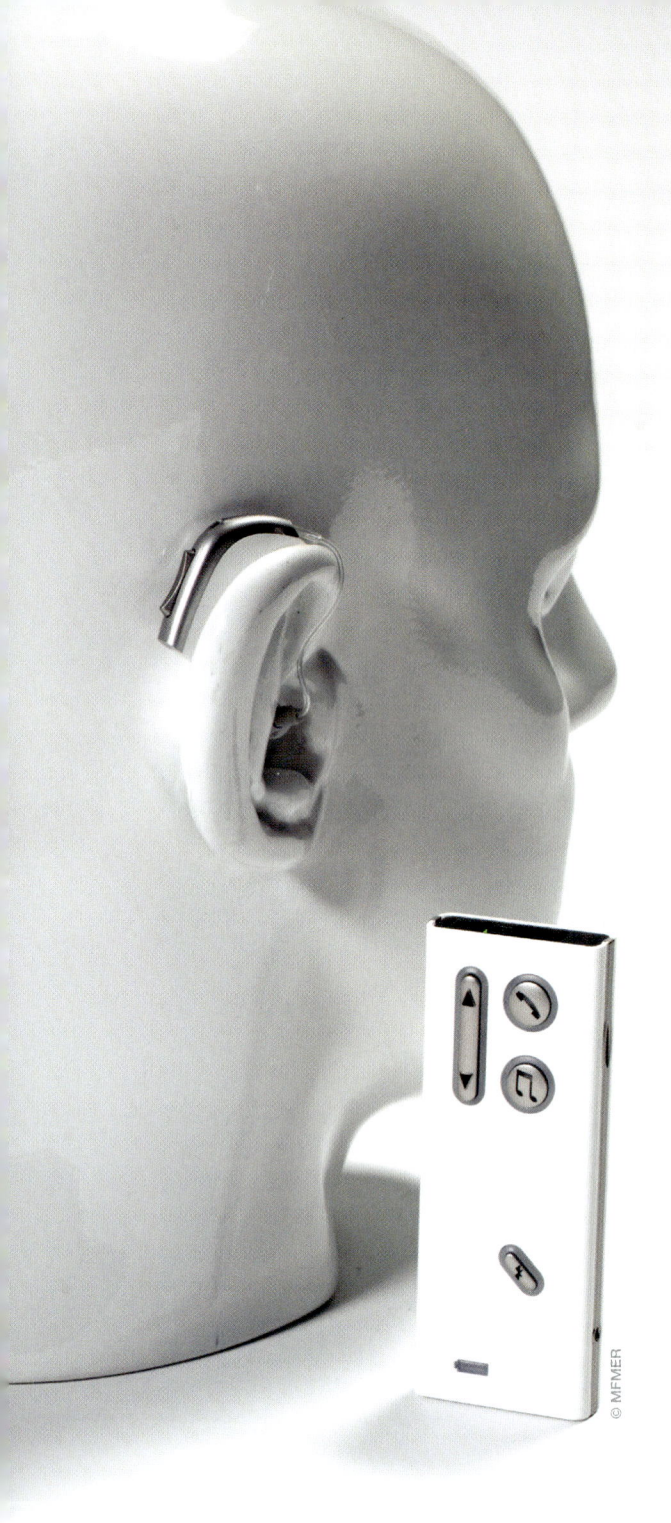

The push of a button on this remote connects your hearing aid to the telephone or allows you to listen to music from your portable music player without any direct hookup.

Hearing aids and cellphones

To make cellphones more accessible, the Federal Communications Commission (FCC) has approved standards for the use of digital wireless devices with hearing aids and cochlear implants in the Hearing Aid Compatibility (HAC) Act of 1988. The standards are meant to designate phones that produce less static and interference and have better telecoil connections.

A HAC-compliant cellphone will be marked with an M or T rating. The M refers to phone use when the hearing aid is set to microphone. Cellphones that work well with hearing aids will have a rating of M3 or M4.

The T refers to phone use when the hearing aid is set to telecoil. If you use a hearing aid or cochlear implant with a telecoil, look for a cellphone with a rating of T3 or T4.

Cellphones that are HAC compliant should be labeled as such. Look for the label in one of these places:

- On a card next to the display phone
- On the phone's package
- In the user manual

If these ratings are not marked on the package, ask your service provider or the device manufacturer. But most likely, if you can't find the label in any of these places, the phone isn't HAC compliant.

Other features you might want to consider in a cellphone include vibrating alerts or a flashing screen, text messaging services, TDD mode, speech-to-text and video streaming.

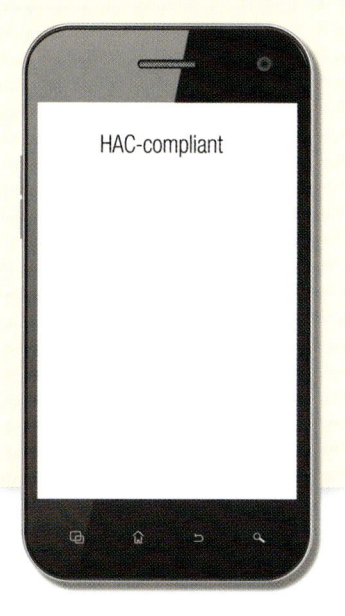

A drawback of this technology is that some cellphones can cause interference with hearing aids — typically resulting in a buzzing sound. However, this is less of a concern with phones that are compatible with hearing aids. See page 195 for more information.

Assistive listening systems

Assistive listening systems improve the sound quality and volume of public address systems for people with hearing loss. One of 3 systems generally will be installed in public places for this purpose: FM, infrared and induction loop.

FM systems

At public speaking events, you may be seated at some distance away and not directly in front of the speaker. The amplification system may be poor quality, and the audience members may move about and talk among themselves. Despite these conditions, you may still be able to hear the speaker clearly with the help of special listening systems, such as an FM system.

You may be familiar with the letters *FM*, which mean "frequency modulation," from tuning your radio to a specific frequency in order to hear your favorite music or talk show. FM listening systems transmit sounds via radio waves, just like a miniature radio station. They operate on special radiofrequencies assigned by the Federal Communications Commission (FCC). FM systems are commonly installed in locations where large audiences gather, such as auditoriums, convention centers, places of worship, museums and theaters.

An FM system consists of two main components: A transmitter and a receiver. The transmitter can broadcast anything from a microphone, radio, television or stereo. It sends an FM signal to a small portable receiver that is tuned to the correct FM frequency.

Receivers come in several forms. Listeners can use a receiver that has volume control and converts the signal to sound via headphones. Another option is to have a receiver attached to a looped cord of wire (neck loop) that converts the FM signal into electromagnetic waves that are picked up by a telecoil in a hearing aid or cochlear implant. Other receivers can be attached to a small adaptor (boot) that attaches to some behind-the-ear hearing aids or cochlear

Assisted listening systems

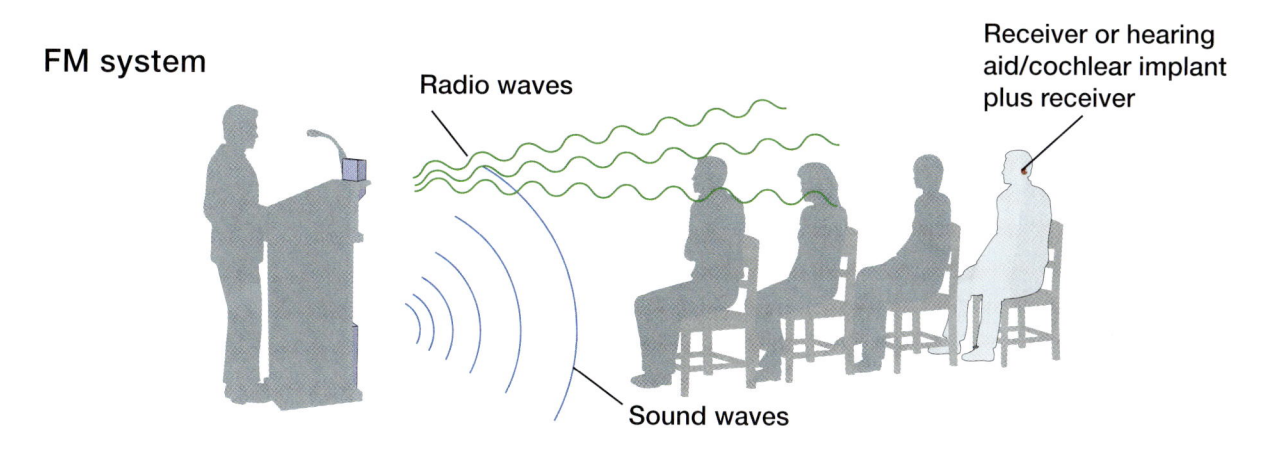

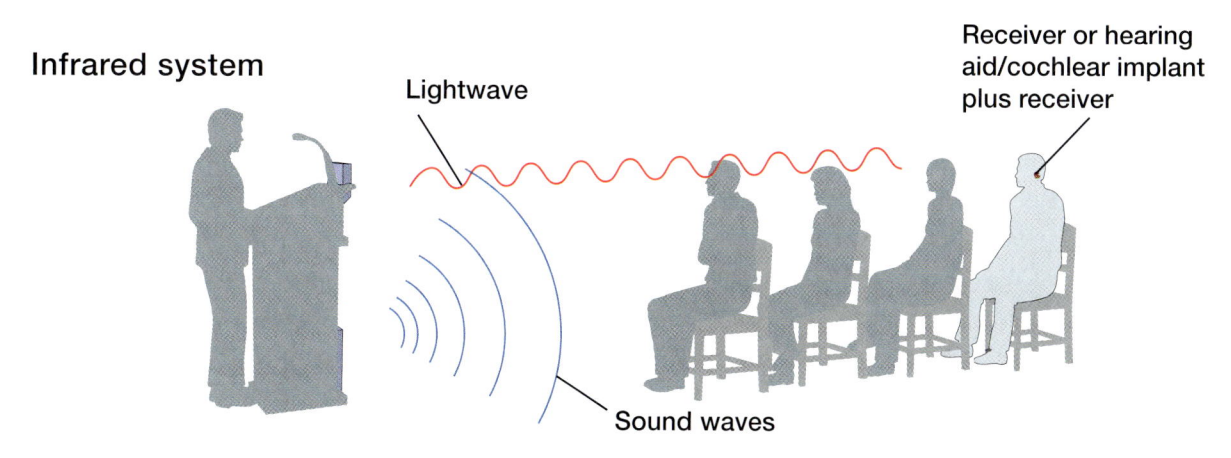

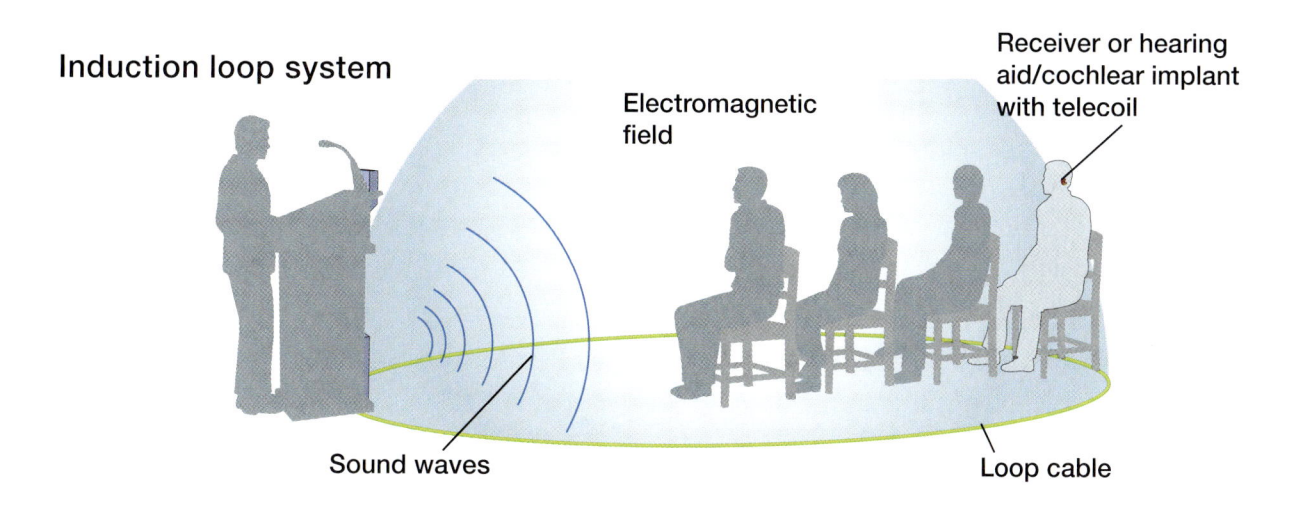

FM system

Radio waves

Receiver or hearing aid/cochlear implant plus receiver

Sound waves

Infrared system

Lightwave

Receiver or hearing aid/cochlear implant plus receiver

Sound waves

Induction loop system

Electromagnetic field

Receiver or hearing aid/cochlear implant with telecoil

Sound waves

Loop cable

Mayo Clinic on Better Hearing and Balance

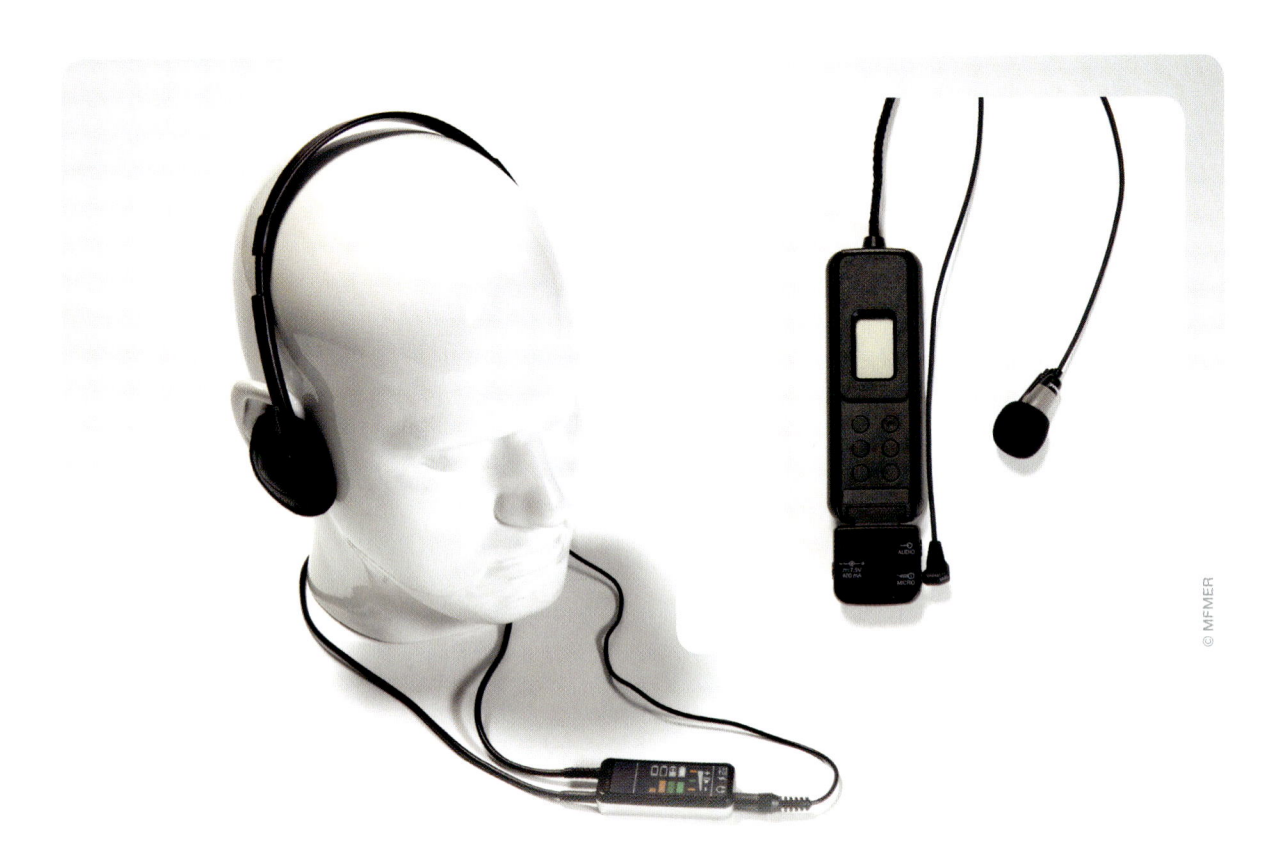

In a setting with a large audience, such as a classroom, an FM system with a transmitter and microphone (right) allows speakers to send their voices directly to you through a receiver that you wear with headphones (left) or hearing aids.

implants and sends the signal directly to the hearing aid or implant. This is known as Direct Audio Input (DAI).

Personal FM systems can be used for one-on-one communication. Composed of a small, portable microphone, receiver and amplifier, they're useful for private conversations in difficult hearing environments such as noisy restaurants or highly reverberant auditoriums. As long as you're tuned to the correct frequency, you can use personal systems while you're walking or in a car, and you can use them to listen to television and radio stations.

A growing number of public buildings, government facilities and business offices are equipped with FM systems to accommodate hearing-impaired visitors. Many schools also are using FM

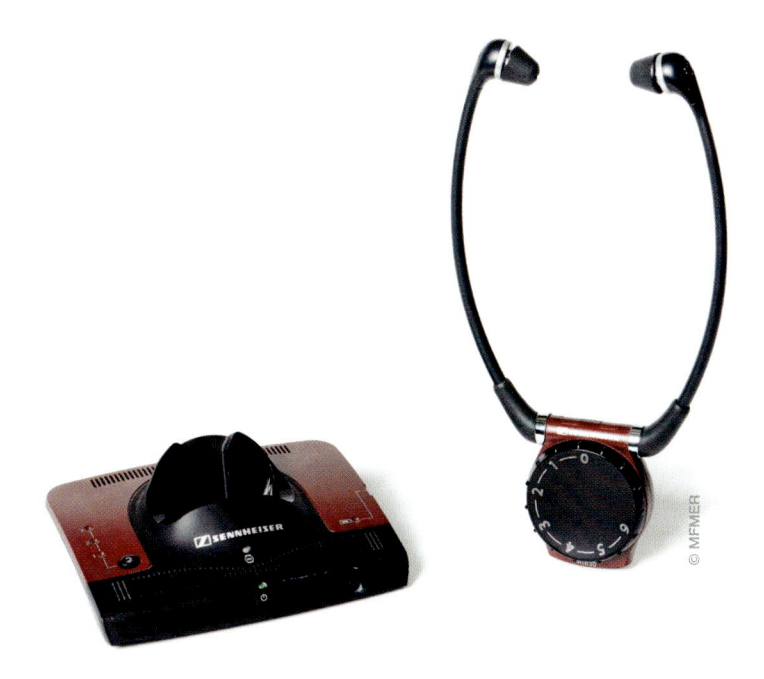

Infrared systems send sounds, for example from a television program, directly to you from a unit that sits on the television (left). A lightweight headset that you wear (right) lets you adjust the device to a volume that you need for hearing while keeping the TV at a volume that's comfortable for others.

technology to assist students with hearing impairment. A newer version of these systems, known as Dynamic FM, further filters the signal and uses directional microphones to reduce noise, among other features.

Infrared systems

Radio waves aren't the only medium available to carry sound in assistive listening systems. Infrared systems transmit sound via lightwaves to receivers worn by hearing-impaired listeners.

Like FM systems, infrared systems are used in locations where hearing is difficult or in situations where large groups of people are gathered. Infrared technology is also commonly available for TV viewing at home.

When this system is used in a large auditorium, an infrared light emitter is plugged into an existing public-address system or sound system. The infrared lightwaves transmit speech or music to receivers that are worn by members of the audience. The receiver may be connected to headphones that

Mayo Clinic on Better Hearing and Balance **199**

Using your hearing aid's telecoil

Many behind-the-ear and in-the-ear hearing aids are equipped with a telecoil (t-coil). The telecoil is helpful for listening on the telephone. Normally, a hearing aid is sensitive to all sound waves. But when the telecoil is turned on, the aid amplifies only electromagnetic waves from the telephone's receiver. This means that the telephone signal is transmitted directly into the hearing aid without any other noise being amplified.

Most phones are compatible with hearing aids, but when you buy a phone, be sure to ask about hearing aid compatibility. If the salesperson doesn't know, try out the phone before buying it. A compatible unit should be labeled HAC on its base. More information about HAC compliance and other standards for mobile phones is on page 197.

The telecoil can also be used with FM systems (see page 196) and induction loop systems (see page 201).

Having a hearing aid with a telecoil broadens your communication options. If your hearing aid has a telecoil and you aren't sure how to use it, consult your audiologist or hearing aid dealer for training.

introduces sound directly to the ear. Or the receiver can be used with a neck loop linked to a hearing aid or cochlear implant equipped with a telecoil.

Using an infrared system with a television allows you to set the TV at a volume that's lower and more comfortable for other listeners. The infrared transmitter sends the TV signal to a personal receiver, which you can adjust to as loud a volume as you need. But your adjustments don't affect the volume level heard by others in the room.

Unlike an FM system, an infrared receiver must be in the transmitter's direct line of broadcast in order to function well. Sunlight can interfere with the signal, so these systems aren't a good choice for outdoor use.

In contrast, because infrared lightwaves are broadcast along a confined path and not emitted in all directions, infrared systems provide more privacy than FM systems do. Infrared systems are often used in courtrooms and government offices and during live performances in theaters and auditoriums.

Induction loop systems

Induction loop systems, also called audio loop systems, transmit sounds using an electromagnetic field created by a loop of wire installed around the listening area. An amplifier and microphone transmit sound via an electric current that flows through the loop. Hearing aids and cochlear implants equipped with telecoils can receive these signals. Separate receivers can be provided to people who don't have the telecoil feature in their hearing aids or cochlear implants.

Induction loop systems can be permanently installed in the floors of large auditoriums or chambers. Portable, temporary loop systems may be set up as needed. Reception with these systems is susceptible to electrical interference. Also, they're not as flexible for personal use as FM systems and infrared systems are.

Captioning

Until the early 1970s, many people with hearing loss weren't able to fully enjoy one of America's favorite pastimes — watching television. In 1972, for the first time, a national TV program — Julia Child's cooking show, *The French Chef* — was broadcast with captions that reflected the audio portion of the show.

Since that broadcast, captions have opened the world of television to people who are deaf or hearing impaired. Hundreds of hours of entertainment, news, public affairs and sports programming are captioned each week on network, public and cable TV.

Similar to movie subtitles, television captions display dialogue as printed words on the screen. Unlike subtitles, captions also indicate sounds such as noise, music and laughter. The text is carefully positioned on the screen to identify who is speaking. Captions are encoded as data within the television signal, ready for immediate broadcast.

Captions may be displayed as open or closed. Open captions appear on all TV screens and can be viewed without a special decoder. Closed captions aren't

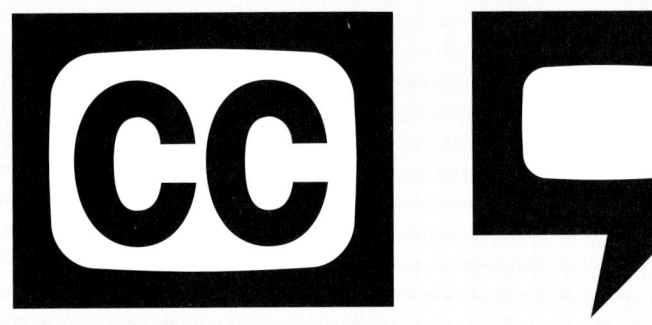

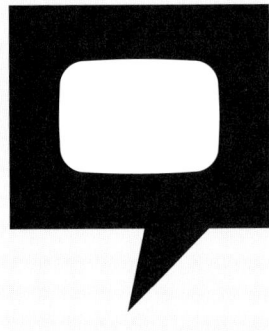

Either of these symbols indicate that a television program is closed-captioned.

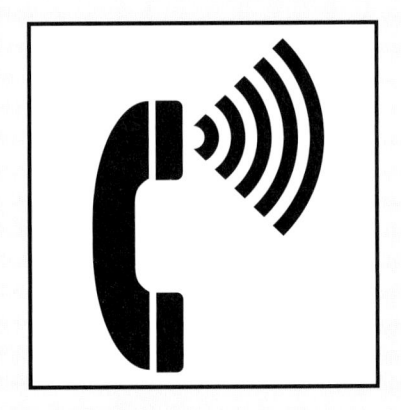

Amplified telephone

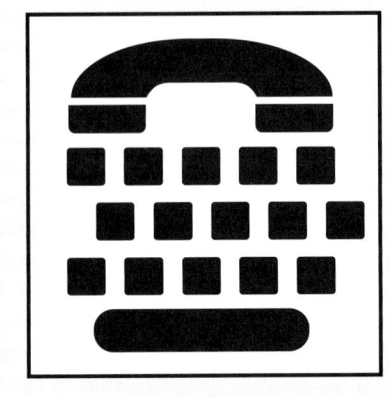

Text telephone

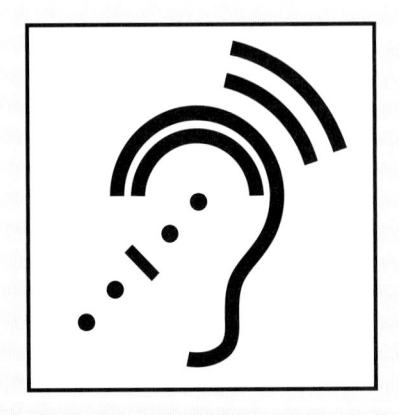

Assistive listening system

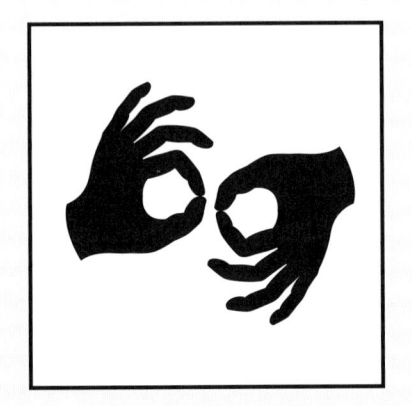

Sign language

When these international symbols appear in public buildings, it means services have been installed for individuals with hearing loss.

Chapter 9: Other options to communicate better

visible on a standard screen. To display the captions, you need a television with a built-in decoder or an added decoder that sits on top of the set.

With either form of decoder, you turn the captions on or off with the touch of a button on the remote control. Since 1993, all television sets with screens 13 inches or larger sold in the United States have built-in decoder circuitry. Because of the widespread availability of closed-captioning, open captions are rarely used.

You can tell if a specific program is closed-captioned when the letters CC appear on the screen, often within a television-shaped symbol. Another symbol shows a small TV screen with a tail at the bottom (see page 202).

Other uses of captioning

Captioning is included on many movies that are for sale or rent on DVD and Blu-ray Disc. It's also featured on many educational and training films.

Captioning is provided for many live events, such as musical and theater performances, lectures, government proceedings, meetings and conferences. Museums and science centers may use captioning in their self-produced films, demonstrations and shows.

Some movie theaters offer a captioning system called Rear Window Captioning. An adjustable transparent plastic panel attaches to the viewer's seat and reflects captions displayed on a panel positioned at the back of the theater.

Alerting devices

Assistive technology can alert you to many special sounds in your environment. Awareness of these sounds is important for your safety and to maintain your independent lifestyle. Sounds that can be signaled include a telephone ring, alarm clock buzz, kitchen timer beep, doorbell chime, a knock at the door, the cry of a baby, and the peal of a smoke alarm or security alarm.

Alerting devices may use one or more of three types of signal to inform you of the sound — an amplified sound, a flashing light or a vibration.

For example, an alarm clock can be wired with a vibrating attachment that's placed under your pillow. At the selected hour, you're gently shaken

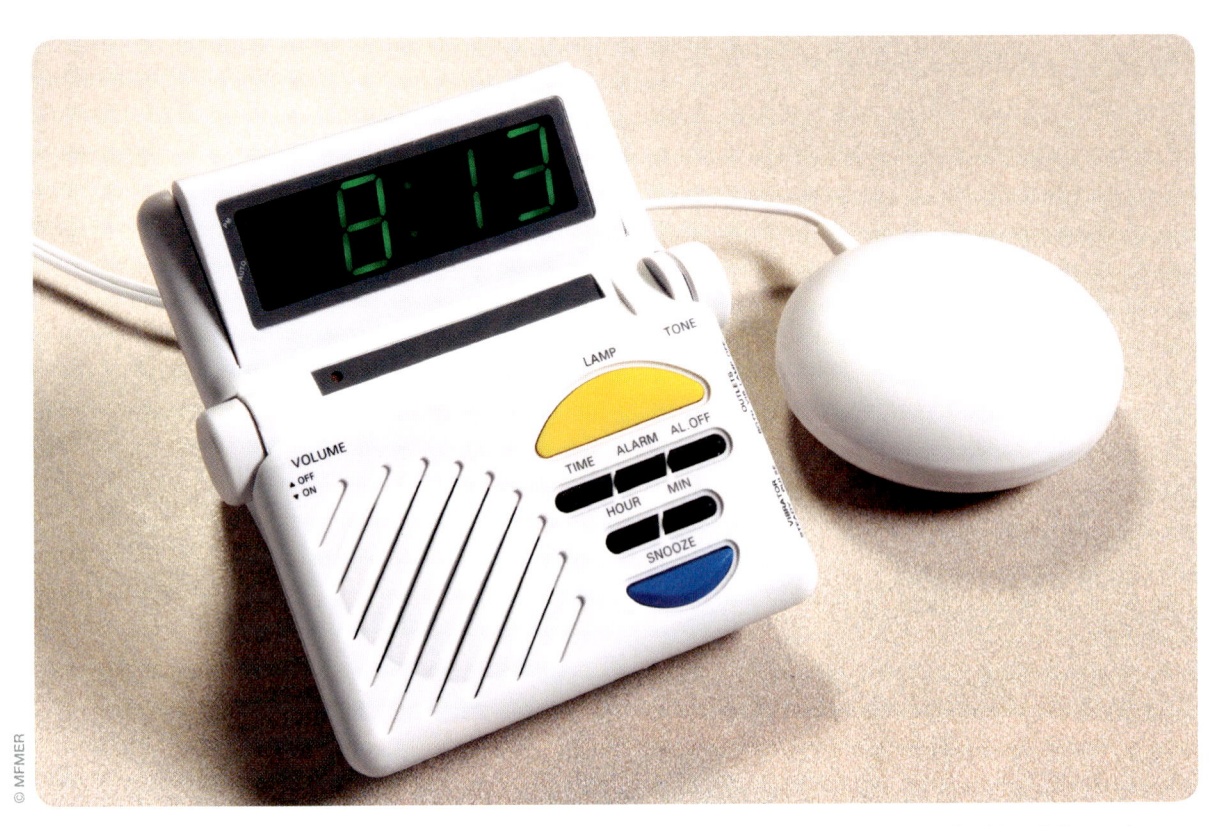

This alarm clock can employ any or all of three options to wake you: a loud sound, a flashing light and a vibrating attachment that can be placed under your pillow to gently shake you.

awake. Another option is an attachment with a flashing light that's plugged into your regular alarm clock.

Devices such as a vibrating pager or wristwatch, or even the vibration setting on a cellphone, can alert you in response to a paging system or time setting.

Alerting systems may be simple or complex. Some multipurpose alarms can use a code to indicate different sounds — for example, a telephone ring might be one light flash, the doorbell three flashes and the smoke alarm a series of on-off flashes. Some systems can be wired for use in several rooms or for transferring from room to room.

Special alerting devices can be used in your vehicle. A siren alert can let you know when an emergency vehicle is approaching. A Blinker Buddy tells you that the turn signal is on with a flashing light and a sound that gets louder the longer the signal remains on.

204 Chapter 9: Other options to communicate better

On the horizon

It wasn't that long ago that hearing aids were just about the only communication aid available for people with hearing loss.

Now, advances in computer engineering and miniaturization are creating new technology and applications. They are also bringing about major improvements to existing devices. And researchers continue to search for new ways to improve people's lives.

Speech recognition systems

One area of research and development is speech recognition, also referred to as voice recognition. Speech recognition allows you to control a computer by speaking to it rather than using a keyboard and mouse. When you speak, your commands appear as text on the computer screen.

The first speech recognition machine was created in 1950. But in 1997, continuous-speech-recognition software became commercially available — which means the machine is able to interpret a voice at a normal conversational rate. These systems are relatively inexpensive and easy to use.

Speech recognition systems can be very useful for someone with hearing impairment. They allow you to capture voices with a microphone and convert what's being said into a visual display on a screen.

Learning to use the software, however, requires some training and patience. You will prepare by entering specialized words into the program and training the system to recognize your voice patterns.

The technology is still not able to handle tricky listening environments. For example, you can't walk into a noisy party, point the microphone in the direction of a speaker and instantly read his or her words on a screen.

The technology is also being explored as a way to help people who rely primarily on speech reading to communicate. As someone speaks, a computer uses speech recognition and other software to create a sequence of visual cues — hand shapes — that help a speech reader distinguish between different speech elements that look similar when spoken. With video equipment, the cues are superimposed over an image of the speaker's face, allowing the speech reader to follow real-time conversation more easily.

Visual communication systems

Visual communication technology has great potential for people with hearing loss, especially those who use sign language as their primary means of communication. This system typically involves the use of video and computer equipment to allow people to communicate in sign language over the phone lines or the Internet.

One computer program under development provides real-time translation of spoken or written English into sign language. The hearing party's words are captured by a microphone or inputted as text and displayed on the recipient's computer screen as a signing figure. Another system provides sign language by way of a computer that's fitted with a digital camera and on-call interpreters.

Many options

Many people with hearing loss aren't aware of the numerous options in technology and computer software that can make communication easier. Assistive listening devices and other communication aids can make a significant difference in easing the daily problems caused by hearing loss. It's worthwhile to explore these options.

Of course, choosing among this ever-changing technology and knowing what might work best for you can be confusing at first. It's all too easy to be overwhelmed or seduced by the gadgetry. If you're not sure where to start, talk to a hearing health professional, such as your audiologist or an ear, nose and throat specialist.

Chapter 10

Problems with balance

The word *dizzy* is used to describe a variety of sensations — an illusion of motion, lightheadedness, weakness, loss of balance, faintness, wooziness and unsteadiness on your feet. You may feel that your surroundings are spinning around you — a condition commonly called vertigo. Imbalance occurs when you have to support yourself or hold on to something in order to maintain your balance.

There are many causes of dizziness, disrupting the complex system of balance in your body. A critical element of this system is the vestibular labyrinth, the main balance organ that — together with the cochlea — is contained in your inner ear. That explains why certain disorders of the inner ear (as discussed in Chapter 4) produce both hearing loss and dizziness as symptoms.

Dizziness is one of the most common reasons why people older than age 65 visit their doctor — right up there with chest pain and fatigue. That's because aging increases your risk of certain conditions that cause dizziness — and especially imbalance. Older adults are also more likely to take medications that can cause dizziness.

Although it may be temporarily disabling, dizziness rarely signals a serious, life-threatening situation.

Doctors often can determine the cause of dizziness, and for most people the signs and symptoms last a short time. Even when no definite cause is found or in cases where the dizziness persists, your doctor can prescribe treatments that usually ease symptoms to a manageable level.

Keeping yourself balanced

Your system of balance allows you to remain upright as you walk and move around or change position, for example, from a sitting to standing position. The system helps keep your vision focused and clear while your head is turning. Good balance also keeps you aware of the position of your head in relation to the ground.

To maintain your balance, your brain must coordinate sensory information coming from your eyes, inner ear, the bottoms of your feet, and major joints such as the ankles, knees and neck. Then the brain signals the muscles throughout your body on how to react and maintain your position.

This same information helps form your perceptions of how you're oriented in space, what direction you're moving in and how fast you're moving.

Your eyes

No matter what position you're in — sitting, standing, lying down or moving — visual signals help you determine where your body is in space. When light hits the photosensitive cells of your retina, it generates electrical impulses that are communicated to the brain through the optic nerve.

Your brain interprets these signals as images. The brain uses the images to calculate, for example, how far your chair seat is above the ground or how far away a car is that's moving in front of you, or how fast you're moving relative to someone walking beside you.

Your nervous system

Millions of nerve cells (neurons) are located in your skin, muscles and joints. When touch, pressure and movement stimulate these cells, they send electrical impulses to your brain about what your body is doing — for example, whether it's lying down on a soft mattress or climbing up a stepladder.

Information about the movement of your neck and your ankles is particularly important for balance because it indicates to your brain which way your head is turned and how steady you are on the ground.

Your vestibular labyrinth

The vestibular labyrinth is your primary balance organ. The brain uses this organ in your inner ear to determine where your head is relative to gravitational space, and whether your head or body is changing its position in space.

Your system of balance

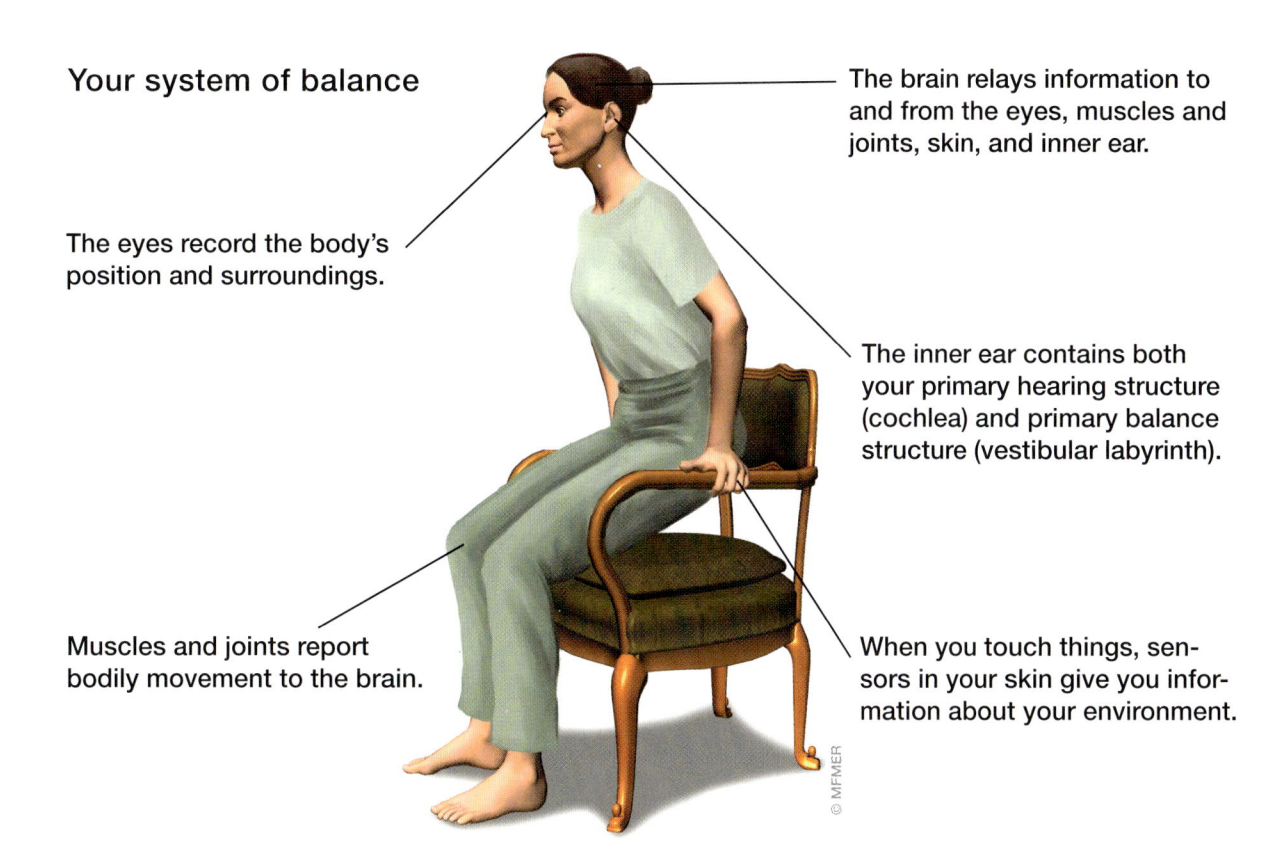

- The brain relays information to and from the eyes, muscles and joints, skin, and inner ear.
- The eyes record the body's position and surroundings.
- The inner ear contains both your primary hearing structure (cochlea) and primary balance structure (vestibular labyrinth).
- Muscles and joints report bodily movement to the brain.
- When you touch things, sensors in your skin give you information about your environment.

Although you're probably not as aware of the vestibular labyrinth as you are of your eyes, your brain relies on its input for balance. This is particularly true when information from the eyes, joints or bottoms of your feet is in some way disrupted.

Problems with dizziness and balance can arise anywhere within this complex, interconnected sensory system. In order for you to be able to maintain your balance across a full range of daily activities, at least two of the three elements — the eyes, musculoskeletal nerves and vestibular labyrinth — must be working well.

For example, closing your eyes in the shower while washing your hair doesn't mean you'll lose your balance. That's because signals from your inner ear and musculoskeletal nerves are helping to keep you upright. However, in addition to having your eyes closed, if your central nervous system can't process the signals properly or if your vestibular labyrinth is not functioning, you may experience dizziness and possibly fall in the shower.

Your vestibular system at work

The vestibular labyrinth is located just behind the cochlea in your inner ear. It consists of three fluid-filled loops called the semicircular canals. The base of each canal widens into a section known as the ampulla, which holds the hair cells that keep your brain informed of the rotational, or turning, motions of your head.

The three semicircular canals are connected to the central structure of the vestibular labyrinth called the vestibule. Within the vestibule are two chambers called the utricle and the saccule. The utricle is the upper chamber connecting all three semicircular canals. The saccule is the lower chamber. These chambers help monitor the position of your head in relation to up-and-down motion and forward and backward motion, such as when you ride in an elevator or a car.

Both the utricle and the saccule contain a patch of sensory hair cells embedded in a gel-like substance. These patches contain tiny particles called otoconia (o-toe-KOE-nee-uh). When you go up in an elevator, the otoconia in the saccule — responsible for detecting vertical movement — are pulled down by gravity. When you move forward in a car, the otoconia in the utricle — responsible for detecting horizontal movement — are pulled backward.

With either action, the otoconia pull the gel-like substance with them. The gel, in turn, stimulates the embedded hair cells, triggering electrical impulses that are sent along the nerve pathways to your brain with information about your vertical and horizontal movements. In similar fashion, impulses from your semicircular canals also provide information about angular changes in the position of your head, such as turning to the left or right.

Your brain responds to these impulses, regardless of what you're doing, by signaling your eyes to move in the opposite direction of your head, keeping the image you're looking at focused on the retina. Your brain also signals the skeletal muscles to react quickly to help you keep your body balanced.

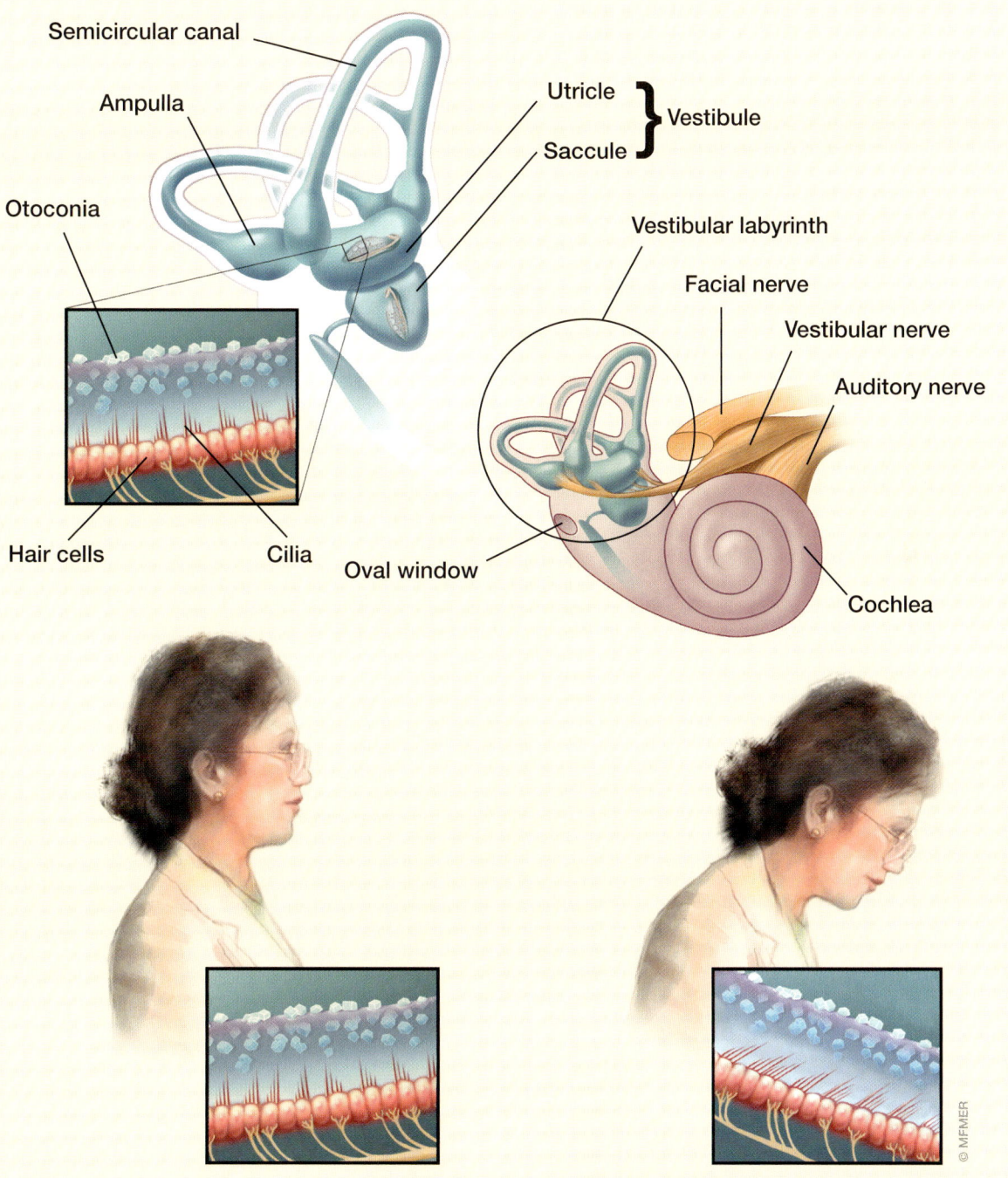

With your head upright, the tiny embedded hairs are perpendicular in relation to the otoconia in your utricle.

If you tilt your head forward, the otoconia are pulled downward with the gel. The embedded hairs shift in the direction of the movement of the otoconia.

Mayo Clinic on Better Hearing and Balance **211**

Causes of dizziness

Everyone has likely experienced brief episodes of dizziness at one point in life. Momentary dizziness is often caused by an abrupt and rapid change in your environment.

Normally, your sense of balance is maintained subconsciously, based on years of practice and on healthy sensory input. For example, a toddler learning to walk is often quite unsteady and frequently loses his or her balance. But as the child gets older, the eye-muscle coordination becomes natural. Soon, walking and running doesn't require a second thought.

You may feel momentarily dizzy when your brain becomes aware of unusual sensory input, such as your first time on board a rocking boat. Another example is when you first get off a treadmill — it often takes a few seconds for you to adjust to the fact that your surroundings now move past you when you walk, in contrast to what happened during your workout.

Dizziness may also be the result of conflicting sensory information. For example, if you're sitting in a movie theater watching the shot of a landscape taken through the window of a speeding train, your eyes will be signaling movement. At the same time, your muscles, nerves and vestibular system indicate you're stationary. This can make you feel momentarily dizzy.

Spinning or sudden movements also cause feelings of dizziness. This happens because there's a brief lag when the fluid in your semicircular canals tries to catch up with the speed of your motion. When you stop moving, the fluid is still in motion for a short time, which makes you dizzy. When the fluid comes to rest, the dizziness generally goes away.

Dizziness caused by these environmental changes generally isn't serious. But sudden, severe attacks or prolonged episodes of dizziness, faintness, lightheadedness or vertigo can be symptoms of an underlying disorder. Sometimes, it's the result of a disruption of your vestibular system. Other causes may include:

- **Low blood pressure.** Low blood pressure can make you feel dizzy, lightheaded or faint when you sit down or stand up too quickly. This is known as orthostatic hypotension (postural hypotension).

- **Poor blood circulation.** Inadequate blood flow to the brain can make you feel lightheaded. Poor blood flow to the inner ear may cause vertigo. Poor circulation may be the result of a heart condition such as blocked arteries or irregular heartbeats (arrhythmia).
- **Multiple sensory deficits.** Lack of input from your eyes, nerves, muscles and joints can make you feel unsteady. Examples include failing vision, nerve damage in your arms and legs (peripheral neuropathy), osteoarthritis, and muscle weakness.
- **Anxiety disorders.** These disorders include panic attacks and a fear of leaving your home or being in large, open spaces (agoraphobia). They can make you feel spaced-out or lightheaded. Even mild forms of situational anxiety can provoke dizziness in some people.
- **Hyperventilation.** Abnormally rapid breathing, which often accompanies anxiety disorders, can make you feel lightheaded.
- **Disorders of the central nervous system.** These include disorders such as multiple sclerosis, tumors and stroke.
- **Migraines.** With or without head pain, migraine events are increasingly recognized as a common cause of dizziness.

Diagnostic tests

If you're experiencing frequent, prolonged or severe episodes of dizziness, bring it to your doctor's attention. You may be asked to undergo several tests that can assess the health of your inner ear and balance system. An audiologist usually performs these tests.

Test results can help determine if one or both ears are affected and how well your inner ear, eyes, muscles and joints work together. The test results may also indicate whether you are a candidate for vestibular and balance rehabilitation therapy.

You'll likely be asked to not eat any food, consume alcohol, and take any sedatives, tranquilizers or pain relievers for 24 hours before testing. You'll also want to wear comfortable clothing, such as pants or a sweat suit, as one of the tests (posturography) requires using a harness.

The tests to diagnose dizziness are simple and nonthreatening. However, they're capable at times of making you feel dizzy, nauseated or anxious. Consult your audiologist with any concerns before, during or after testing. The examination may include one or more of the following tests:

> ### Should you be concerned about dizziness?
>
> Generally, any unexplained recurrent or severe spell of dizziness warrants a visit to your doctor. Although it's uncommon for dizziness to signal a serious illness, see your doctor immediately if you experience dizziness or vertigo with any of the following:
>
> - New, different or severe headache
> - Blurred vision or double vision
> - Hearing loss
> - Speech impairment
> - Leg or arm weakness
> - Loss of consciousness
> - Falling or difficulty with walking
> - Numbness or tingling
> - Chest pain or rapid or slow heart rate
>
> These signs and symptoms may signal the development of a more serious problem, such as a brain tumor, stroke, Parkinson's disease, multiple sclerosis or heart disease.

Hearing test

Because the cochlea and vestibular labyrinth are both contained in the inner ear, problems with one of these structures often accompany problems with the other.

The results of a hearing test may reveal something about your problems with balance. For a description of the standard hearing test, see Chapter 2.

Nystagmography

Nystagmography is actually a battery of tests that evaluates the interaction between your inner ear and your eye muscles — an interaction known as the vestibuloocular reflex.

Electronystagmography (ENG) is performed using electrodes to collect the information. Videonystagmography (VNG) uses tiny video cameras.

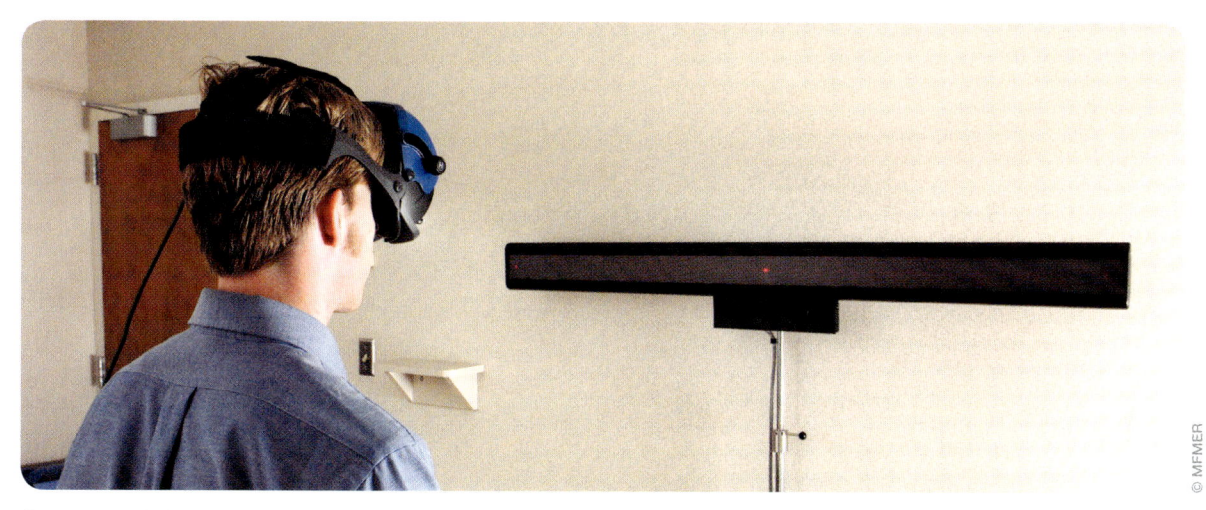

One part of videonystagmography involves following a pinpoint of light with your eyes as it moves across a horizontal electronic bar. This test evaluates how well the brain portions of your balance system control eye movements when your inner ear is not involved.

Whenever you turn your head, your inner ear signals the brain regarding this movement. The brain, in turn, signals your eye muscles in the vestibulo-ocular reflex. Essentially, your eyes will move in the opposite direction that you turn your head, permitting you to keep an object in a steady field of vision.

ENG and VNG detect periods of uncontrolled, back-and-forth eye movements (nystagmus). Nystagmus (nis-TAG-mus) may indicate a disorder or injury that's disrupting the vestibuloocular reflex. The tests are performed to study dizziness and vertigo.

For VNG tests, you may be asked to wear special goggles equipped with tiny infrared cameras that continually track the movement of your eyes (shown above). If the eye movements are found to occur without any stimuli — for example, without you changing the position of your head — you may be experiencing nystagmus.

For ENG tests, instead of goggles, electrodes are taped at locations around your eyes to record the activity.

In order for the examiner to determine how well your eye movements will respond to signals from your inner ear, you may be asked to:

- Stare continuously at a fixed point of light or a spot

Mayo Clinic on Better Hearing and Balance

- Follow a point of light with your eyes as it moves back and forth along a horizontal bar
- Follow rotating points of light with your eyes
- Lie in different positions while your eye movements are recorded

Another test, known as the caloric test, involves warm water, cool water or air being circulated through a soft tube placed in your ear canal. The audiologist will observe your eye movements as these different temperatures stimulate the inner ear.

Dix-Hallpike test

The Dix-Hallpike test can determine whether certain movements of your head trigger a form of vertigo known as benign paroxysmal positional vertigo (BPPV). BPPV is characterized by sudden, short bursts of vertigo (see page 220).

You'll start the test sitting on an examining table. The audiologist may study your eyes directly for the eye movements (nystagmus) characteristic of BPPV. Or you may be asked to wear special goggles equipped with cameras that display the eye movements on a video screen. Then specific steps will occur:

- The audiologist moves your head to the right or the left at an angle of about 45 degrees.
- You move from a sitting position to lying down with your head extended over the edge of the table but still at the same angle and supported by the audiologist.
- The audiologist closely observes the movement of your eyes. If nystagmus occurs, it will indicate the location of the problem.

This procedure is done for both ears. If you have BPPV, you'll probably experience vertigo after two to 10 seconds of changing position. The sensation may last for 30 seconds to one minute. The direction of the nystagmus when you experience vertigo usually determines which ear is affected.

The canalith repositioning procedure is usually successful in treating BPPV (see page 222).

Rotation tests

Rotation tests also detect your vestibuloocular reflex, but they tend to be more sensitive to inner ear problems. For example, they can monitor your control of eye movements while you're taking medications that may damage the inner ear (ototoxic medications) — which typically affect both ears. Not everyone will undergo rotation tests during a vestibular exam.

During one form of rotation testing, your audiologist may use electrodes or goggles equipped with infrared cameras to monitor your eye movements as your body is rotated in different directions and at various speeds. For safety, you're strapped into the chair with a harness and your head is secured against a headrest.

Typically, the testing room is darkened and your audiologist is seated at a computer console just outside the door. A microphone and headset allow you to maintain contact with the audiologist. Often, the computer-controlled chair moves very slowly in a full circle. At faster speeds, it moves back and forth in a very small arc as your eye movements are recorded.

Rather than spinning the chair, the audiologist may have you focus on an object and voluntarily move your head from side to side or up and down for brief periods. Simplifying the test more, your audiologist may watch your eye movements while he or she manually moves your head or slowly spins you in a swivel chair.

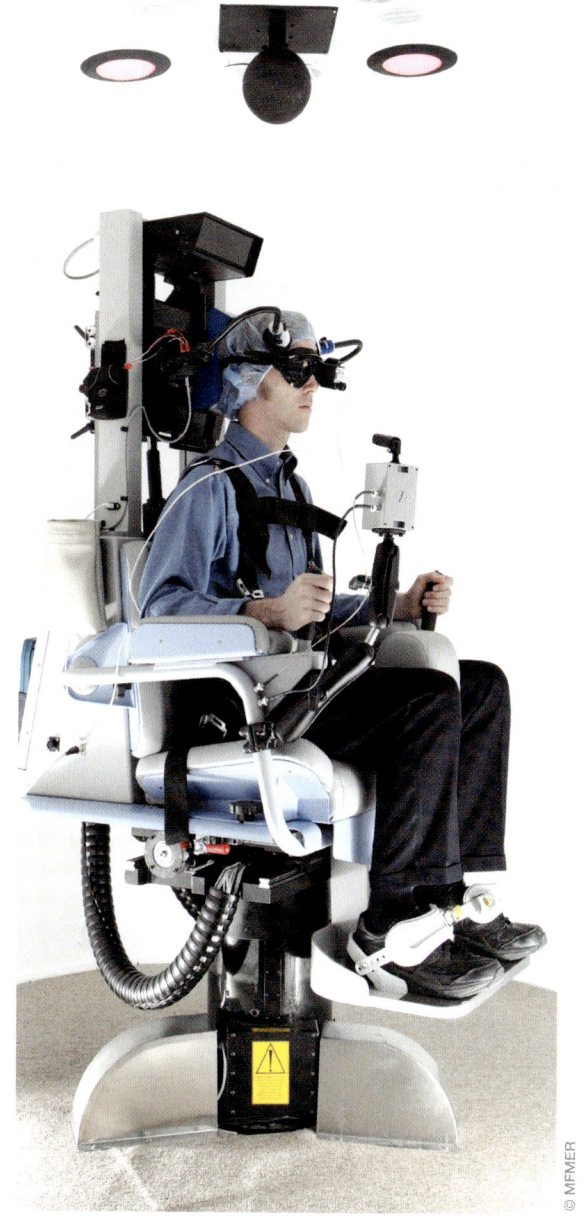

During a rotation test, you'll sit in a rotary chair in a darkened room. The audiologist will monitor your eye movements while your body is rotated in the computer-controlled chair in different directions and at different speeds.

Mayo Clinic on Better Hearing and Balance **217**

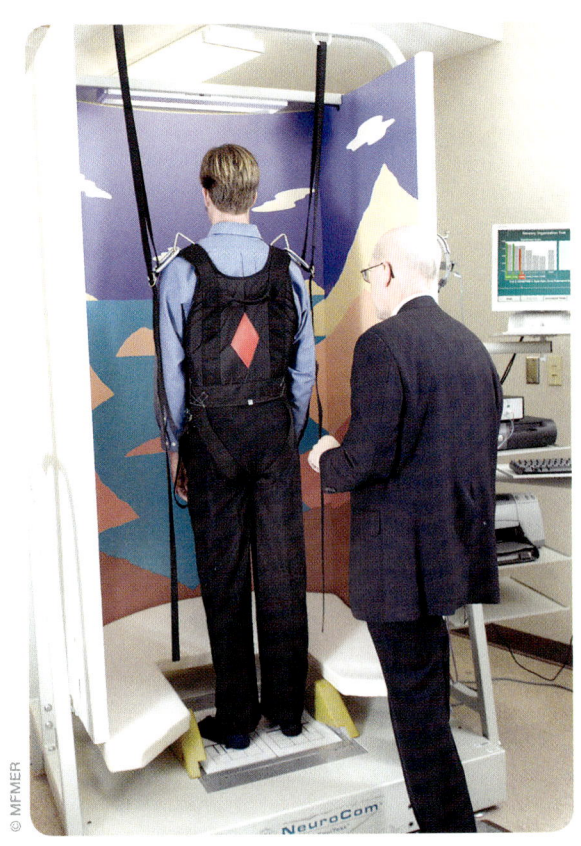

Posturography measures how well you maintain your balance when your sensory systems are slightly altered. A platform detects changes in how you distribute your weight as you stand.

Posturography

Posturography tests your ability to integrate the sensory information coming from different elements of your balance system: your eyes, the vestibular system in your inner ear, your muscles and joints, and the bottoms of your feet. The exam reveals which elements of the system you've come to rely on most for balance — either on their own or in combination with other elements.

To start the test, you'll be asked to remove your shoes and stand on a platform that detects changes in how you distribute your weight as you stand. This will help calculate the sway movements of your body to stay balanced. Wear comfortable clothes because you'll be slipping into a safety harness to make sure you don't fall. The audiologist will be standing close behind you in case you need some assistance to stabilize yourself.

During testing, varying conditions are created by altering one of your sensory systems. For example, you may be asked to remain balanced while your eyes are closed, or the platform you're standing on will no longer be stable and is set to rock with your body movements. The testing determines how well you're able to adjust to the changing circumstances.

Vestibular evoked myogenic potential

Vestibular evoked myogenic potential (VEMP) allows the audiologist to evaluate specific parts of the inner

Chapter 10: Problems with balance

ear — the saccule and utricle, which are contained in the vestibular labyrinth (see page 210). Specifically, this test measures a neurological pathway between the inner ear and the brain known as the vestibulo-collic reflex.

You start the test either seated or, in most cases, reclined at an angle. Several electrodes are taped to two large muscles in your neck and just under each eye. Earphones are worn to deliver loud sounds to one ear or both ears. For part of the test, you'll be asked to contract the muscles of your neck, usually by simultaneously lifting and turning your head or, if sitting, by pressing your head against your hand or a semi-inflated blood pressure cuff that's held in your hand. During another part of the test, you'll be asked to look upward toward your forehead.

VEMP testing is useful for the detection of perilymph fistulas, particularly superior semicircular canal dehiscence (see page 230). Research also suggests that VEMP testing may help diagnose Meniere's disease (see page 223).

Other tests

Magnetic resonance imaging (MRI) can reveal a variety of abnormalities — such as tumors — that may affect brain structures. Computerized tomography (CT) scans may be used to check for bone fractures or other skull abnormalities.

Blood tests may be used to check for an underlying infection. And since blood pressure and circulation can affect dizziness, cardiovascular tests may be done to check the health of your heart and blood vessels.

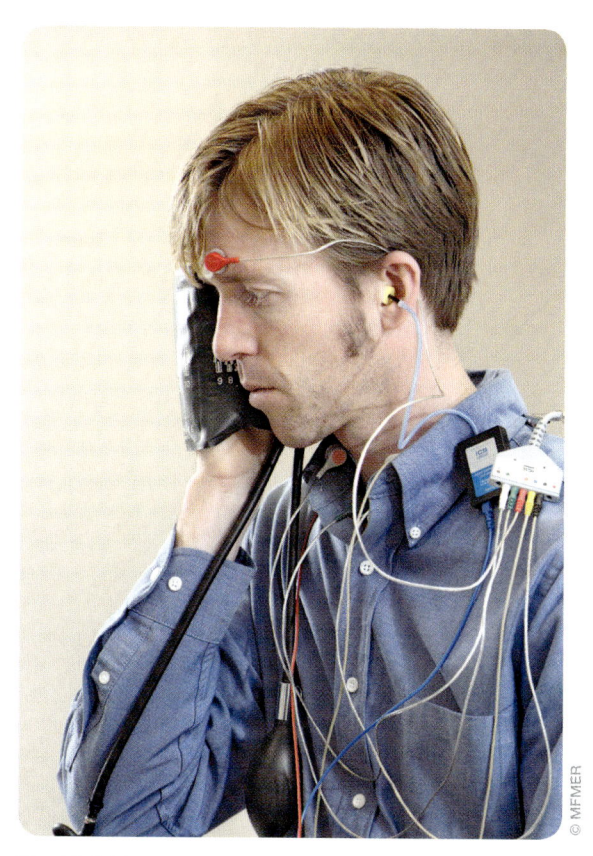

For VEMP testing, you press a semifilled blood pressure cuff against your cheek to cause contractions of your neck muscles.

Vestibular disorders

Dizziness and, especially, vertigo — the sensation that your surroundings are whirling or spinning — are commonly associated with vestibular disorders. The problem may arise from an infection in the inner ear or on the auditory nerve. It may also result from loose otoconia in the vestibular labyrinth (see page 210).

If you have a vestibular disorder, you may also experience nausea or vomiting, changes in heart rate and blood pressure, fear, anxiety, and even panic. These effects may make you feel tired, depressed and lacking focus.

Most of the time, the vestibular problem is benign — which means it isn't life-threatening — and your doctor can prescribe ways to manage the condition. Some common vestibular disorders are described below:

Benign paroxysmal positional vertigo

Benign paroxysmal (buh-NINE par-ok-SIZ-mul) positional vertigo is commonly known by the abbreviation BPPV. This condition is a common cause of vertigo and more likely to occur in older adults.

BPPV is characterized by sudden, short bursts of vertigo — usually lasting less than a minute — that typically occur after you turn or change the position of your head. You may feel as if you're spinning or floating. Your eyes move back and forth involuntarily (nystagmus) while this happens. You may also experience nausea with rare occasions of vomiting, and lingering fatigue. Vertigo associated with BPPV may come and go unpredictably for weeks or even years.

Although the cause is unknown, BPPV is considered a mechanical problem of the balance system — and not a neurological problem with the sensory hair cells in the vestibular labyrinth or with the vestibular nerve. Sometimes a blow to the head precedes the condition, but BPPV may also occur spontaneously as a natural result of aging or from damage to the balance organ.

Regardless of the cause, scientists have learned that the tiny otoconia that are normally located in the utricle of the vestibular labyrinth break loose. Most often, these loose pieces accumulate in one of the semicircular canals.

Certain movements — such as rolling over in bed, sitting up or bending forward — move the particles. This movement disturbs the fluid of the inner ear, which causes the hair cells in the canals to bend, setting off brief episodes of vertigo.

With the assistance of an audiologist, a simple procedure may be all it takes to manage BPPV. The canalith repositioning procedure involves maneuvers for positioning the head (shown on page 222). The goal is to progressively move the misplaced otoconia out of the canal to an open area near the utricle.

It may be necessary to repeat the procedure several times in a single visit before the feeling of vertigo is eliminated. Afterward, you'll need to keep your head upright for the rest of the day to help ensure that the particles stay out of the canal.

The canalith repositioning technique can be highly effective. However, a recurrence of vertigo frequently happens in the first year following a successful maneuver. If the symptoms do return, repeating the procedure usually helps. Therefore, it's important that individuals are instructed to perform the movements on their own to effectively manage the condition.

Migraine-related dizziness

While the most common disorder for dizziness in adults is BPPV, the second most common is migraine-related dizziness (vertiginous migraine).

Migraines have recently been recognized to involve dizziness. The dizziness can take any form — spinning, unsteadiness, lightheadedness, spontaneous or motion provoked. This means that the form of dizziness isn't very helpful in determining whether migraine could be the source of the dizziness. The dizziness that accompanies migraines is episodic, and may not always occur with a headache.

Newly established criteria suggest that in order for migraine to be considered as a cause for the dizziness the person must first meet the criteria for migraines set forth by the International Classification of Headache Disorders. Then more than half of the dizziness events must carry with them a migraine or other migraine symptoms (such as increased sensitivity to light), even without a headache.

Migraine-related dizziness is commonly confused with Meniere's disease (see page 223). Part of the challenge is that migraines are much more common

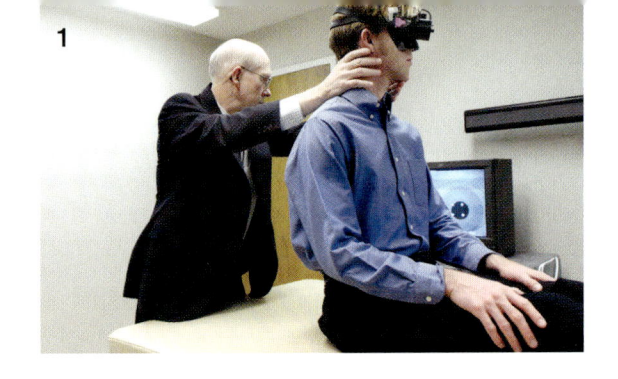

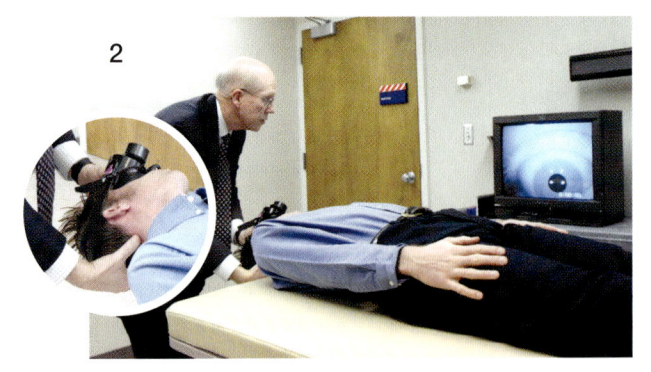

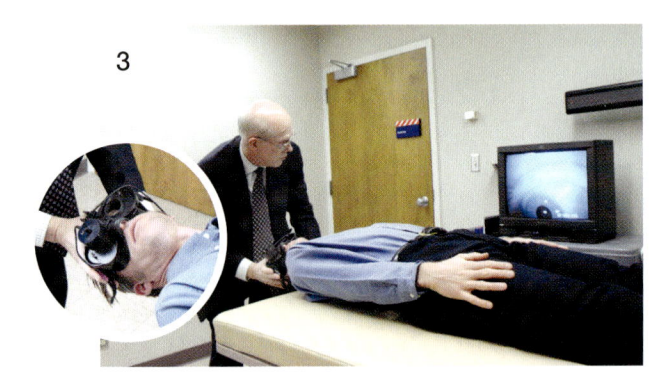

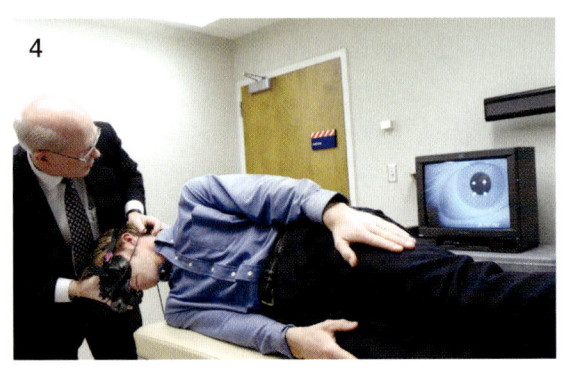

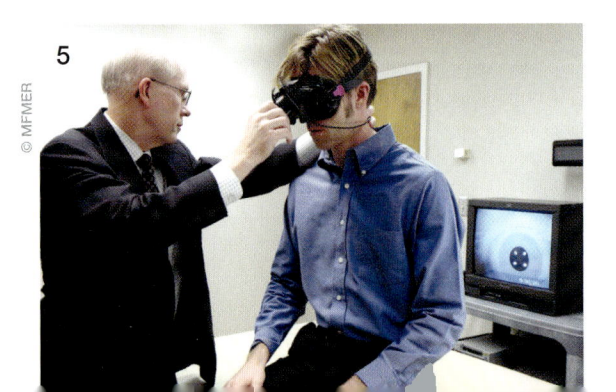

To help relieve BPPV, your audiologist may help you perform a series of maneuvers known as the canalith repositioning procedure. Each step is held for about 30 seconds. This example is for BPPV on your left side.

1. Start in a seated position with your head turned at a 45-degree angle to the left.

2. Move to a reclining position while your head is kept at the same angle. The audiologist supports your head as it extends over the edge of the table.

3. Still reclined, turn your head to the right.

4. Roll over on your side. Your head is angled slightly as you look down at the floor.

5. Return carefully to a sitting position with your chin tilted down.

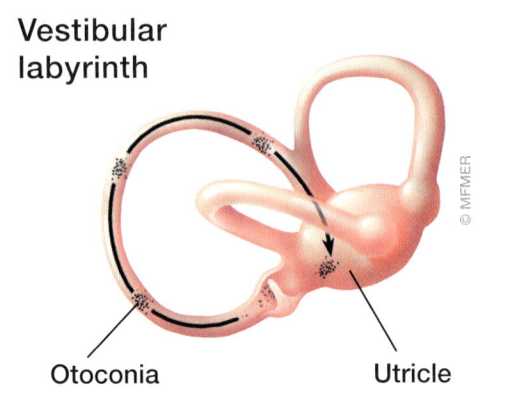

Vestibular labyrinth

Otoconia   Utricle

As you work through the procedure, the loose otoconia return to the area of the utricle.

in people with Meniere's disease than they are in the general population. Both disorders can cause similar symptoms in the same person and can confuse the diagnosis.

Migraine-related dizziness is treated by getting the migraines under control. A variety of medications may be used to prevent and treat migraines. Other helpful strategies include getting adequate sleep, practicing relaxation techniques, and watching your diet and lifestyle for migraine triggers to avoid.

Chronic subjective dizziness syndrome

Another cause of dizziness is chronic subjective dizziness syndrome (CSD), a condition commonly associated with migraines and anxiety. This persistent dizziness typically occurs with movement and is made worse by complex visual environments (such as the grocery store), visual motion (such as a movie), visual patterns and focused visual tasks (such as reading).

CSD is a conditioned response that develops out of the fear and anxiety that may result when dizziness occurs from another cause. Medications used to treat anxiety or depression may help control the condition, as can vestibular and balance therapy.

Meniere's disease

Meniere's (meh-NAYRZ) disease can affect adults at any age but is most likely to occur between 20 and 60 years of age. It's characterized by sudden attacks of vertigo, which may last anywhere from 20 minutes to several hours, but not longer than 24 hours.

The vertigo may make you feel nauseated or cause you to vomit. Other signs and symptoms of the condition include hearing loss, tinnitus and the feeling of a plugged ear. Vertigo is usually the worst symptom. You may be extremely sensitive to head movement, and the feeling of imbalance may continue from one to two days.

Attacks may occur as frequently as every day or as infrequently as once a year. Between attacks, you usually feel back to normal. Although your ability to hear typically fluctuates with the attacks, the degree of hearing loss may gradually worsen. Meniere's disease usually affects only one ear, although it may affect both ears in about 25 to 30 percent of cases.

Surgery for vestibular disorders

Vertigo and other symptoms of vestibular disorders are most often treated with medications or through rehabilitation therapy, but surgery also may be an option. Which option is decided on will depend on the frequency and severity of your symptoms, the amount of hearing you've retained, your overall health and your wishes.

Some of the more common surgical procedures used for vestibular disorders include:

- Patching a tear in either the oval window or the round window leading from the middle ear to the inner ear (perilymph fistula).
- Placing tissue over a tear at the top of one of the semicircular canals or blocking the canal (superior semicircular canal dehiscence).
- Draining excess fluid (endolymph) from the endolymphatic sac that's located near the mastoid bone behind your ear. This is called endolymphatic decompression surgery.
- Cutting the vestibular nerve (vestibular nerve section) at a location before it joins with the auditory nerve. This procedure can potentially eliminate vertigo while preserving your hearing. It may be a reasonable option for a younger person with severe symptoms of Meniere's disease and no other significant medical problems.
- Destroying the inner ear (labyrinthectomy). This is a relatively simple operation with fewer risks than in vestibular nerve section. Because the procedure involves destruction of the labyrinth, it's usually reserved for those who have no usable hearing in the affected ear. After surgery, the brain gradually adjusts, compensating for the loss of the balance mechanism in one ear by relying on the functioning mechanism of the other ear. Vestibular and balance therapy can help hasten this compensation process.

The cause of Meniere's disease is unknown, but scientists believe it's associated with fluctuations in the volume of fluid in the inner ear, as well as with the content of the fluid.

Treating Meniere's disease involves taking medications to manage the dizziness and nausea and consuming a low-salt diet. Limiting your salt intake can help decrease the level of fluid in your body — and possibly the level in your inner ear — and decrease the frequency of attacks. Your doctor also may prescribe a diuretic to help you accomplish this.

If you experience frequent episodes of vertigo, your doctor may inject a small quantity of an antibiotic called gentamicin into your middle ear. Gentamicin is capable of causing inner ear damage, but in controlled amounts can reduce the activities of your vestibular system and control vertigo while leaving hearing intact. If dizziness is so severe that it inhibits your daily life, inner ear surgery also may be an option.

Labyrinthitis

Labyrinthitis is an inflammation of the inner ear — also known as the labyrinth — affecting both your balance and your hearing. The inflammation often follows the development of a bacterial ear infection or a viral upper respiratory illness. It may also occur after head trauma, or by itself with no other associated illness.

Signs and symptoms of labyrinthitis include sudden, intense vertigo that may last for several days, nausea and vomiting, nystagmus, hearing loss, and tinnitus. If the inflammation is associated with a bacterial infection, you may experience a total loss of hearing in the affected ear.

Most of the time, the dizziness will go away on its own after a few weeks. Nevertheless, it's still important that you consult your doctor. Not making rapid head movements during the first few days you experience symptoms can help keep them under control. However, it's important to get back to normal functioning and movement as soon as possible.

If the problem underlying labyrinthitis is a bacterial one, the doctor will likely prescribe antibiotics to help get rid of the infection. Steroids may be given if there's no evidence of infection. If the condition is diagnosed within 72 hours of onset, the doctor may prescribe antiviral drugs.

Your doctor may also recommend medications to relieve dizziness and nausea. In some cases, a brief hospitalization is necessary due to the risk of dehydration from severe vomiting. Vestibular and balance rehabilitation will often help you manage symptoms associated with imbalance and movement sensitivity.

Vestibular neuronitis

The symptoms of vestibular neuronitis are similar to labyrinthitis — both conditions cause a sudden onset of vertigo in addition to nausea, vomiting and nystagmus. Indeed, the two medical terms are sometimes — mistakenly — used interchangeably.

Both conditions may be caused by a viral infection, but whereas labyrinthitis is an infection of the inner ear, vestibular neuronitis is an infection of the vestibular nerve that connects the inner ear to the brain. Labyrinthitis may cause hearing loss, and vestibular neuronitis does not.

Signs and symptoms of vestibular neuronitis may last from several days to weeks, being severe at first and then gradually improving. Often, vestibular neuronitis will develop after a cold or other upper respiratory viral infection.

Most people recover completely from the neuronitis, although some may experience mild imbalance after the infection has been resolved.

Your doctor may prescribe medications to suppress the vertigo and nausea and steroids such as prednisone to help reduce inflammation from the infection. Your doctor may also prescribe vestibular and balance rehabilitation to help in your recovery (see page 231).

Reactions to medications

The action of certain medications can damage the organs of hearing and balance in your inner ear. For this reason, these medications are considered ototoxic (*oto-* means "ear"). A list of common ototoxic drugs is in Chapter 4.

The effects of these medications, which can range from mild to severe, often depend on the doses you're taking and the length of time you take them, as well as factors such as your kidney and liver functions. Signs and symptoms of ototoxicity include:

- Onset of tinnitus in one or both ears
- Worsening of existing tinnitus
- A feeling that one or both ears are plugged

- Loss of hearing or worsening of existing hearing loss
- Blurred vision when you move your head
- Loss of balance

Make sure that your doctor is aware of any balance or hearing problem whenever you go for a medical visit. Report if you're experiencing balance problems after taking certain medications. This could help you avoid unnecessary exposure to ototoxic drugs.

Imbalance may persist following use of some medications. Vestibular and balance rehabilitation can teach you how to adjust to and cope with the ongoing loss of balance (see page 231).

The use of alcohol also can cause vertigo and nystagmus, but these symptoms are temporary and will disappear once the alcohol's effects have subsided. However, the effects of alcohol can last up to 24 hours. Prolonged alcohol abuse can damage parts of your brain and result in permanent issues with imbalance.

Acoustic neuroma

An acoustic neuroma, also known as a vestibular schwannoma, is a slow-growing, benign tumor that develops on what's known as the eighth cranial nerve. This nerve is made up of the vestibular nerve and auditory nerve together.

An acoustic neuroma develops as a result of overproduction of certain cells, known as Schwann cells, that cover the nerves (see the illustration on page 90). What causes the overproduction of cells is unknown.

Hearing loss in one ear and tinnitus are common signs and symptoms of the disorder. As the tumor grows, it can affect other nerves that lead to your face, causing facial numbness and facial weakness. Although the vestibular nerve and blood supply to the balance organ are involved, the tumor grows slowly enough that imbalance and vertigo are rare symptoms.

Despite slow growth, it's possible for an acoustic neuroma to grow big enough to push up against the brainstem and interfere with life-sustaining functions. Your doctor may detect the acoustic neuroma with the use of magnetic resonance imaging (MRI).

An acoustic reuroma can be removed surgically or successfully treated with radiation therapy.

Fall prevention: Tips to prevent falls

As you get older, physical changes and health conditions make falls more likely. In fact, falls are a leading cause of injury among older adults. Still, fear of falling doesn't need to rule your life. Instead, consider these simple fall-prevention strategies.

1. **Make an appointment with your doctor**
   Begin your fall-prevention plan by making an appointment with your doctor. Be prepared to answer questions such as:

- **What medications are you taking?** Make a list of your prescription and over-the-counter medications and supplements, or bring them with you to the appointment. Your doctor can review your medications for side effects and interactions that may increase your risk of falling.
- **Have you fallen before?** Write down the details, including when, where and how you fell. Details such as these may help your doctor identify specific fall-prevention strategies.
- **Could your health conditions cause a fall?** Be prepared to discuss your health conditions and how comfortable you are when you walk. Your doctor may evaluate your muscle strength, balance and walking style (gait) as well.

2. **Keep moving**
   Physical activity can go a long way toward fall prevention. With your doctor's OK, consider activities such as walking, water workouts or tai chi. Such activities improve strength, balance, coordination and flexibility.

If you avoid physical activity because you're afraid of falling, tell your doctor. He or she may recommend carefully monitored exercise programs or refer you to a physical therapist. The physical therapist can create a custom exercise program aimed at improving your balance, flexibility, muscle strength and gait.

3. **Wear sensible shoes**
   Consider changing your footwear as part of your fall-prevention plan. High heels, floppy slippers and shoes with slick soles can make you slip, stumble and fall. So can walking in your stocking feet.

4. Remove home hazards

Take a look around your home. Your living room, kitchen, bedroom, bathroom, hallways and stairways may be filled with hazards. To make your home safer:

- Remove boxes, newspapers, electrical cords and phone cords from walkways.
- Move coffee tables, magazine racks and plant stands from high-traffic areas.
- Secure loose rugs with double-faced tape, tacks or a slip-resistant backing.
- Store clothing, dishes, food and other necessities within easy reach.
- Immediately clean up spilled liquids, grease or food.
- Use nonskid floor wax.
- Use nonslip mats in your bathtub or shower.

5. Light up your living space

Keep your home brightly lit to avoid tripping on objects that are hard to see. Also:

- Place night lights in your bedroom, bathroom and hallways.
- Place a lamp within reach of your bed for middle-of-the-night needs.
- Make clear paths to light switches that aren't near room entrances. Consider trading traditional switches for glow-in-the-dark or illuminated switches.
- Turn on the lights before going up or down stairs.
- Store flashlights in easy-to-find places in case of power outages.

6. Use assistive devices

Your doctor might recommend using a cane or walker to keep you steady. Other assistive devices can help, too. For example:

- Handrails for both sides of stairways
- Nonslip treads for bare-wood steps
- A raised toilet seat or one with armrests
- Grab bars for the shower or tub
- A sturdy plastic seat for the shower or tub — plus a hand-held shower nozzle

If necessary, ask your doctor for a referral to an occupational therapist. He or she can help you brainstorm other fall-prevention strategies.

Perilymph fistula

Perilymph fistula refers to the leakage of perilymph, a fluid from the inner ear, into the air-filled middle ear. The leakage occurs through a small tear in either the oval window or round window, which are thin membranes separating the middle ear and inner ear.

The condition most commonly results from trauma to the head but also may be caused by rapid changes in atmospheric pressure — such as that experienced while scuba diving or doing airplane maneuvers. It may also occur due to extreme exertion — such as that needed for heavy lifting or childbirth.

The condition is controversial because the holes or defects in the membrane are so small and exceedingly difficult to detect — which can often can make diagnosis difficult.

Signs and symptoms of perilymph fistula may include vertigo, imbalance, nausea and vomiting. A fistula may also lead to tinnitus and hearing loss.

Bed rest and avoiding sudden movements often allow the rupture to heal on its own. If this doesn't work, surgery may be performed to repair the tiny opening.

Superior semicircular canal dehiscence

Superior semicircular canal dehiscence (SSCD) is a type of perilymph fistula involving an abnormal opening in the inner ear. But with SSCD, the opening is at the top of one of the semicircular canals of the vestibular labyrinth, where there's a lack of bone covering the canal.

The primary symptom associated with SSCD is dizziness when straining — for example, when lifting something heavy — or when hearing loud noises such as dog barks. The condition may involve a specific type of hearing loss.

While not easy to diagnose, SSCD is far less controversial than is an oval or round window fistula. That's because the opening on the semicircular canal can be detected with a CT scan or from certain audiological tests. Surgery can often repair the defect, relieving dizziness and returning your hearing to normal levels.

Dizziness in children

Children of all ages can have problems with dizziness and balance. While not as common as in adults, children may be affected by many of the same disorders. The most common disorder in children is migraine-related dizziness. In younger children, accumulation of fluid in the middle ear also is a common cause of dizziness.

The child's description of his or her dizziness, along with any observations that can be provided by parents or other caregivers are key parts of an evaluation. All of the tests used to evaluate dizziness in adults can be used for children, with modifications — such as the child sitting on his or her parent's lap during the rotary chair test — if necessary. A hearing evaluation will also be completed.

Treatment of dizziness in children also is similar to that used for adults. For migraine issues, there is a higher reliance on diet control, but medications can be used when needed.

Vestibular rehabilitation

Dizziness and vertigo frequently go away on their own. But sometimes they persist. If you experience dizziness, vertigo, or other signs and symptoms of a vestibular disorder that disrupt your life for several weeks or more, your doctor may refer you to a physical therapist for vestibular and balance rehabilitation.

This is an effective therapeutic program that uses physical exercise to decrease your symptoms and help you regain your sense of balance. Vestibular and balance rehabilitation is frequently recommended after inner ear surgery.

Adapting to change

The goals of this therapy are to stay active and to learn to maintain your everyday routine despite the balance concerns. This effort will help the normal mechanisms within your brain and central nervous system and your musculoskeletal system adapt to the changes you're experiencing. This adaptation is known as compensation.

When your vestibular system is damaged, your brain receives conflicting messages about movement and your body's position in space. That causes the dizziness or vertigo. You may try to avoid rapid movements at first in order to avoid these symptoms. But remaining relatively inactive for long periods of time doesn't stimulate your brain to change and adapt.

Balance exercises

Balance exercises can help you maintain your balance — and confidence — at any age. If you're an older adult, balance exercises are especially important because they can help you prevent falls and maintain your independence.

Nearly any activity that keeps you on your feet and moving, such as walking, can help you maintain good balance. You can also include specific balance exercises in your daily routine. Try balancing on one foot while waiting in line, or stand up and sit down without using your hands.

If you have severe balance problems or an orthopedic condition, get your doctor's OK before doing balance exercises.

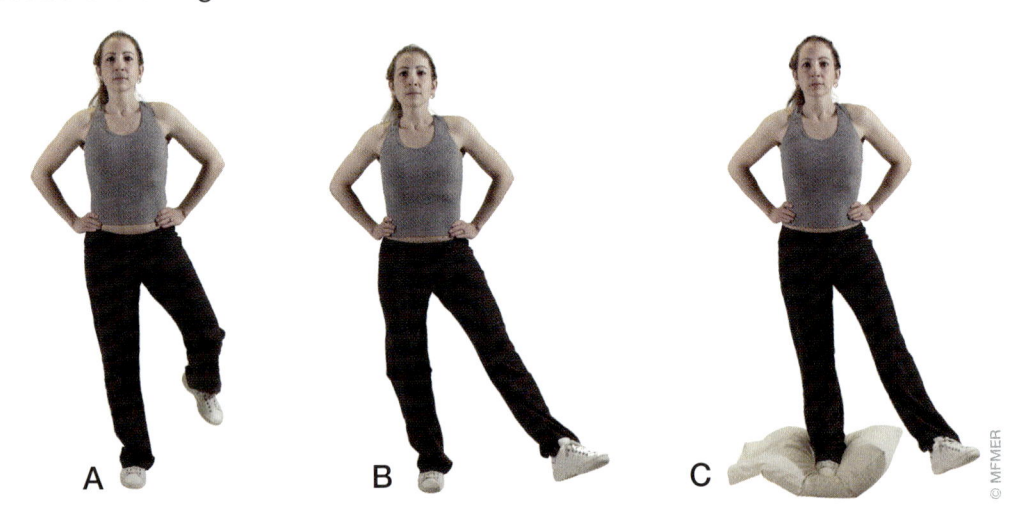

Single-leg balance
1. Stand with your feet hip-width apart and your weight equally distributed on both legs. Place your hands on your hips. Lift your left leg off the floor and bend it back at the knee (A).
2. Hold the position as long as you can maintain good form, up to 30 seconds.
3. Return to the starting position and repeat on the other side. As your balance improves, increase the number of repetitions.
4. For variety, reach out with your foot as far as possible without touching the floor (B).
5. For added challenge, balance on one leg while standing on a pillow or other unstable surface (C).

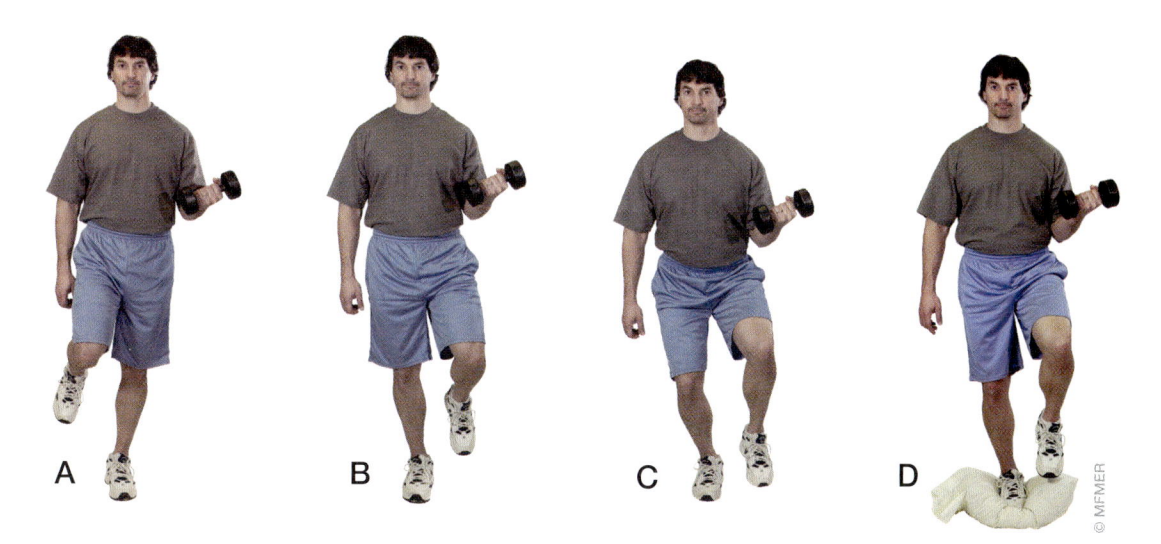

Bicep curls for balance

1. Stand with your feet hip-width apart and your weight equally distributed on both legs. Hold the dumbbell in your left hand with your palm facing upward. Lift your right leg off the floor and bend it back at the knee (A).
2. Hold the position as long as you can maintain good form, up to 30 seconds.
3. Return to the starting position and repeat on the other side (B). As your balance improves, increase the number of repetitions.
4. For added challenge, balance on the leg opposite the weight (C) or while standing on a pillow or other unstable surface (D).

Weight shifts

1. Stand with your feet hip-width apart and your weight equally distributed on both legs (A).
2. Shift your weight to your right side, then lift your left foot off the floor (B).
3. Hold the position as long as you can maintain good form, up to 30 seconds.
4. Return to the starting position and repeat on the other side. As your balance improves, increase the number of repetitions.

Mayo Clinic on Better Hearing and Balance **233**

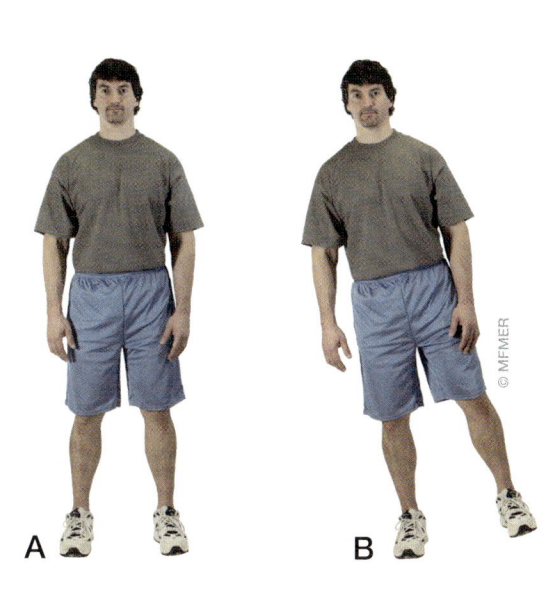

Adaptation often occurs naturally with experience, as you move around and carry out daily activities. In order for your brain to adapt, it needs to continue receiving signals from the balance organs — even if the signals are abnormal. Eventually, your brain resets itself to other sources of sensory input.

For example, if your inner ear on the left side stops functioning, your balance system may gradually switch to a heavier reliance on the organs of your right ear. When compensation is complete, you'll rarely notice the dizziness and vertigo anymore.

Anti-vertigo medications are important for relieving acute spells of dizziness, but long-term therapeutic use of these drugs is discouraged. That's because these medications are mostly sedative in nature and may, in the long run, delay the ability of your brain to compensate.

At times, the signs and symptoms of a balance disorder become chronic, which increases your risk of falling and injuring yourself. In older adults, falls are a major cause of disability and death. Thus, vestibular and balance rehabilitation can be an important factor in the prevention of falls. See pages 228-229 for other information on fall prevention.

What's in a program?

A vestibular and balance rehabilitation program generally starts with a thorough assessment of signs and symptoms and underlying conditions. This allows a physical therapist to design an exercise program customized to your needs. The assessment typically includes:

- Musculoskeletal evaluation to assess your strength, coordination and flexibility skills
- Balance and gait assessments that are compared with those of others in your age group and that test the interaction of your balance organs
- Questions about the frequency and severity of your symptoms, when and where they occur, and what factors might make them worse
- Rating your level of dizziness and vertigo as you change in and out of various positions
- Assessment of your ability to control eye movement while your head is in motion

With a better understanding of your situation, the therapist can help you set goals for the therapy, such as improving your eye movement control and increasing your activity levels. The therapist can also advise you on how to accomplish these goals.

Typically, your therapist will recommend a number of exercises that you can do at home, in between visits to the physical therapy center. For example, you may be requested to do exercises in which you focus on a visual target 5 to 10 feet away while moving from a sitting position to a standing position and back again with your eyes open. You may then be asked to repeat the procedure with your eyes closed.

Other simple exercises may include watching a target at arm's length and moving your head quickly to the right and left while keeping the target in focus. This activity can be repeated several times a day.

At first, these exercises may make you dizzy, and you usually start out doing only a few repetitions at a time. Soon, your brain will become accustomed to the movements — it will find ways to compensate for your vestibular injury. You'll gradually increase the duration and intensity of the exercises. As you continue your program, the dizziness and vertigo will begin to fade away.

You also may be given exercises to increase your strength and coordination of muscle responses — to improve your balance control. This might include a daily walking program.

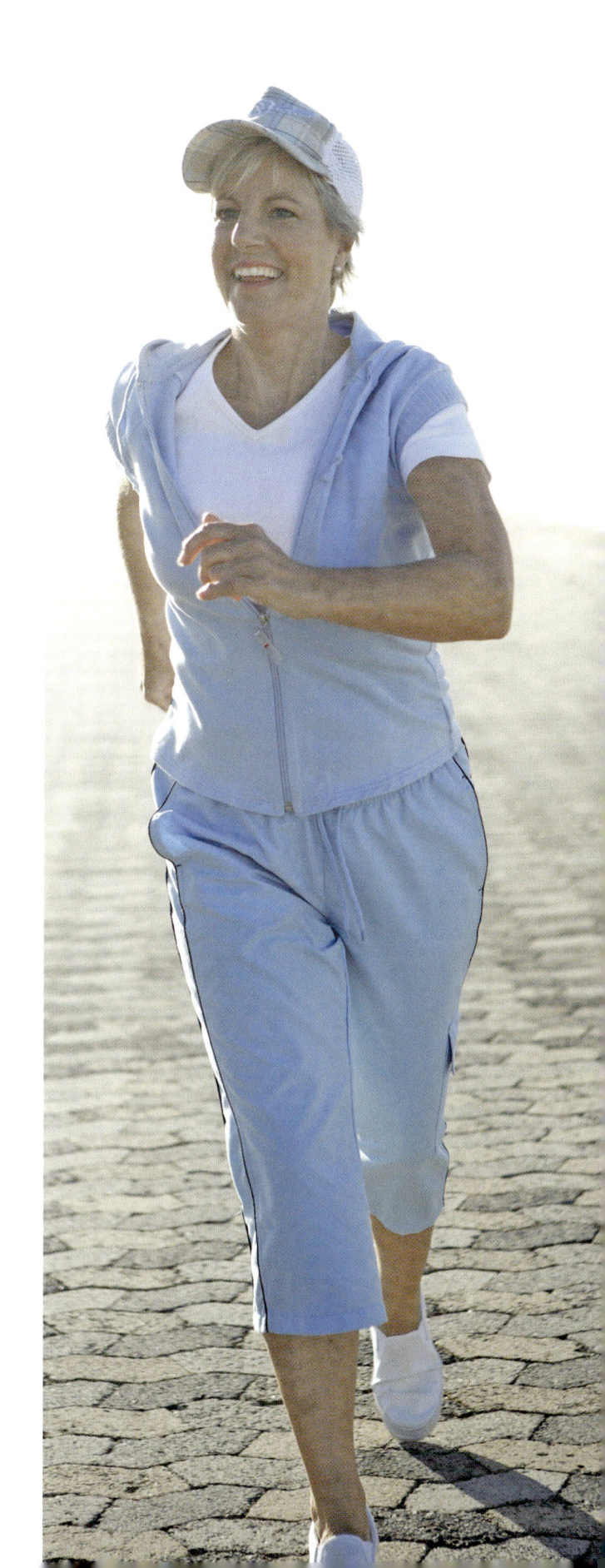

The best general suggestion is getting back to your normal, active daily routine as quickly as you can.

Staying active

Even after you finish a formal therapy program, it's important to stay physically active. If your body goes through a period of inactivity, such as during a bout with the flu or after minor surgery, your brain may forget some of its compensation methods.

To correct this, you'll need to retrain your balance system. This can be done by regularly performing the exercises that were initially prescribed to you, until the dizziness and vertigo go away. Generally, the signs and symptoms will recede more quickly the second time around.

For many individuals, tai chi has been helpful as a way of maintaining leg strength and balance after vestibular compensation is complete. It's often included as part of an active therapy program — but talk to your doctor before starting any exercise program.

Additional resources

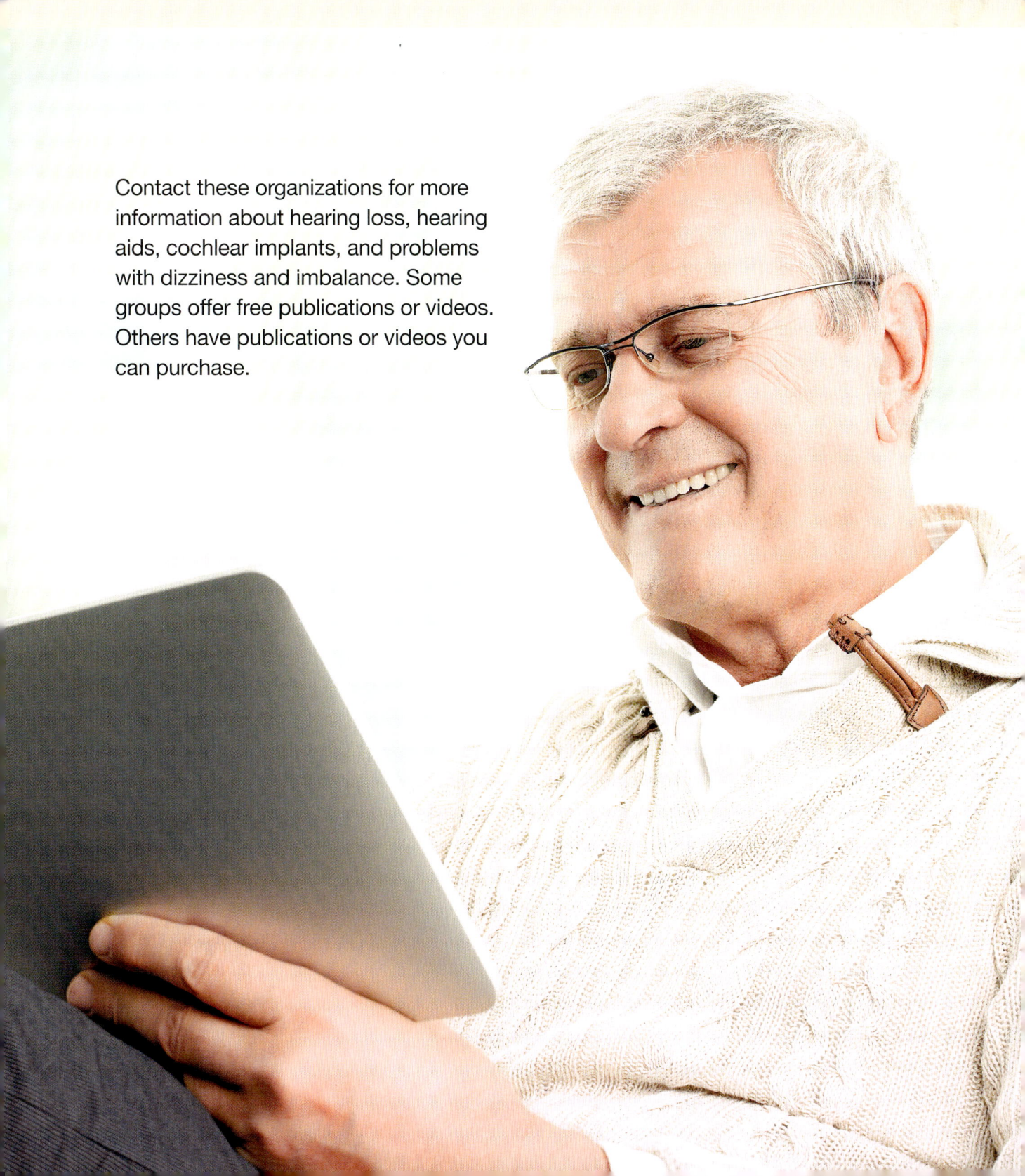

Contact these organizations for more information about hearing loss, hearing aids, cochlear implants, and problems with dizziness and imbalance. Some groups offer free publications or videos. Others have publications or videos you can purchase.

Alexander Graham Bell Association for the Deaf and Hard of Hearing
3417 Volta Place NW
Washington, DC 20007
202-337-5220 or 202-337-5221 (TTY)
www.agbell.org

American Academy of Audiology
11480 Commerce Park Drive, Suite 220
Reston, VA 20191
800-222-2336
www.audiology.org

American Academy of Otolaryngology — Head and Neck Surgery
1650 Diagonal Road
Alexandria, VA 22314-2857
703-836-4444
www.entnet.org

American Association of People with Disabilities
2013 H Street NW, Fifth Floor
Washington, DC 20006
202-457-0046 or 800-840-8844
www.aapd.com

American Auditory Society
P.O. Box 779
Pennsville, NJ 08070
877-746-8315
www.amauditorysoc.org

American Hearing Research Foundation
310 W. Lake St., Suite 111
Elmhurst, IL 60126
630-617-5079
www.american-hearing.org

American Society for Deaf Children
800 Florida Ave. NE, No. 2047
Washington DC, 20002-3695
800-942-2732
www.deafchildren.org

American Speech-Language-Hearing Association
2200 Research Blvd.
Rockville, MD 20850-3289
800-638-8255 or 301-296-5650 (TDD)
www.asha.org

American Tinnitus Association
P.O. Box 5
Portland, OR 97207-0005
503-248-9985 or 800-634-8978
www.ata.org

Association of Late-Deafened Adults
8038 Macintosh Lane, Suite 2
Rockford, IL 61107
815-332-1515 or 866-402-2532
www.alda.org

Better Hearing Institute
1444 I Street NW, Suite 700
Washington, DC 20005
202-449-1100
www.betterhearing.org

Canine Companions for Independence
P.O. Box 446
Santa Rosa, CA 95402-0446
866-224-3647 or 800-572-2275
www.caninecompanions.org

Center for Hearing and Communication
50 Broadway, Sixth Floor
New York, NY 10004
917-305-7700 or 917-305-7999 (TDD)
www.chchearing.org

Children of Deaf Adults (CODA) International
P.O. Box 902067
Sandy, UT 84090
www.coda-international.org

The Children's Hearing Institute
380 Second Ave., Ninth Floor
New York, NY 10010
646-438-7819
www.childrenshearing.org

Dangerous Decibels
Oregon Health & Science University
Oregon Hearing Research Center, NRC-04
3181 S.W. Sam Jackson Park Road
Portland, OR 97239
503-494-0670
www.dangerousdecibels.org

Hands & Voices
P.O. Box 3093
Boulder, CO 80307
303-492-6283 or 866-422-0422
www.handsandvoices.org

Hearing Health Foundation
363 Seventh Ave., 10th Floor
New York, NY 10001-3904
866-454-3924 or 888-435-6104 (TDD)
www.hearinghealthfoundation.org

Hearing Loss Association of America
7910 Woodmont Ave., Suite 1200
Bethesda, MD 20814
301-657-2248
www.hearingloss.org

International Hearing Society
16880 Middlebelt Road, Suite 4
Livonia, MI 48154
734-522-7200
www.ihsinfo.org

National Association of the Deaf
8630 Fenton St., Suite 820
Silver Spring, MD 20910-3819
301-587-1788 or 301-587-1789 (TDD)
www.nad.org

National Center for Rehabilitative Auditory Research
Portland VA Medical Center
3710 S.W. U.S. Veterans Hospital Road, 95-NCRAR
Portland, OR 97239
503-220-8262, ext. 54525
www.ncrar.research.va.gov

National Institute on Deafness and Other Communication Disorders
National Institutes of Health
31 Center Drive, MSC 2320
Bethesda, MD 20892-2320
800-241-1044 or 800-241-1055 (TDD)
www.nidcd.nih.gov

Paws With A Cause
4646 S. Division
Wayland, MI 49348
800-253-7297
www.pawswithacause.org

Vestibular Disorders Association
5018 N.E. 15th Ave.
Portland, OR 97211
800-837-8428
www.vestibular.org

Index

A

access, hearing loss and, 112–114
acoustic neuroma
  closed-skull procedure, 91
  defined, 90, 227
  development of, 227
  illustrated, 90
  removal of, 90–91, 227
  See also inner ear problems
acoustic reflex, 22
acoustic reflex test, 44–45
activation, cochlear implant
  complete programming, 179
  process, 177–178
  tuning speech processor and, 178–179
  waiting time for, 177
acute ear infection, 64–67
ADA (Americans With Disabilities Act), 114, 184
adaptation to change, 231–234
adults
  hearing exams, 33
  recommended screening schedule, 34
air conduction, 42
ALDs. *See* assistive listening devices

alerting devices, 203–204
American Sign Language (ASL), 125
Americans With Disabilities Act (ADA), 114, 184
amplifiers
  hearing aid, 137
  telephone, 189
amplitude, sound, 18, 19
antibiotics
  for chronic ear infections, 68
  ruptured eardrum, 63
anxiety
  defined, 118
  disorders, 213
  signs and symptoms, 119
ASL (American Sign Language), 125
assertive communication, 119–120
assistive listening devices (ALDs)
  acoustic difficulties and, 184–185
  buying, 187
  defined, 185–186
  distance and, 184
  functioning of, 187
  with hearing aids or cochlear implants, 188
  noise and, 184
  personal amplifiers, 186
  reverberation and, 184
  transmitter/receiver, 187
  uses for, 186–187
  in the workplace, 114

See also communication technologies
assistive listening systems
  defined, 196
  FM, 196–199
  illustrated, 197
  induction loop, 201
  infrared, 199–201
audiograms
  defined, 49–51
  horizontal lines, 51
  illustrated, 50
  Meniere's disease, 88
  noise-induced hearing loss, 81
  otosclerosis, 74
  of presbycusis, 79
  sound representation on, 51
  speech spectrum and, 52–54
  understanding, 49–53
  vertical lines, 51
audio input, hearing aid, 148
audiological evaluation, cochlear implants, 174
audiological exams
  air conduction, 42
  audiometry and, 41, 42
  benefits of, 41–42
  defined, 41
  speech reception test, 43
  word recognition test, 43–44
  See also hearing exams
audiologists
  defined, 31

audiologists (cont.)
   education, 31–32, 149
   finding, 149
audiometry, 41, 42
auditory nerve fibers, cochlear implants and, 171
auditory brainstem response test, 44–46
aural rehabilitation
   defined, 128
   goal of, 129
   sessions, 131
   software programs, 131
   steps, 129
   See also support
autoimmune inner ear disease
   corticosteroids, 94
   defined, 92
   hearing loss in, 92
   signs and symptoms, 92–94
   treatment options, 94
   See also inner ear problems

B

background noise, controlling, 158
BAHA (bone-anchored hearing aid), 143–144
balance
   exercises, 232–233
   eyes and, 208
   maintaining, 208–211
   nervous system and, 208
   system illustration, 209
   vestibular labyrinth and, 208–209, 210–211
balance problems
   diagnostic tests and, 213–219
   Dix-Hallpike test and, 216
   dizziness and, 212–213
   fall prevention and, 228–229
   hearing test and, 214
   nystagmography and, 214–216
   overview of, 207
   posturography and, 218
   rotation tests and, 216–217
   vestibular disorders, 220–231
   vestibular evoked myogenic potential (VEMP) and, 218–219
barotrauma
   causes of, 63–64
   defined, 62
   treatment, 64
batteries, hearing aid
   dead or defective, 159–160
   door, opening when not in use, 162
   in hearing aid illustration, 137
   illustrated, 159
behavioral observation audiometry, 49
behind-the-ear (BTE) aids, 140–142
benign paroxysmal positional vertigo (BPPV), 220–221
benign tumors, 61
bicep curls for balance, 233
binaural hearing, 20
blood circulation, poor, 213
blood tests, 219
Bluetooth interface, hearing aid, 148
bone-anchored hearing aid (BAHA), 143–144
bone conduction devices
   BAHA, 143–144
   defined, 143
   magnetic, 144
   in-the-mouth, 144
BPPV (benign paroxysmal positional vertigo), 220–221
brain, sound pathway to, 22–23, 24
BTE (behind-the-ear) aids, 140–142

C

CA (communication assistant), 190-192
canalith repositioning, 222
candidates, cochlear implants, 167–171
Canine Companions for Independence (CCI),128
captioned service, 192
captioned telephones, 191
captioning
   defined, 200
   open vs. closed, 201–203

symbols, 202
uses for, 203
care and handling, cochlear implants, 178
care providers
    audiologists, 31–32
    exams, scheduling, 32
    neurotologists, 31
    otolaryngologists, 30–31
    working together, 32
CCI (Canine Companions for Independence), 128
cellphones, hearing aids and, 195
central nervous system disorders, 213
cerumen, 13
children
    behavioral observation audiometry, 48
    cochlear implants and, 169–170 173, 180
    conditioned play audiometry, 48, 49
    dizziness in, 230–231
    hearing aids for, 150–151
    hearing loss in, 32–33
    hearing tests for, 47–49
    immunizations and, 86–87
    inner ear infection (otitis media), 66
    purchasing hearing aids for, 150
    recommended screening schedule, 34
    screening, 32

visual reinforcement audiometry, 48, 49
cholesteatoma
    defined, 70
    signs and symptoms, 70–71
    treatment, 71
chronic ear infection
    defined, 67–68
    fluid, draining, 69
    signs and symptoms, 68
    treatment, 68–69
chronic subjective dizziness (CSD) syndrome, 223
CIC (completely-in-the-canal) aids, 139–140
cilia, 15, 22
cleaning hearing aids, 162
cochlea
    chambers, 15
    defined, 15
    duct, 15
    hair cells, 15–17
    illustrated, 16
    See also inner ear
cochlear implants
    activation of, 177–179
    adjusting to, 179–181
    auditory nerve fibers and, 171
    benefits of, 164, 172–173
    candidates for, 167–171
    care and handling, 178
    in children, 169–170, 173, 180
    components illustration, 168
    contributing factors, 171–172

    Deaf community and, 169
    defined, 163
    duration of hearing loss and, 171
    electrodes, 167
    first sounds, 179
    function illustration, 166
    functioning of, 165–167
    hearing aids vs., 164–165
    hearing with, 164
    history of, 163–164
    implant procedure, 173–179
    listening situations and, 179
    meningitis and, 176
    microphone, 165
    motivation and, 171–172
    positivity and, 181–182
    programming schedule, 180
    quality of life and, 164
    receiver-stimulator, 167
    rehabilitation training and education, 180
    speech processor, 167
    support services, 179
    support system, 182
    technology improvement, 163–164
cognitive behavioral therapy, in managing tinnitus, 105
communication
    assertive, 119–120
    effective, 119
    with hearing aids, tips for, 157–158

communication (cont.)
   with hearing-impaired person, 122
communication assistant (CA), 190–192
communication technologies
   alerting devices, 203
   assistive listening devices, 184–188
   assistive listening systems, 196–201
   captioning, 201–204
   on the horizon, 295–296
   multipurpose devices, 193–194
   overview of, 183–184
   speech recognition systems, 205
   telephone devices, 188–193
   text messaging, 194–196
   visual communication systems, 206
   See also cochlear implants; hearing aids
complementary and alternative treatments, in managing tinnitus, 107–108
completely-in-the-canal (CIC) aids, 139–140
computerized tomography (CT) scans, 68, 219
conditional play audiometry, 48, 49
conductive hearing loss
   defined, 23, 55
   muffled sounds, 55
   reversal of, 55

congenital hearing problems
   defined, 94
   factors causing, 94–95
   hearing loss, 94
conventional hearing aids
   behind-the-ear (BTE), 140–142
   in-the-canal (ITC), 140
   completely-in-the-canal (CIC), 139–140
   functioning of, 139
   open fit, 142–143
   receiver-in-the-canal (RIC), 142
corticosteroids, 94
costs, hearing aid, 154
CSD (chronic subjective dizziness syndrome), 223
cued speech, 124–125
cysts, 71

D

Deaf community, cochlear implants and, 169
deafness, sudden, 85–86
decibels, 21
denial, hearing loss, 113
depression, 118
directional microphones, 147
Dix-Hallpike test, 216
dizziness
   causes of, 207, 212–213
   in children, 230–231
   concern about, 214
   diagnostic tests, 213–219

   migraine related, 221–223
   See also balance problems
dogs, hearing, 126–128
drug therapy, in managing tinnitus, 105

E

ear
   as acoustic devices, 12–13
   foreign objects in, 58–59
   inner, 15–17, 22–25
   middle, 13–15, 70–76
   outer, 13, 14, 56–61
   parts of, 13
   structure of, 12–16
   trauma to, 62
ear, nose and throat (ENT) specialists, 173
ear candling, 58
ear discomfort, with hearing aids, 160
eardrum
   barotrauma, 63–64
   defined, 13
   problems, 61–64
   ruptured, 62–63
   in sound pathway, 20–21
ear infection
   acute, 64–67
   chronic, 67
   ruptured eardrum and, 62
ear-level FM systems, 149
ear-water drying drops, 61
earwax blockage
   ear candling and, 58
   hearing loss due to, 57

treatment, 56–58
electrodes, cochlear implants, 167
electronics, hearing aid, 145–147
electronystagmography (ENG), 214–215
emotional effects
   anxiety, 118–119
   depression, 118
employees
   recommended screening schedule, 34
   screening, 33–36
employment and hearing loss
   ADA and, 114
   assistive listening devices, 114
   for deaf or severely hearing impaired, 114
   quality of life and, 114–116
   in the workplace, 115
ENG (electronystagmography), 214–215
environment
   listening, 120–121
   planning for, 121
eustachian tube, 13–15
evaluating information, 130
eyes, in balance system, 208, 209

F

fall prevention, 229–229
federal government resources, 132

feedback, hearing aid, 159
fitting hearing aids, 153-154
FM systems
   defined, 196
   function illustration of, 197
   illustrated, 198
   personal, 198
   in public locations, 198–199
   use with hearing aids or cochlear implants, 196
   See also assistive listening systems
foreign objects in ear, 58–59
frequencies, sound
   audible to humans, 18
   basilar membrane and, 22
   defined, 18
   hearing loss in, 54
   as sound wave property, 18

G

gene therapy, 96
glomus jugulare, 71–72
glomus tympanicum, 71–72
groups, support, 131

H

hair cell regeneration, 95
head trauma, 87
hearing, protecting, 54, 106
Hearing Aid Compatibility (HAC) Act, 195
hearing aids
   adjustment to, 133–134
   amplifier, 137
   audio input, 148

batteries, 137, 159–160
behind-the-ear (BTE), 140–142
benefits of using, 133, 136
Bluetooth interface, 148
bone conduction devices, 143–144
buying, 149–154
in-the-canal (ITC), 140
cellphones and, 195
for children, 150–151
cleaning, 162
cochlear implants versus, 164–165
common problems, 158–161
completely-in-the-canal (CIC), 139–140
conventional, 139–143
costs, 154
directional microphones, 147
ear discomfort, 160
ear-level FM systems, 149
electronics, 145–147
feedback, 159
fitting, 153-154
function of, 133
how they work, 136–138
illustrated, 137
implantable aids, 144–145
listening differences with, 136–138
maintenance, 161–162
with maskers, 104
microphone, 137
moisture and, 160

Mayo Clinic on Better Hearing and Balance   **245**

hearing aids (cont.)
- motivation as success key, 134
- open fit, 142–143
- parts of, 137
- priorities, setting, 134–136
- program button, 137
- readjustment, 155–157
- receiver-in-the-canal (RIC), 142
- remote control, 148
- remote microphones, 148
- resistance to, 135
- satisfaction, increasing, 134
- selection criteria, 145–149
- sound collection, 136
- speaker, 137
- styles, 134, 138–145
- styles illustration, 141
- technology, 12, 133
- telecoils, 147–148, 200
- tips for better communication, 157–158
- trade-offs, 134
- two versus one, 138
- wax blockage and, 160
- wearing, 154–160

hearing dogs
- accompanying owners, 127
- function of, 126
- organizations, 128

hearing evaluations, 153

hearing exams
- acoustic reflex test, 44–45
- adults, 33
- audiogram, 49–53
- audiological, 40–44
- auditory brainstem response test, 45–46
- in balance problem diagnosis, 214
- behavioral observation audiometry, 49
- children, 32–33
- conditional play audiometry, 48, 49
- employees, 33–36
- in hearing aid buying process, 153
- medical evaluation, 37–40
- otoacoustic emissions test, 46–47
- preliminary, with primary doctor, 29
- receiving, 29–54
- schedule recommendations, 34
- scheduling, 32
- tests for children, 47–49
- tympanometry, 44
- typical, 36–39
- visual reinforcement audiometry, 48, 49

hearing-impaired people, communication with, 122

hearing level, measurement of, 21

hearing loss
- addressing, 28
- age and, 11–12
- in children, 32–33
- compensating for, 25–28
- conductive, 23, 55
- congenital hearing problems, 94
- consequences of, 12
- denial, 113
- due to earwax blockage, 56–58
- emotional effects, 118–119
- frequencies, 54
- as gradual, 112
- levels of, 42
- living with, 111–132
- masking of, 25–28
- mixed, 25
- noise-induced, 80–85
- questions to help recognize, 26
- recognizing signs of, 26
- refusal to acknowledge, 12, 25, 54
- sensorineural, 23–25, 77
- social isolation from, 11
- statistics, 11
- subjective tinnitus, 101
- support, finding, 128–132
- symmetrical, 53
- types of, 23–25

Hearing Loss Association of America (HLAA), 112

hearing protectors, 83–85

hyperacusis, 101

hyperventilation, 213

I

identity, hearing loss and, 117–118

imaging tests, 40

implantable aids, 144–145
implant procedure
    activation, 177–179
    audiological evaluation, 173–174
    complications from surgery, 176–177
    cost of, 174
    imagery, 173–174
    incision healing time, 177
    medical evaluation, 173–174
    meningitis and, 176
    pre-implantation, 173–175
    psychological evaluation, 175
    surgery, 175–177
    surgery doctor, 173
    See also cochlear implants
induction loop systems, 197, 201
infants and toddlers
    recommended screening schedule, 34
    screening, 32–33
    See also children
information, evaluating, 130
infrared systems
    advantages/disadvantages, 200–201
    defined, 199
    function illustration of, 197
    using, 200
    See also assistive listening systems
inner ear
    cilia, 15, 22

cochlea, 15–17
    damage to, 23–25
    defined, 15
    illustrated, 16
    sound pathways into, 22
    vestibular labyrinth, 17
    vibrations, 22
inner ear problems
    acoustic neuroma, 90–91
    autoimmune disease, 92–94
    congenital, 94–95
    gene therapy and, 96
    hair cell regeneration, 95
    head trauma, 87
    labyrinthitis, 89
    Meniere's disease, 87–89
    noise-induced hearing loss, 80–85
    presbycusis, 78–80
    reaction to medications, 91–92
    research, 95
    sudden deafness, 85–86
    viral infections, 86–87
international symbols, 202
in-the-canal (ITC) aids, 140
in-the-mouth bone conduction, 144
isolation, 116–117

J

jaw disorders, 102

L

laboratory tests, 40
labyrinthitis, 89, 225–226

lip reading. *See* speech reading
listening environment, 120–121
living with hearing loss
    access, 112–114
    emotional effects, 118–119
    employment, 114–116
    overview of, 111
    quality of life, 112–119
    relationships, 116–118
    social interaction, improving, 119–128
    support, finding, 128–132
low blood pressure, as dizziness cause, 212

M

magnetic bone conduction, 144
maintenance, hearing aid, 161–162
masking sources, 104–105
medical evaluation
    cochlear implants, 173–175
    imaging tests, 40
    laboratory tests, 40
    medical history and, 37
    otoscopy, 39
    physical exam, 37–39
    tuning fork test, 39–40
medications
    ototoxic, 91–92, 93
    reactions to, 91–92, 226–227
    subjective tinnitus, 101–102

Meniere's disease
- attacks, 87, 223
- audiogram, 88
- defined, 87, 223
- treatment, 89, 225
- as vestibular disorder, 223–225

meningitis, cochlear implants and, 176

microphones, cochlear implants, 165

microphones, hearing aid
- directional, 147
- illustrated, 137
- remote, 148

middle ear
- cholesteatoma, 70–71
- cysts and tumors, 71–72
- defined, 13
- eardrum, 20–21
- eustachian tube, 13–15
- illustrated, 14
- ossicles, 13
- ossicular chain disruption, 75–76
- otosclerosis, 72–75
- problems, 64–76
- sound pathways into, 20–22
- vibrations, 20–21

middle ear infection
- in children, 67
- defined, 65
- illustrated, 64
- pain, easing, 66
- signs and symptoms, 65–66
- treatment, 66–67

migraine-related dizziness, 221–223

migraines, 213

mixed hearing loss, 25

moisture, hearing aids and, 160

motivation
- cochlear implants and, 171–172
- hearing aids and, 134

multipurpose communication devices, 193–194

music therapy, in managing tinnitus, 105

N

National Institute on Deafness and Other Communication Disorders, 26

nervous system, balance and, 208

neurotologists, 31

noise
- distracting, moving away from, 121
- sound levels of, 83

noise-induced hearing loss
- audiogram, 81
- causes of, 80
- defined, 80
- personal listening devices and, 84
- prevention, 83
- statistics, 82–83

nystagmography, 214–216

O

objective tinnitus, 100

Occupational Safety and Health Administration (OSHA), 33

open-fit aids, 142–143

Organ of Corti, 15, 77

ossicles, 13

ossicular chain disruption
- defined, 75–76
- surgery, 76
- treatment, 76

ossiculoplasty, 76

otitis media
- in children, 67
- chronic, 67–69
- defined, 65
- illustrated, 65
- pain, easing, 66
- signs and symptoms, 65–66
- treatment, 66–67

otoacoustic emissions test, 46–47

otoconia, 210

otolaryngologists, 30–31, 173

otosclerosis
- audiogram, 74
- defined, 72
- hearing loss, 72–73
- treatment, 73–75

otoscope, 38

otoscopy, 39

ototoxic medications, 91–92, 93

outer ear
    benign tumors, 61
    cerumen, 13
    defined, 13
    eardrum, 13
    earwax blockage, 56–58
    foreign objects in, 58–59
    illustrated, 14
    pinna, 13
    problems, 56–61
    sound pathways into, 20
    swimmer's ear, 59–61

P

Paws with a Cause, 128
perilymph fistula, 230
personal amplifiers, 186
personal listening devices, 84
physical activity, in vestibular rehabilitation, 236
physical exam, 37–39
pinna, 13
positioning yourself, 120–121
positive attitude, cochlear implants and, 181–182
posturography, 218
presbycusis
    audiogram, 79
    compensation for, 80
    defined, 78
    in sensorineural hearing loss, 77
    with tinnitus, 79
problems, hearing aid
    batteries, 159–160
    ear discomfort, 160
    feedback, 159
    moisture, 160
    troubleshooting questions, 158
    wax blockage, 160
program button, hearing aid, 137
psychological evaluation, cochlear implants, 175
purchasing hearing aids
    through audiologists, 149
    buying process, 149, 152–154
    caution, 149
    for children, 150
    costs, 154
    fitting and, 153-154
    hearing aid selection, 153
    hearing evaluation and, 153
    hearing exams and, 152-153
    options, 152-153
    tips for, 152
    trial period, 154

Q

quality, sound, 18–20
quality of life
    access, 112–114
    cochlear implants and, 164
    emotional effects, 118–119
    employment, 114–116
    relationships, 116–118
    See also living with hearing loss
questions
    hearing aid troubleshooting, 158
    recognizing hearing loss, 26
    tinnitus, 103

R

reactions to medications, 91–92, 226–227
receiver-in-the-canal (RIC) aids, 142
receiver-in-the-ear (RITE) aids, 142
receiver-stimulator, cochlear implants, 167
relationships and hearing loss
    identity, 117–118
    isolation, 116–117
    quality of life and, 116–118
remote control, hearing aid, 148
remote microphones, 148
repetitive transcranial magnetic stimulation (rTMS), 108
resistance to hearing aids, 135
resources
    federal government, 132
    state, 132
    types of, 131–132
RIC (receiver-in-the-canal) aids, 142
rotation tests, 216–217
rTMS (repetitive transcranial magnetic stimulation), 108

ruptured eardrum
    ear infection and, 62
    trauma to the ear and, 62
    treatment, 62–63

S

screening. *See* hearing exams
sensorineural, 77
sensorineural hearing loss
    causes of, 163
    defined, 23–25, 77
    example, 25
    factors, 77–78
    hair cell damage, 165
    presbycusis, 77, 78–80
sign language
    as complete language, 125
    defined, 125
    learning, 126
    sight and, 126
single-leg balance, 232
social interaction
    assertive communication, 119–120
    cued speech, 124–125
    hearing dogs, 126–128
    with hearing-impaired person, 122
    improving, 119–128
    listening environment, 120
    sign language, 125–126
    speech reading, 123–124
sound
    characteristics of, 17–20
    differences between, 17–18
    frequencies, 18

intensity of, 18
knowledge and recognition of, 23
noise levels and, 83
occurrence of, 17
timbre of, 18–20
sound pathways
    binaural hearing, 20
    to the brain, 22–23
    defined, 20
    illustrated, 24
    inner ear, 22
    middle ear, 20–22
    outer ear, 20
sound pressure level (SPL)
    defined, 18
    measurement of, 21
sound waves
    amplitude, 19
    frequency, 19
    properties of, 19
    through air, 17
    through fluid, 17
speaker, hearing aid, 137
speech processor, cochlear implants, 167
speech reading
    defined, 123
    factors contributing to, 123
    learning, 123
    tips for, 124
speech reception test, 43
speech recognition systems, 205
speech recognition threshold (SRT), 43
speech spectrum, 54

squamous cell carcinoma, 72
SSCD (superior semicircular canal dehiscence), 230
SSNHL (sudden sensorineural hearing loss), 85–86
stapedotomy, 73
state resources, 132
subjective tinnitus
    causes of, 102
    defined, 100
    hearing loss, 101
    jaw disorders, 102
    medications, 101–102
sudden deafness, 85–86
sudden sensorineural hearing loss (SSNHL), 85–86
superior semicircular canal dehiscence (SSCD), 230
support
    aural rehabilitation, 128–131
    cochlear implants and, 182
    finding, 128–132
    groups, 131
    information, evaluating, 130
    resources, 131–132
surgery
    cochlear implants, 175–177
    ossiculoplasty, 76
    risks, 76
    tympanomastoidectomy, 69
    for vestibular disorders, 224
swimmer's ear
    causes of, 59–60
    defined, 59

illustrated, 59
treatment, 60–61
symmetrical hearing loss, 53

T

talking face to face, 158
TDD, or text telephone, 190
telecoils, 147–148, 200
telecommunication relay service (TRS)
    captioned service, 192
    communication assistant (CA), 190–192
    defined, 190
    text-to-voice, 192
    using, 190
    video relay service (VRS), 192
telephone devices
    adapters, 189
    built-in amplifiers, 189
    defined, 188
    for hearing impairment, 191
    ringers, 190
    TRS and, 190–192
    See also communication technologies
text messaging, 194–196
text telephone, or TDD, 190
timbre, 18–20
tinnitus
    in association with ear disorders, 97
    causes of, 98, 99
    cognitive behavioral therapy for, 105
    complementary, alternative and new treatments for, 107–108
    defined, 78, 97
    diagnosis, 102–103
    doctor questions about, 103
    drug therapy for, 105
    experience of, 97
    frequency and intensity determination, 103
    hearing aids with maskers for, 104
    hyperacusis and, 101
    impact on people's lives, 97
    managing, 98, 102–103, 104–108
    masking sources, 104–105
    mechanisms triggering, 98
    music therapy for, 105
    objective, 100
    presbycusis with, 78
    self-help tips for, 106
    subjective, 100–102
    TRT, 105–107
    types, 99–102
tinnitus retraining therapy (TRT)
    defined, 107
    goal of, 107
    treatment, 107
trauma to the ear, 62
trial period, hearing aids, 154
tumors, benign, 61
tuning forks, 38
tuning fork test, 39–40
tympanomastoidectomy, 69
tympanometry, 44, 45

V

VEMP (vestibular evoked myogenic potential), 218–219
vestibular disorders
    acoustic neuroma, 227
    benign paroxysmal positional vertigo (BPPV), 220–221
    chronic subjective dizziness syndrome, 223
    labyrinthitis, 225–226
    Meniere's disease, 223–225
    migraine-related dizziness, 221–223
    perilymph fistula, 230
    reactions to medications, 226–227
    superior semicircular canal dehiscence (SSCD), 230
    surgery for, 224
    vestibular neuronitis, 226
    See also balance problems
vestibular evoked myogenic potential (VEMP), 218–219
vestibular labyrinth
    balance problems and, 209
    defined, 17, 208–209
    functioning of, 210–211
    location of, 210
vestibular neuronitis, 226
vestibular rehabilitation
    adapting to change, 231–234
    assessment, 234

vestibular rehabilitation (cont.)
    exercise recommendation, 235
    physical activity and, 236
    program, 234–236
videonystagmography (VNG), 214–215
video relay service (VRS), 192
viral infections, 86–87
visual communication systems, 206
visual reinforcement audiometry, 48, 49
voice-carry-over (VCO), 192
VRS (video relay service), 192

W

wax blockage, 160
wearing hearing aids
    adaptation to, 154-155
    background noise and, 158
    comfort level, building, 157
    help, asking for, 158
    practicing, 155-156
    readjustment, 155–157
    talking face to face and, 158
    tips for better communication, 157–158
weight shifts, 233
word recognition test, 43–44

Housecall

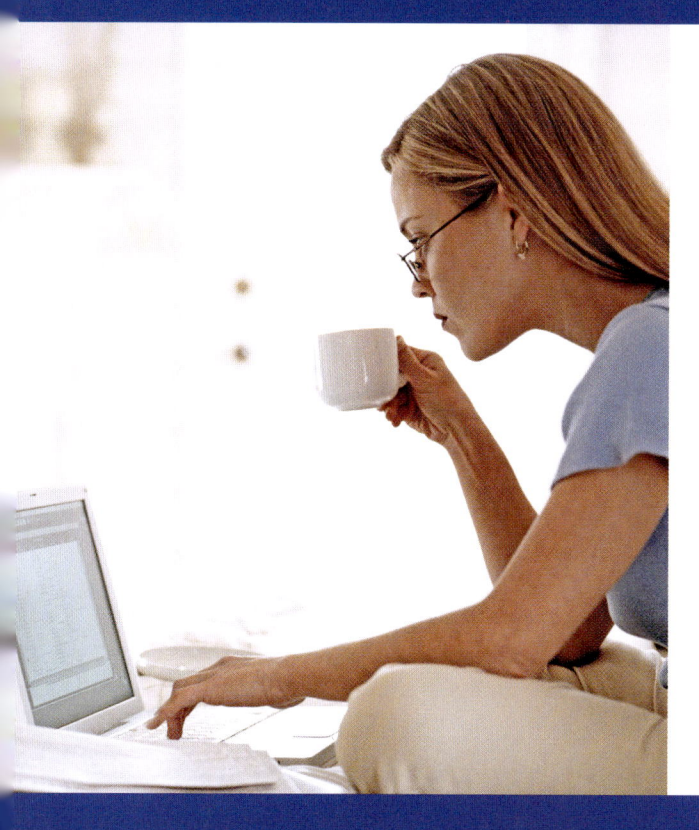

MAYO CLINIC

What our readers are saying ...

"I depend on **Mayo Clinic Housecall** more than any other medical info that shows up on my computer. Thank you so very much."

"Excellent newsletter. I always find something interesting to read and learn something new."

"**Housecall** is a must read – keep up the good work!"

"I love **Housecall**. It is one of the most useful, trusted and beneficial things that come from the Internet."

"The **Housecall** is timely, interesting and invaluable in its information. Thanks much to Mayo Clinic for this resource!"

"I enjoy getting the weekly newsletters. They provide me with friendly reminders, as well as information/conditions I was not aware of."

Get the latest health information direct from Mayo Clinic ... Sign up today, it's FREE!

Mayo Clinic Housecall is a FREE weekly e-newsletter that offers the latest health information from the experts at Mayo Clinic. Stay up to date on topics that are current, interesting, and most of all important to your health and the health of your family.

What you get
- Weekly top story
- Additional healthy highlights
- Answers from the experts
- Quick access to trusted health tools
- Featured blogs
- Health tip of the week
- Special offers

Don't wait ... Join today!
MayoClinic.com/Housecall/Register

We're committed to helping you enjoy better health and get the most out of life every day. We hope you decide to become part of the Mayo Clinic family, where you can always count on receiving an interesting mix of health information from a trusted source.

More great Mayo Clinic publications

Visit **www.store.MayoClinic.com** for reliable Mayo Clinic publications to help with your top health interests.

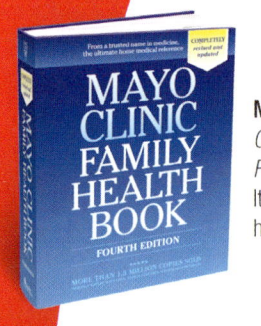

Mayo Clinic Family Health Book
Completely revised and updated Fourth Edition
It's your owner's manual for the human body.

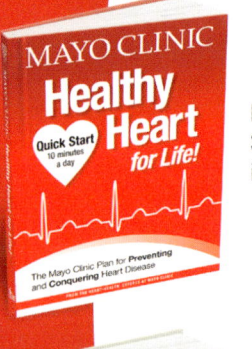

Mayo Clinic Healthy Heart for Life
Start improving your heart health in as little as 10 minutes a day.

The Mayo Clinic Diet
#1 New York Times Best Seller
The last diet you'll ever need!

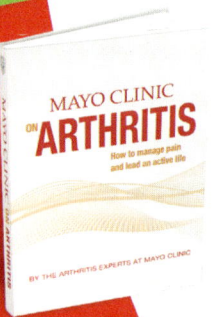

Mayo Clinic on Arthritis
Better medications, improved treatments and self-care tips to lead a more active, comfortable life.

Many more popular titles to choose from ...

- Mayo Clinic on Healthy Aging
- Mayo Clinic on Alzheimer's Disease
- The Mayo Clinic Breast Cancer Book
- Mayo Clinic Essential Diabetes Book
- The Mayo Clinic Diabetes Diet
- The Mayo Clinic Diabetes Diet Journal
- Mayo Clinic on Digestive Health
- Mayo Clinic Fitness for EveryBody
- Fix-It And Enjoy-It Healthy Cookbook
- Mayo Clinic Guide to Your Baby's First Year
- Mayo Clinic Guide to a Healthy Pregnancy
- Mayo Clinic on Better Hearing and Balance
- Mayo Clinic 5 Steps to Controlling High Blood Pressure
- Mayo Clinic Book of Home Remedies
- Mayo Clinic on Managing Incontinence
- The Mayo Clinic Kids' Cookbook
- The New Mayo Clinic Cookbook
- The Mayo Clinic Diet Journal
- Mayo Clinic Guide to Preventing and Treating Osteoporosis
- Mayo Clinic Essential Guide to Prostate Health
- Mayo Clinic Guide to Better Vision

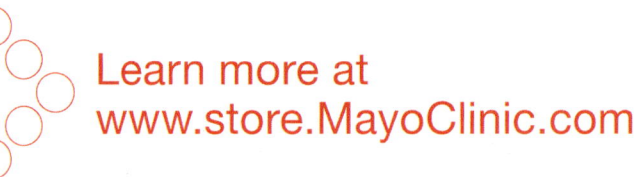

Learn more at www.store.MayoClinic.com